ACP | MKSAP® 18

Medical Knowledge Self-Assessment Program®

Dermatology

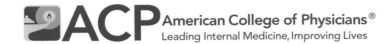

ACP American College of Physicians®
Leading Internal Medicine, Improving Lives

Welcome to the Dermatology Section of MKSAP 18!

In these pages, you will find updated information on approaches to various diseases and therapeutic principles in Dermatology. Included are more than **200** color images of dermatologic disease. We review rashes and other eruptions, skin and nail infections, neoplasms, pruritus and urticaria, autoimmune bullous diseases, and other clinical challenges. All of these topics are uniquely focused on the needs of generalists and subspecialists *outside* of Dermatology.

The core content of MKSAP 18 has been developed as in previous editions—all essential information that is newly researched and written in 11 topic areas of internal medicine—created by dozens of leading generalists and subspecialists and guided by certification and recertification requirements, emerging knowledge in the field, and user feedback. MKSAP 18 also contains 1200 all-new peer-reviewed, psychometrically validated, multiple-choice questions (MCQs) for self-assessment and study, including 72 in Dermatology. MKSAP 18 continues to include *High Value Care* (HVC) recommendations, based on the concept of balancing clinical benefit with costs and harms, with associated MCQs illustrating these principles and HVC Key Points called out in the text. Internists practicing in the hospital setting can easily find comprehensive *Hospitalist*-focused content and MCQs, specially designated in blue and with the 🄷 symbol.

If you purchased MKSAP 18 Complete, you also have access to MKSAP 18 Digital, with additional tools allowing you to customize your learning experience. MKSAP Digital includes regular text updates with new, practice-changing information, 200 new self-assessment questions, and enhanced custom-quiz options. MKSAP Complete also includes more than 1200 electronic, adaptive learning–enhanced flashcards for quick review of important concepts, as well as an updated and enhanced version of Virtual Dx, MKSAP's image-based self-assessment tool. As before, MKSAP 18 Digital is optimized for use on your mobile devices, with iOS- and Android-based apps allowing you to sync between your apps and online account and submit for CME credits and MOC points online.

Please visit us at the MKSAP Resource Site (mksap.acponline.org) to find out how we can help you study, earn CME credit and MOC points, and stay up to date.

On behalf of the many internists who have offered their time and expertise to create the content for MKSAP 18 and the editorial staff who work to bring this material to you in the best possible way, we are honored that you have chosen to use MKSAP 18 and appreciate any feedback about the program you may have. Please feel free to send any comments to mksap_editors@acponline.org.

Sincerely,

Patrick Alguire

Patrick C. Alguire, MD, FACP
Editor-in-Chief
Senior Vice President Emeritus
Medical Education Division
American College of Physicians

Dermatology

Committee

Bryan E. Anderson, MD, Section Editor[1]
Professor of Dermatology
Department of Dermatology
Vice Chair, Department of Dermatology
Penn State University Hershey Medical Center
Hershey, Pennsylvania

Galen T. Foulke, MD[2]
Assistant Professor of Dermatology
Department of Dermatology
Penn State University Hershey Medical Center
Hershey, Pennsylvania

M. Yadira Hurley, MD[2]
Professor of Dermatology and Pathology
Interim Associate Chairman
Director of Dermatopathology, Department of Dermatology
Saint Louis University School of Medicine
St. Louis, Missouri

Jeremy Jackson, MD[2]
Associate Professor of Dermatology
Department of Dermatology
University of Mississippi Medical Center
Brandon, Mississippi

Charlene Lam, MD, MPH[2]
Assistant Professor of Dermatology
Department of Dermatology
Penn State University Hershey Medical Center
Hershey, Pennsylvania

Editor-in-Chief and Deputy Editor

Patrick C. Alguire, MD, FACP[2]
Senior Vice President Emeritus, Medical Education
American College of Physicians
Philadelphia, Pennsylvania

Dermatology Reviewers

Dennis W. Boulware, MD, FACP[1]
Robert D. Cho, MD, FACP[1]
Elie G. Dib, MD, FACP[1]
Karli Edholm, MD, FACP[1]
Bonnie P. Hannah, MD, FACP[1]
Alan T. Kaell, MD, FACP[1]
Ateeq U. Rehman, MBBS, FACP[1]

Hospital Medicine Dermatology Reviewers

Sumit Mamun, MBBS, FACP[1]
Daniel L. Wagstaff, MD, FACP[1]

Dermatology ACP Editorial Staff

Randy Hendrickson[1], Production Administrator/Editor, Self-Assessment and Educational Programs
Margaret Wells[1], Director, Self-Assessment and Educational Programs
Becky Krumm[1], Managing Editor, Self-Assessment and Educational Programs

ACP Principal Staff

Davoren Chick, MD, FACP[2]
Senior Vice President, Medical Education

Patrick C. Alguire, MD, FACP[2]
Senior Vice President Emeritus, Medical Education

Sean McKinney[1]
Vice President, Medical Education

Margaret Wells[1]
Director, Self-Assessment and Educational Programs

Becky Krumm[1]
Managing Editor

Valerie Dangovetsky[1]
Administrator

Ellen McDonald, PhD[1]
Senior Staff Editor

Megan Zborowski[1]
Senior Staff Editor

Randy Hendrickson[1]
Production Administrator/Editor

Julia Nawrocki[1]
Digital Content Associate/Editor

Linnea Donnarumma[1]
Staff Editor

Chuck Emig[1]
Staff Editor

Jackie Twomey[1]
Staff Editor

Joysa Winter[1]
Staff Editor

Kimberly Kerns[1]
Administrative Coordinator

---

1. Has no relationships with any entity producing, marketing, reselling, or distributing health care goods or services consumed by, or used on, patients.

2. Has disclosed relationship(s) with any entity producing, marketing, reselling, or distributing health care goods or services consumed by, or used on, patients.

Disclosure of relationships with any entity producing, marketing, reselling, or distributing health care goods or services consumed by, or used on, patients.

Patrick C. Alguire, MD, FACP
Royalties
UpToDate

Davoren Chick, MD, FACP
Royalties
Wolters Kluwer Publishing
Consultantship
EBSCO Health's DynaMed Plus
Other: Owner and sole proprietor of Coding 101 LLC; research consultant (spouse) for Vedanta Biosciences Inc.

Galen Foulke, MD
Research Grants/Contracts
Boehringer Ingelheim, HedgePath Pharmaceuticals Inc., Novartis, Resolve Therapeutics LLC

M. Yadira Hurley, MD
Honoraria
Castle Biosciences Inc.
Research Grants/Contracts
Abbott, AbbVie, Actelion, Amgen, Anacor Pharmaceuticals Inc., AstraZeneca, Centocor Ortho Biotech Inc., Genentech Inc., Novartis, Pfizer Inc., Regeneron Pharmaceuticals Inc., XOMA Corp.
Speakers Bureau
Actelion Pharmaceuticals Ltd.

Jeremy Jackson, MD
Speakers Bureau
AbbVie, Actelion Pharmaceuticals Ltd., Celgene Inc., Novartis, Sun Pharmaceuticals Industries Ltd.
Research Grants/Contracts
ActelionPharmaceuticals Ltd., Novartis

Charlene Lam, MD, MPH
Research Grants/Contracts
HedgePath Pharmaceuticals Inc.

Acknowledgments

The American College of Physicians (ACP) gratefully acknowledges the special contributions to the development and production of the 18th edition of the Medical Knowledge Self-Assessment Program® (MKSAP® 18) made by the following people:

Graphic Design: Barry Moshinski (Director, Graphic Services), Michael Ripca (Graphics Technical Administrator), and Jennifer Gropper (Graphic Designer).

Production/Systems: Dan Hoffmann (Director, Information Technology), Scott Hurd (Manager, Content Systems), Neil Kohl (Senior Architect), and Chris Patterson (Senior Architect).

MKSAP 18 Digital: Under the direction of Steven Spadt (Senior Vice President, Technology), the digital version of MKSAP 18 was developed within the ACP's Digital Products and Services Department, led by Brian Sweigard (Director, Digital Products and Services). Other members of the team included Dan Barron (Senior Web Application Developer/Architect), Chris Forrest (Senior Software Developer/Design Lead), Kathleen Hoover (Senior Web Developer), Kara Regis (Manager, User Interface Design and Development), Brad Lord (Senior Web Application Developer), and John McKnight (Senior Web Developer).

The College also wishes to acknowledge that many other persons, too numerous to mention, have contributed to the production of this program. Without their dedicated efforts, this program would not have been possible.

MKSAP Resource Site (mksap.acponline.org)

The MKSAP Resource Site (mksap.acponline.org) is a continually updated site that provides links to MKSAP 18 online answer sheets for print subscribers; access to MKSAP 18 Digital; Board Basics® e-book access instructions; information on Continuing Medical Education (CME), Maintenance of Certification (MOC), and international Continuing Professional Development (CPD) and MOC; errata; and other new information.

International MOC/CPD

For information and instructions on submission of international MOC/CPD, please go to the MKSAP Resource Site (mksap.acponline.org).

Continuing Medical Education

The American College of Physicians is accredited by the Accreditation Council for Continuing Medical Education (ACCME) to provide continuing medical education for physicians.

The American College of Physicians designates this enduring material, MKSAP 18, for a maximum of 275 *AMA PRA Category 1 Credits*™. Physicians should claim only the credit commensurate with the extent of their participation in the activity.

Up to 16 *AMA PRA Category 1 Credits*™ are available from July 31, 2018, to July 31, 2021, for the MKSAP 18 Dermatology section.

Learning Objectives

The learning objectives of MKSAP 18 are to:

- Close gaps between actual care in your practice and preferred standards of care, based on best evidence
- Diagnose disease states that are less common and sometimes overlooked and confusing
- Improve management of comorbid conditions that can complicate patient care
- Determine when to refer patients for surgery or care by subspecialists
- Pass the ABIM Certification Examination
- Pass the ABIM Maintenance of Certification Examination

Target Audience

- General internists and primary care physicians
- Subspecialists who need to remain up to date in internal medicine
- Residents preparing for the certifying examination in internal medicine
- Physicians preparing for maintenance of certification in internal medicine (recertification)

ABIM Maintenance of Certification

Check the MKSAP Resource Site (mksap.acponline.org) for the latest information on how MKSAP tests can be used to apply to the American Board of Internal Medicine (ABIM) for Maintenance of Certification (MOC) points following completion of the CME activity. Successful completion of the CME activity, which includes participation in the evaluation component, enables the participant to earn up to 275 medical knowledge MOC points in the ABIM's MOC program. It is the CME activity provider's responsibility to submit participant completion information to ACCME for the purpose of granting ABIM MOC credit.

Earn Instantaneous CME Credits or MOC Points Online

Print subscribers can enter their answers online to earn instantaneous CME credits or MOC points. You can submit your answers using online answer sheets that are provided at mksap.acponline.org, where a record of your MKSAP 18 credits will be available. To earn CME credits or to apply for MOC points, you need to answer all of the questions in a test and earn a score of at least 50% correct (number of correct answers divided by the total number of questions). Please note that if you are applying for MOC points, you must also enter your birth date and ABIM candidate number.

Take either of the following approaches:

1. Use the printed answer sheet at the back of this book to record your answers. Go to mksap.acponline.org, access the appropriate online answer sheet, transcribe your answers, and submit your test for instantaneous CME credits or MOC points. There is no additional fee for this service.
2. Go to mksap.acponline.org, access the appropriate online answer sheet, directly enter your answers, and submit your test for instantaneous CME credits or MOC points. There is no additional fee for this service.

Earn CME Credits or MOC Points by Mail or Fax

Pay a $20 processing fee per answer sheet and submit the printed answer sheet at the back of this book by mail or fax, as instructed on the answer sheet. Make sure you calculate your score and enter your birth date and ABIM candidate number, and fax the answer sheet to 215-351-2799 or mail the answer sheet to Member and Customer Service, American College of Physicians, 190 N. Independence Mall West, Philadelphia, PA 19106-1572, using the courtesy envelope provided in your MKSAP 18 slipcase. You will need your 10-digit order number and 8-digit ACP ID number, which are printed on your packing slip. Please allow 4 to 6 weeks for your score report to be emailed back to you. Be sure to include your email address for a response.

If you do not have a 10-digit order number and 8-digit ACP ID number, or if you need help creating a username and password to access the MKSAP 18 online answer sheets, go to mksap.acponline.org or email custserv@acponline.org.

Disclosure Policy

It is the policy of the American College of Physicians (ACP) to ensure balance, independence, objectivity, and scientific rigor in all of its educational activities. To this end, and consistent with the policies of the ACP and the Accreditation Council for Continuing Medical Education (ACCME), contributors to all ACP continuing medical education activities are required to disclose all relevant financial relationships with any entity producing, marketing, re-selling, or distributing health care goods or services consumed by, or used on, patients. Contributors are required to use generic names in the discussion of therapeutic options and are required to identify any unapproved, off-label, or investigative use of commercial products or devices. Where a trade name is used, all available trade names for the same product type are also included. If trade-name products manufactured by companies with whom contributors have relationships are discussed, contributors are asked to provide evidence-based citations in support of the discussion. The information is reviewed by the committee responsible for producing this text. If necessary, adjustments to topics or contributors' roles in content development are made to balance the discussion. Further, all readers of this text are asked to evaluate the content for evidence of commercial bias and send any relevant comments to mksap_editors@acponline.org so that future decisions about content and contributors can be made in light of this information.

Resolution of Conflicts

To resolve all conflicts of interest and influences of vested interests, ACP's content planners used best evidence and updated clinical care guidelines in developing content, when such evidence and guidelines were available. All content underwent review by peer reviewers not on the committee to ensure that the material was balanced and unbiased. Contributors' disclosure information can be found with the list of contributors' names and those of ACP principal staff listed in the beginning of this book.

Hospital-Based Medicine

For the convenience of subscribers who provide care in hospital settings, content that is specific to the hospital setting has been highlighted in blue. Hospital icons (🏥) highlight where the hospital-only content begins, continues over more than one page, and ends.

High Value Care Key Points

Key Points in the text that relate to High Value Care concepts (that is, concepts that discuss balancing clinical benefit with costs and harms) are designated by the HVC icon [HVC].

Educational Disclaimer

The editors and publisher of MKSAP 18 recognize that the development of new material offers many opportunities for error. Despite our best efforts, some errors may persist in print. Drug dosage schedules are, we believe, accurate and in accordance with current standards. Readers are advised, however, to ensure that

the recommended dosages in MKSAP 18 concur with the information provided in the product information material. This is especially important in cases of new, infrequently used, or highly toxic drugs. Application of the information in MKSAP 18 remains the professional responsibility of the practitioner.

The primary purpose of MKSAP 18 is educational. Information presented, as well as publications, technologies, products, and/or services discussed, is intended to inform subscribers about the knowledge, techniques, and experiences of the contributors. A diversity of professional opinion exists, and the views of the contributors are their own and not those of the ACP. Inclusion of any material in the program does not constitute endorsement or recommendation by the ACP. The ACP does not warrant the safety, reliability, accuracy, completeness, or usefulness of and disclaims any and all liability for damages and claims that may result from the use of information, publications, technologies, products, and/or services discussed in this program.

Publisher's Information

Disclaimer Regarding Direct Purchases from Online Retailers

CME and/or MOC for MKSAP 18 is available only if you purchase the program directly from ACP. CME credits and MOC points cannot be awarded to those purchasers who have purchased the program from non-authorized sellers such as Amazon, eBay, or any other such online retailer.

Unauthorized Use of This Book Is Against the Law

publication for his or her own exclusive use. Send requests in writing to MKSAP® Permissions, American College of Physicians, 190 N. Independence Mall West, Philadelphia, PA 19106-1572, or email your request to mksap_editors@acponline.org.

MKSAP 18 ISBN: 978-1-938245-47-3
(Dermatology) ISBN: 978-1-938245-49-7

Printed in the United States of America.

For order information in the U.S. or Canada call 800-ACP-1915. All other countries call 215-351-2600, (Monday to Friday, 9 AM – 5 PM ET). Fax inquiries to 215-351-2799 or email to custserv@acponline.org.

Errata

Errata for MKSAP 18 will be available through the MKSAP Resource Site at mksap.acponline.org as new information becomes known to the editors.

Table of Contents

Approach to the Patient with Dermatologic Disease

Morphology 1
Physical Examination 2
Diagnostic Tests for Skin Disorders 2

Therapeutic Principles in Dermatology

General Considerations 3
Topical Glucocorticoids 3
Topical Antifungal Agents 4
Topical Immunomodulators 4
Topical Retinoids 4
Topical Antibiotics 4
Phototherapy 4

Common Rashes

Eczematous Dermatoses 4
   Atopic Dermatitis 4
   Contact Dermatitis 5
   Lichen Simplex Chronicus 6
   Intertrigo 6
   Hand Dermatitis 7
   Xerotic Eczema 7
   Nummular Eczema 8
   Stasis Dermatitis 8
Papulosquamous Dermatoses 8
   Psoriasis 8
   Lichen Planus 9
   Pityriasis Rosea 10
   Seborrheic Dermatitis 10
Miliaria 11
Transient Acantholytic Dermatosis 11

Disorders of Pigmentation

Vitiligo 12
Melasma 13

Drug Reactions 14

Acneiform Eruptions

Acne 17
Rosacea 19
Hidradenitis Suppurativa 21

Common Skin Infections

Bacterial Skin Infections 21
   Folliculitis 21
   Abscesses/Furuncles/Carbuncles 22
   Methicillin-Resistant *Staphylococcus aureus*
   in Hospitalized Patients 23
   Impetigo 23
   Cellulitis/Erysipelas 24
   Pitted Keratolysis 25
   Erythrasma 25
Superficial Fungal Infections 25
   Tinea 25
   Pityriasis Versicolor 27
   Candidiasis 28
Viral Skin Infections 28
   Herpes Simplex Virus 28
   Varicella/Herpes Zoster 29
   Warts 30
   Molluscum Contagiosum 31

Infestations

Scabies 31
Lice 31
Bed Bugs 32

Bites and Stings

Spiders 33
Hymenoptera 33
Worms 34
Fleas 34

Cuts, Scrapes, and Burns

Cuts and Scrapes 34
Burns 34

Common Neoplasms

Benign Neoplasms 35
   Seborrheic Keratosis 35
   Melanocytic Nevi 35
   Dysplastic Nevi 35
   Halo Nevi 36
   Sebaceous Hyperplasia 36

Callus/Corns 36
Acrochordon (Skin Tags) 37
Cherry Angiomas 37
Dermatofibroma 37
Solar Lentigines and Ephelides 37
Hypertrophic Scars and Keloids 37
Pyogenic Granulomas 38
Epidermal Inclusion Cysts 38
Lipomas 39
Digital Myxoid Cysts 39
Xanthoma 39
Neurofibromas 39
Precancerous and Cancerous Neoplasms 39
Basal Cell Carcinoma 39
Actinic Keratosis 41
Squamous Cell Carcinoma 41
Keratoacanthoma 42
Malignant Melanoma 42

Pruritus 44

Urticaria 45

Autoimmune Bullous Diseases 46

Cutaneous Manifestations of Internal Disease
Rheumatology 50
Lupus Erythematosus 50
Dermatomyositis 53
Sclerosing Disorders 54
Rheumatoid Arthritis 55
Vasculitis 56
Nephrology 57
Calciphylaxis 57
Kyrle Disease 57
Nephrogenic Systemic Fibrosis 58
Gastroenterology 58
Pyoderma Gangrenosum 58
Dermatitis Herpetiformis 59
Porphyria Cutanea Tarda 59
Hematology/Oncology 60
Sweet Syndrome 61
Amyloidosis 61
Endocrinology 62
Eruptive Xanthomas 62
Acanthosis Nigricans 62

Necrobiosis Lipoidica 63
Pretibial Myxedema 63
Infectious Disease 63
Pulmonary 64

Dermatologic Emergencies
Retiform Purpura 64
Erythema Multiforme 65
Stevens-Johnson Syndrome and Toxic
Epidermal Necrolysis 66
Drug Hypersensitivity Syndrome
(or DRESS Syndrome) 67
Acute Generalized Exanthematous Pustulosis 68
Erythroderma 68

Hair Disorders
Hypertrichosis/Hirsutism 69
Alopecia 70
Nonscarring Localized and
Generalized Alopecia 70
Scarring Localized and Generalized Alopecia 72

Nail Disorders
Infection 73
Paronychia 73
Inflammatory Dermatosis 73
Ingrown Toenail 75
Melanonychia 75
Squamous Cell Carcinoma 76

Disorders of the Mucous Membranes
Melanotic Macule 76
Amalgam Tattoo 76
Leukoplakia and Erythroplakia 76
Oral Candidiasis 77
Aphthous Ulcers 77
Lichen Planus 77
Actinic Cheilitis and Squamous Cell Carcinoma 78
Lichen Sclerosus 78
Black Hairy Tongue 78
Geographic Tongue 78

Foot and Lower Leg Ulcers
Venous Stasis Ulcers 79
Arterial Insufficiency Ulcers 79
Neuropathic Ulcers 80
Other Causes of Lower Extremity Ulcers 80

Dermatologic Conditions of Pregnancy and Aging

Pregnancy and Lactation 81
Aging 81
    Infection 84
    Chronic Wounds/Poor Wound Healing 84

Bibliography 85

Self-Assessment Test 89

Index 149

Dermatology High Value Care Recommendations

The American College of Physicians, in collaboration with multiple other organizations, is engaged in a worldwide initiative to promote the practice of High Value Care (HVC). The goals of the HVC initiative are to improve health care outcomes by providing care of proven benefit and reducing costs by avoiding unnecessary and even harmful interventions. The initiative comprises several programs that integrate the important concept of health care value (balancing clinical benefit with costs and harms) for a given intervention into a broad range of educational materials to address the needs of trainees, practicing physicians, and patients.

HVC content has been integrated into MKSAP 18 in several important ways. MKSAP 18 includes HVC-identified key points in the text, HVC-focused multiple choice questions, and, for subscribers to MKSAP Digital, an HVC custom quiz. From the text and questions, we have generated the following list of HVC recommendations that meet the definition below of high value care and bring us closer to our goal of improving patient outcomes while conserving finite resources.

High Value Care Recommendation: A recommendation to choose diagnostic and management strategies for patients in specific clinical situations that balance clinical benefit with cost and harms with the goal of improving patient outcomes.

Below are the High Value Care Recommendations for the Dermatology section of MKSAP 18.

- There is a generic equivalent in each class of topical glucocorticoids.
- Cost-effective treatment of hand dermatitis includes topical emollients such as petrolatum and minimizing hand washing (see Item 54).
- Combined topical glucocorticoids and antifungal agents should be avoided.
- Use plain petrolatum in place of topical antibiotics on clean wounds.
- Over-the-counter treatment of seborrheic dermatitis includes selenium sulfide or zinc pyrithione shampoos.
- Discontinuation of the causative drug is the first step in treating drug reactions.
- Topical antibiotics should not be used as monotherapy for acne.
- The diagnosis of folliculitis can be made from the clinical presentation.
- Pruritus may persist for weeks after eradication of scabies and does not require retreatment.
- Most "spider bites" are actually misdiagnosed folliculitis or furuncles.
- Excision of dysplastic nevi is reserved for lesions that are changing in size and color, are symptomatic, or stand out from other nevi.
- Evaluation for urticaria is not recommended unless history suggests a specific cause.
- A gluten-free diet is first-line treatment for dermatitis herpetiformis.
- All forms of lupus benefit from sun avoidance and a broad-spectrum sunscreen.
- Heliotrope rash and Gottron papules are pathognomonic for dermatomyositis.
- Löfgren syndrome is pathognomonic for sarcoidosis.
- Do not screen for susceptibility to Stevens-Johnson syndrome and toxic epidermal necrolysis with HLA-B*1502 and HLA-B*5801.
- To avoid unnecessary treatment, obtain culture or microscopic confirmation of onychomycosis.
- Treatment of eczema, venous insufficiency, and interdigital tinea infection can decrease the risk of recurrent cellulitis (see Item 20).
- Routine systemic antibiotics are not indicated for venous stasis ulcers.
- Actinic purpura is a normal sign of aging and requires no additional testing.

Dermatology

Approach to the Patient with Dermatologic Disease

General internists, in their day-to-day clinical interactions, will often be called upon to evaluate dermatologic problems. A thorough understanding of the skin and its associated structures is required (**Figure 1**).

Morphology

Morphology of skin lesions can be categorized as primary or secondary. Primary skin lesion morphology is the appearance of a rash or growth in its initial or unaltered state. Dermatologic conditions can be categorized as growths or rashes. Growths are localized areas of abnormal skin, whereas rashes are more widespread in appearance. Over time, with itching or rubbing, secondary skin changes may occur.

Table 1 lists primary and secondary skin lesions. Other important characteristics of skin lesions include color, distribution, grouping, and configuration. Rather than focusing initially on identification of specific rashes and their characteristics, a differential diagnosis should be developed based on morphologic features of the primary skin disease. For example, a linear pattern is often seen in contact dermatitis, a grouped pattern is seen in herpes viral infections, and tinea infections are often annular.

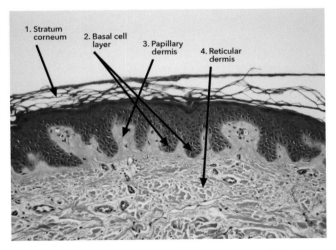

FIGURE 1. Structure of the skin showing: (1) Stratum corneum; (2) Basal cell layer; (3) Papillary dermis; and (4) Reticular dermis.

TABLE 1. Types of Skin Lesions	
Primary Skin Lesions	**Characteristics**
Macule	Small flat discoloration of the skin typically <1 cm in diameter
Patch	Flat discoloration of the skin >1 cm in diameter often with surface change, such as scale
Papule	Small <1 cm elevation of the skin, solid in nature
Plaque	Flat-topped "plateau-like" elevation of the skin >1 cm in diameter
Nodule	Space-occupying lesion within the dermis; larger than a papule and located deeper
Cyst	Fluid-filled nodule containing fluid that is expressible
Vesicle	Small clear fluid-filled blister <1 cm
Bulla	Larger clear fluid-filled blister >1 cm
Pustule	Vesicle filled with purulent material
Atrophy	Loss of one or more portions of the skin
Burrow	Serpiginous epidermal streaking/disruption caused by scabies mite
Comedo	Noninflammatory lesion caused by keratin debris within the sebaceous gland/hair follicle orifice; can be open or closed
Telangiectasia	Visibly dilated, but not palpable, blood vessel in the epidermis
Wheal/Hive	Transient, edematous, erythematous papule or plaque
Secondary Skin Lesions	**Characteristics**
Crust	Dried serous fluid commonly derived from blisters or pustules; often moist and yellow or brown
Excoriation	Defect in the epidermis often caused by scratching
Fissure	Linear break in the epidermis, usually along skin lines on the palms or soles
Lichenification	Visible thickening of the stratum corneum resulting in accentuation of the normal skin lines
Scale	Thickened stratum corneum; often dry and white or gray
Ulcer	Full-thickness destruction of the epidermis into the underlying dermis

Physical Examination

No standardized method has been developed for how to best perform a full-body skin examination, but experts agree that patients should be fully undressed and covered with an examination gown. Attempting to perform a full-body skin examination by having patients lift their shirt or roll up their sleeves is insufficient. Proper lighting is essential, as side lighting can often detect subtle elevations of the skin. A systematic approach is recommended. One method is to start with the head and neck, working down to the torso, upper extremities, and lower extremities. Care should be taken to ensure that the digits, umbilicus, and scalp are thoroughly examined. A full-body skin examination should take 2 minutes. The routine skin examination may be incorporated into the complete physical examination by assessing the torso when auscultating the heart and lungs, the arms while checking blood pressure and pulse, and the back while listening to the lungs. The skin examination is a good time to reinforce ultraviolet light protection techniques and review the signs and symptoms of skin cancer (see Common Neoplasms). The most recent U.S. Preventive Services Task Force (USPSTF) statement found insufficient evidence to screen adults for skin cancer, including persons with increased risk of skin cancer.

Rashes in persons with skin of color may be harder to detect since the pink-red color that is a sign of inflammation can be more subtle on darker skin. Persons with skin of color often have normal variations in skin color with areas of hyperpigmentation along the gingiva and lines of demarcation on the trunk and extremities. Scrapes, bug bites, or acne often heal with hyperpigmentation. Areas of active inflammation from seborrhea, eczema, or psoriasis may develop hyper- or hypopigmentation.

Diagnostic Tests for Skin Disorders

Diagnostic tools and tests that may augment the physical examination include preparation of specimens using potassium hydroxide (KOH), wet mounting, or Tzanck preparations; and use of a Wood lamp or a dermatoscope to visualize lesions. These techniques and tools are easy to use and have minimal equipment requirements; however, skill and experience are necessary for accurate and reliable interpretation.

If tinea or candida is suspected, a scraping of the skin at the leading edge of the rash is done. The scale is placed on a microscope slide, and KOH is applied to the specimen. The presence of branching hyphae indicates tinea, whereas the presence of pseudohyphae indicates candida. Similarly, a wet mount is done when evaluating for scabies. In this case, mineral oil is used in place of KOH. Mineral oil will allow the scabies mite to stay alive and will aid in detection.

A Wood lamp is an inexpensive ultraviolet light that can be used to evaluate hypo- and depigmentation as seen in vitiligo. It can also detect skin fluorescence associated with erythrasma and the urine fluorescence in patients with porphyria cutanea tarda. The Tzanck preparation can detect multinucleated giant cells within a blister cavity, thus determining a herpes viral infection. The Tzanck preparation does not distinguish between members of the herpes virus family. A hand-held microscope, called a dermatoscope, is a tool used predominately to help with the evaluation of pigmented skin lesions.

In addition, no office is complete without a camera and the capability to store photographs. Serial photographs can be used to follow the progress or improvement of a rash, to follow changes in a pigmented nevus, or to document the location of biopsy sites for proper location.

The clinician must determine whether a patient has a dermatologic emergency or urgency that requires immediate intervention or referral. **Table 2** describes situations that mandate immediate intervention or referral to a specialist.

KEY POINTS

- Rather than focusing initially on identification of specific rashes and their characteristics, a differential diagnosis should be developed based on morphologic features of the primary skin disease.
- The best method to evaluate dermatologic conditions is the full-body examination.

TABLE 2. Dermatologic Emergencies
Widespread erythema or erythroderma (drug eruption, bacterial toxin-mediated disease, severe psoriasis)
High fever and widespread rash (severe drug eruptions, rickettsial diseases)
Diffuse peeling or sloughing of skin (toxic epidermal necrolysis, infection)
Dark, dusky, purple areas of painful skin (impending skin loss from infection or severe drug eruption)
Mucosal inflammation, erosions, or ulceration (severe drug eruption, autoimmune blistering disease with high risk of morbid scarring)
Widespread blistering (autoimmune blistering disease, infection, severe drug eruption)
Purpura, particularly "retiform" or lacey, patterned purpura (vasculitis, vasculopathy, infection, autoimmune disease)
Broad areas of exquisitely painful skin out of proportion to clinical examination findings (necrotizing fasciitis)
Angulated purpura of the distal extremities (sepsis, autoimmune phenomena)
Palpable purpura (small vessel vasculitis from infection, medications, or autoimmune reactions)
Immunosuppressed, particularly patients with neutropenia, with skin lesions of unknown cause in the setting of fever, particularly red or purple nodules (skin signs of infection in immunosuppressed hosts)
Purple or necrotic skin lesions in immunosuppressed hosts (angioinvasive fungal infection)
Rapidly growing lesions in immunosuppressed hosts (infection, malignancy)
Worrisome pigmented lesions warrant urgent (not emergent) referral and evaluation (melanoma)

Therapeutic Principles in Dermatology

General Considerations

The effectiveness of a topical medication depends largely on its ability to be absorbed through the skin. Absorption is dependent on the chemical structure of the medication, its concentration, skin hydration, skin thickness, and the delivery vehicle.

In general, ointments have a higher potency than creams, which in turn have a higher potency than solutions or suspensions. The various vehicles that are available are listed in Table 3. Creams rub in and dissipate without leaving a residue, and patients tend to favor their use. The alcohol content and drying nature of gels can cause burning and stinging on non-intact skin. An occlusive vehicle such as an ointment increases penetration, but adherence may be low because of its greasy feel.

Table 4 outlines the various categories of topical medications, including those most frequently used and the indications for which they are used.

Topical Glucocorticoids

Topical glucocorticoids are used for their anti-inflammatory effects. Because they are applied directly to the area of involvement, systemic adverse effects are minimized. Topical glucocorticoids are classified by their potency level. One should become comfortable with one in each class from weak to ultra-potent. There is a generic equivalent in each class, allowing for a cost-effective approach (**Table 5**).

In general, twice-daily dosing is the most common dosing schedule, and the medication should be applied in a thin film. A rule of thumb is that 30 grams of a topical glucocorticoid will be enough to cover the entire surface of a 70 kg adult, once. Proportionately less is needed for smaller areas.

Topical glucocorticoids may cause striae, easy bruising, atrophy, and telangiectasia. Side effects are most frequently seen when using higher potencies for longer periods of time; in areas of thin skin (such as the face); skin folds; or when used under occlusion. Use of glucocorticoids around the eyes can exacerbate glaucoma and cause cataracts.

TABLE 3. Vehicles for Topical Medications

Vehicle	Characteristics
Cream	Equal mixture of oil and water with a smooth texture and whitish in color
	Easily rubs in and leaves minimal residue
	High patient preference because of aesthetic feel and appearance
Foam	Preparation that merges a gas (propane or butane) with the medication
	Allows the medication to be dispersed within a field of minute bubbles
	Used predominantly in terminal-hair–bearing skin
Gel	Semisolid vehicle with alcohol base
	Drying in nature
	Irritating to broken skin due to alcohol content
Lotion	Thicker in nature than a solution due to its increased emollient properties
	Base is typically water
	Easy to apply on large areas
Ointment	Oil in water mixture with a transparent clear appearance and greasy/oily texture
	Most occlusive of the vehicles
	Highest viscosity
	Difficult to use under clothing, on hands/fingers of an active person
Patch	Unique vehicle that is applied to skin
	Standardized method of releasing medication over time
Powder	Solid particulate preparation
	Typically used in skin folds to aid in moisture control and to reduce skin-on-skin friction
Solution	The active medication is suspended in a water or alcohol base
	Viscosity of water, easy to apply to scalp/hair-bearing areas
Suspension	Oil and water mixture that separates when allowed to sit
	Must be shaken thoroughly before use

TABLE 4. Frequently Used Topical Medications

Medication	Indications
Topical glucocorticoids	Inflammatory dermatoses
Topical antifungals	Cutaneous fungal infections
Terbinafine, nystatin, econazole, miconazole, ciclopirox, clotrimazole	
Topical retinoids	
Tretinoin, adapalene	Acne
Tazarotene	Psoriasis
Topical antibiotics	
Mupirocin, neomycin, bacitracin	Antibacterial agents
Erythromycin, clindamycin	Acne
Metronidazole	Rosacea
Topical chemotherapy	
5-fluorouracil	Actinic keratosis
Antiparasitic	
Permethrin	Scabies
Vitamin D analogues	
Calcipotriene	Psoriasis

TABLE 5.	Potency and Examples of Topical Glucocorticoids
Potency	**Glucocorticoid**
Weak	Hydrocortisone 1.0% or 2.5%
Low	Desonide 0.05%
	Triamcinolone acetonide 0.025%
	Fluocinolone acetonide 0.01%
Medium	Triamcinolone acetonide 0.1%
	Fluocinolone acetonide 0.025%
	Betamethasone valerate 0.1%
	Fluticasone propionate 0.05%
	Hydrocortisone butyrate 0.1%
	Hydrocortisone valerate 0.02%
High	Betamethasone dipropionate 0.05%
	Fluocinonide 0.05%
	Halcinonide 0.1%
	Amcinonide 0.1%
	Desoximetasone 0.25%
	Triamcinolone acetonide 0.5%
Ultra	Augmented betamethasone dipropionate 0.05%
	Clobetasol propionate 0.05%
	Halobetasol propionate 0.05%
	Diflorasone diacetate 0.05%
	Flurandrenolide tape

Topical Antifungal Agents

Topical antifungal agents are used to treat tinea or candida infections. Topical azole antifungal agents are suitable for treatment of localized infection, whereas oral agents are used to treat recurrent, recalcitrant, or widespread disease.

Topical glucocorticoids are frequently commercially combined with topical antifungal agents (clotrimazole-betamethasone). These combinations should be avoided. The use of a combination drug can worsen some tinea infections and when used in the groin area has a high risk of causing striae.

Topical Immunomodulators

Topical immunomodulators (tacrolimus ointment and pimecrolimus cream) can be used in place of topical glucocorticoids on the face, in skin folds, or in occlusive areas of the body (axilla/groin) for an extended period of time without the development of atrophy, striae, and telangiectasia. These medications have a black box warning for the rare development of skin cancer and cutaneous lymphoma.

Topical Retinoids

Topical retinoids are used frequently in the treatment of acne and psoriasis. They are vitamin A analogues with effects on keratinocyte proliferation and differentiation. Use should be avoided in pregnancy due to the risk of teratogenicity.

Topical Antibiotics

Clindamycin and erythromycin are two topical antibiotics used in the treatment of acne. They are well tolerated and have few to no side effects. Bacterial resistance has been shown to occur when using the agents as solo therapy. The combination of benzoyl peroxide and a topical antibiotic has shown to limit bacterial resistance. Over-the-counter combination antibiotics are used frequently. They typically have minimal side effects. The most frequent side effect is allergic contact dermatitis. This is seen with neomycin and bacitracin.

Phototherapy

When taken 2 hours before ultraviolet A (UVA) light exposure, oral psoralen increases the absorption of UVA. Historically, the combination of psoralen plus UVA (PUVA) phototherapy for the treatment of psoriasis has been shown to be effective but significantly increased the risk for developing skin cancer. Newer phototherapy units using a narrow band of ultraviolet B (UVB) has been shown to be safe and effective with a much smaller risk of skin cancer.

KEY POINTS

- Topical glucocorticoids can avoid the adverse effects of systemic glucocorticoid therapy but can cause striae, easy bruising, atrophy, and telangiectasia.
- There is a generic equivalent in each class of topical glucocorticoids, allowing for a cost-effective approach. **HVC**
- Combined topical glucocorticoids and antifungal agents should be avoided. **HVC**

Common Rashes

Eczematous Dermatoses

Eczematous dermatoses are common inflammatory conditions that present as pruritic, erythematous patches or plaques that may show weeping or dry scaling at various stages. These dermatoses lead to impaired skin barrier function, often allowing for secondary bacterial infections.

Treatment includes avoidance of known triggers, use of mild cleansers followed by immediate application of fragrance-free emollients and topical anti-inflammatory medications.

Atopic Dermatitis

Atopic dermatitis commonly presents on the face and flexural surfaces, such as the popliteal and antecubital fossae (**Figure 2**). Excoriations and thickening (lichenification) of the skin from scratching often accompany other signs of the atopic triad (allergic rhinitis, asthma, and eczema). The pathogenesis is

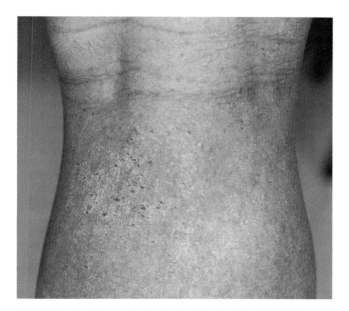

FIGURE 2. Atopic dermatitis showing skin thickening (lichenification) due to scratching and dry scaling in the popliteal flexure.

thought to be caused by a mutation in filaggrin, a protein in the epidermis important in the barrier function of the skin. Affected skin is often secondarily infected by *Staphylococcus aureus* due to a decrease in antimicrobial peptides. The use of fragrance-free, non–soap-based cleansers and moisturizers along with topical glucocorticoids is the primary treatment.

Topical calcineurin inhibitors, such as tacrolimus and pimecrolimus, are steroid-sparing agents useful for areas such as the face and skin folds where permanent atrophy from long-term or potent topical glucocorticoid use is a concern.

Contact Dermatitis

Pathophysiology and Evaluation

There are two types of contact dermatitis: allergic and irritant. Allergic contact dermatitis is a type IV, T-cell–mediated, delayed hypersensitivity reaction. On re-exposure to a specific allergen, sensitized T-cells trigger an inflammatory cascade, leading to an eczematous eruption at the site of contact; rarely, a widespread eruption (id reaction) may occur. Irritant contact dermatitis is more common than allergic contact dermatitis and is not immune mediated. Irritant contact dermatitis occurs from direct damage to the skin from harsh chemicals, soaps, or detergents.

Discovering the cause of contact dermatitis is essential to its treatment and prevention. A detailed history can help identify the cause, but often epicutaneous patch testing is needed to identify the source (**Figure 3 A** and **Figure 3 B**). For patch testing, a number of standardized chemicals are applied to the skin and removed 48 hours later. Evaluation is performed at the time of patch removal and again 5 to 7 days later to assess for redness and eczematous reaction at any of the sites. Because allergies can develop over time, a long history of using a

product without a problem does not exclude that product as a potential trigger.

Common Causes of Allergic Dermatitis

Urushiol, the allergen that is a common cause of allergic contact dermatitis, is found in plants such as poison ivy, oak, and sumac, which are members of the genus *Toxicodendron* (formerly *Rhus*). Clinically, it presents with intensely pruritic, often linear, vesicular papules, plaques, and vesicles (**Figure 4**). Lesions can present at different locations at different times up to 14 days after exposure in sensitized patients. Fluid from vesicles and blisters is not antigenic. After exposure, patients should remove any contaminated clothing and gently wash the skin with soap and water. It is critical for those sensitive to these antigens to avoid inhaling any smoke resulting from the unintentional or inadvertent burning of these plants as the smoke contains allergenic plant particles.

Nickel, another common allergen, is commonly found in everyday items such as jewelry, zippers, cell phones, and even medical devices. Eczematous dermatitis of the lower abdomen is a common presentation of a nickel allergy from a snap or

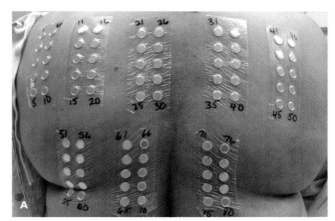

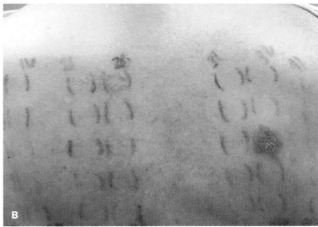

FIGURE 3. (*A*) Epicutaneous patch testing is commonly applied to the back to evaluate for allergic contact dermatitis. (*B*) The erythematous patch identified 48 hours after epicutaneous patch testing indicates a positive reaction to a specific allergen (methylisothiazolinone).

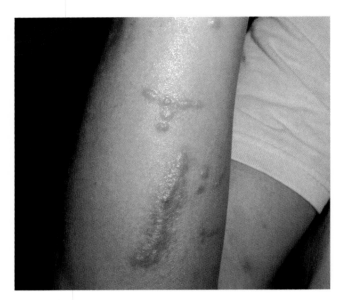

FIGURE 4. Linear erythematous plaques and vesicles are commonly seen in allergic contact dermatitis from poison ivy.

belt buckle. Patients may use a commercially available nickel test kit to identify items that contain nickel.

Fragrances are also common allergens found in many cosmetic products, moisturizers, and detergents. They may also be present as flavoring agents of toothpastes, mouthwashes, and food beverages.

Neomycin and bacitracin are commonly used for wound care. They can cause an allergic contact dermatitis that mimics a wound infection. Given the prevalence of sensitivity to these products, patients should use plain petrolatum in place of topical antibiotics to aid healing of clean wounds.

Almost all household cleansers and personal hygiene products contain preservatives that can produce allergic contact dermatitis. Certain occupations also are at increased risk of allergic contact dermatitis (**Table 6**).

KEY POINT

HVC • Use plain petrolatum in place of topical antibiotics to aid healing of clean wounds and avoid developing allergic contact dermatitis.

Treatment of Contact Dermatitis

Avoidance of the causative agent is preventive and curative. Topical glucocorticoids are used while the patient and clinician work together to identify and eliminate the source. Severe allergic contact eruptions may necessitate a 2- to 3-week taper of systemic glucocorticoids. Because of the risk of rebound dermatitis, shorter courses of systemic glucocorticoids are not recommended.

Lichen Simplex Chronicus

Lichen simplex chronicus is a condition caused by repetitive scratching or rubbing. Predisposing conditions include atopic

dermatitis, xerosis, and psychiatric conditions such as obsessive-compulsive disorder. Lichen simplex chronicus manifests as thickened plaques with erythema and hyperpigmentation (**Figure 5**). Exaggerated skin markings are seen on the surface of the skin as well. Common sites include the genitals, back of the neck, wrists, ankles, and lower legs. Lichen simplex chronicus is treated with moisturizers, high and ultrapotent topical glucocorticoids, and intralesional glucocorticoid injections.

Intertrigo

Intertrigo is dermatitis involving adjacent skin folds (axillary, inframammary, abdominal, and inguinal) (**Figure 6**). Predisposing conditions include obesity, friction, occlusion, and factors that interfere with immune response, such as

TABLE 6. Common Contact Allergens	
Contact Allergens	**Occupations/Exposures**
Benzophenones	Sunscreens (contact and photocontact dermatitis)
Balsam of Peru	Common fragrance in personal care products and foods
Methacrylate	Dental fillings, cement for joint replacement (orthopedic surgeons and dentists)
Methylisothiazolinone	Baby wipes, personal care products
Paraphenylenediamine	Permanent hair dye
Formaldehyde and formaldehyde-releasing preservatives (Quaternium-15)	Cosmetics and personal care products
Rubber accelerators (carba mix, thiurams, benzothiazoles)	Shoe and glove dermatitis; common in health care workers
Cocamidopropyl betaine	Personal care products (shampoos)

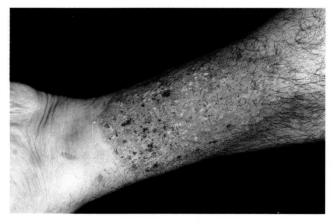

FIGURE 5. As atopic dermatitis becomes chronic, the skin becomes lichenified with accentuated skin lines (lichen simplex chronicus) and, particularly in dark skin, hyperpigmented.

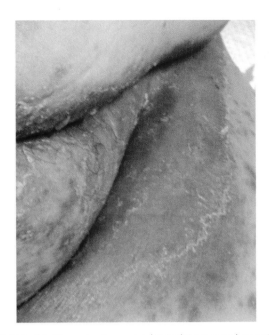

FIGURE 6. Intertrigo, a chronic recurrent skin condition seen in obese patients, is caused by moist conditions in skin fold areas and is worsened by heat and exercise. The rash is confined to the intertriginous areas and does not extend beyond these boundaries. Secondary infection with *Candida* may occur, as with this patient. Clues to *Candida* infection include small red papules on the periphery of the rash.

diabetes mellitus. Intertrigo presents with erythematous, macerated plaques. Secondary infection with *Candida* is common and may be suspected by the presence of multiple small red papules and pustules that surround the main rash (satellite pustules).

Treatment of intertrigo consists of drying the area and use of agents such as antifungal powder, to reduce moisture and maceration and to prevent secondary yeast infection. Short courses of low-potency topical glucocorticoids may be added to treat the associated inflammation. If secondary *Candida* infection is suspected, concomitant treatment with topical antifungal agents can be added.

Hand Dermatitis

Hand dermatitis often results from a combination of causes such as excessive hand washing, contact dermatitis, atopic dermatitis, or dyshidrotic eczema (pompholyx). It is most commonly seen in patients who hold jobs involving frequent or prolonged exposure to water, chemicals, and occlusive gloves (health care, house cleaning, food preparation, hairstyling). It is characterized by pruritic, erythematous plaques on the palmar and dorsal hands, which can lead to fissuring and lichenification over time (**Figure 7**). Dyshidrotic eczema presents with vesicles on the palms and sides of the fingers.

The differential diagnosis of hand eczema includes tinea, psoriasis, and scabies. The entire body should be examined for other rashes that may help differentiate hand dermatitis from these other rashes. If tinea is suspected, the feet should be

examined for tinea pedis and onychomycosis (two feet-one hand syndrome).

Treatment includes topical emollients such as petrolatum. A potent topical glucocorticoid may be necessary during flares. Triggers should be identified and avoided, and hand washing minimized. White cotton glove liners are recommended inside of rubber gloves when working with chemicals and water.

Xerotic Eczema

Also called eczema craquelé or asteatotic eczema, xerotic dermatitis is often seen on the lower extremities of older persons. Dry weather and excessive bathing are known inciting factors. The lesions are erythematous with plate-like cracked scale, often resembling a dried up creek bed (**Figure 8**). Although aging is the most common cause, hypothyroidism or medications such as diuretics may be implicated.

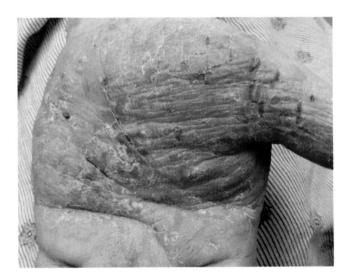

FIGURE 7. Hand dermatitis with findings of palmar edema, erythema, desquamation, and fissuring.

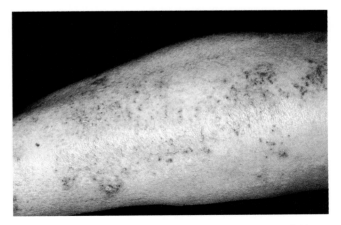

FIGURE 8. Severe xerotic eczema is characterized by redness and a "tile-like" pattern on dry skin (xerosis) with evidence of trauma from scratching. This typically occurs during midwinter in northern climates.

Treatment consists of thick emollients and potent topical glucocorticoids for a 2- to 3-week course.

Nummular Eczema

Nummular eczema, also called discoid eczema, is characterized by coin-shaped, pruritic, scaly plaques (**Figure 9**). This form of eczema is common on the extremities. The round shape may lead to confusion between this form of eczema and other conditions, such as tinea corporis, nummular psoriasis, or contact dermatitis. Tinea corporis often has a partially cleared center and scaling at the periphery. Psoriasis is often located on the elbows, knees, scalp, or intergluteal cleft and has larger, thicker white scale. Contact dermatitis may be suggested by location on the body that matches contact with a potential allergen.

Potent topical glucocorticoids and emollients are the preferred treatment.

Stasis Dermatitis

Stasis dermatitis, which can be very pruritic and erythematous, is common in patients with chronic lower extremity edema, most commonly secondary to venous stasis (**Figure 10**). Symptoms are often bilateral with medial distal leg predominance, although it may be unilaterally symptomatic. Dependent edema, hyperpigmentation, and dilated veins are common associated findings. Symptoms can be managed topically with glucocorticoids and emollients, but the condition will not significantly improve until the edema is addressed

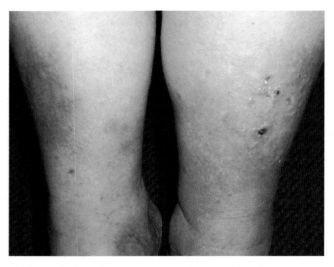

FIGURE 10. Stasis dermatitis characterized by edema, bilateral erythematous patches, weeping vesicles, ankle varicosities, and hyperpigmentation.

with leg elevation and compression stockings. Because of a similar clinical presentation, stasis dermatitis can be misdiagnosed as cellulitis; however, cellulitis is usually unilateral, more acute in onset, and often associated with pain, leukocytosis, and occasionally fever.

KEY POINTS

- Allergic contact dermatitis is a type IV T-cell–mediated delayed hypersensitivity reaction and is best diagnosed with epicutaneous patch testing.
- Hand dermatitis is characterized by pruritic, erythematous plaques on the hands and results from a combination of causes, such as excessive hand washing, contact dermatitis, atopic dermatitis, or dyshidrotic eczema (pompholyx).
- Stasis dermatitis is sometimes misdiagnosed as cellulitis; however, cellulitis is usually unilateral, more acute in onset, and often associated with pain, leukocytosis, and occasionally fever.

HVC

Papulosquamous Dermatoses

Papulosquamous dermatoses are characterized by scaly papules and plaques caused by inflammation of the epidermis.

Psoriasis

Psoriasis is a chronic, inflammatory dermatosis, typically presenting with thick, well-demarcated erythematous plaques with overlying silvery scale (**Figure 11**). It affects approximately 2% to 4% of the population. The incidence peaks at age 30 to 39 years and again around 60 years. Disease severity can range drastically with some patients having only one plaque to an erythrodermic presentation involving more than 90% of the body surface area. Psoriasis has many clinical presentations,

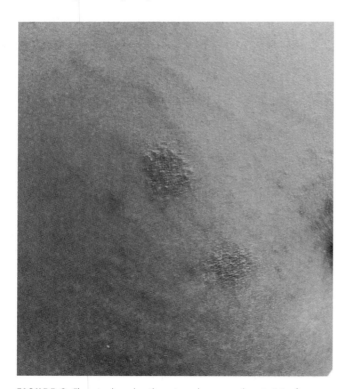

FIGURE 9. The coin-shaped erythematous plaques are characteristic of nummular dermatitis.

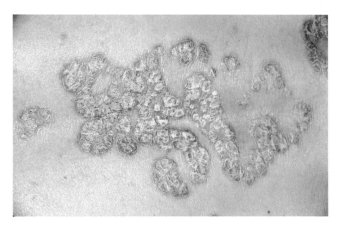

FIGURE 11. Psoriasis presents as well-demarcated, erythematous, polymorphous plaques with silvery scale.

the most common being plaque psoriasis, or psoriasis vulgaris. Nail psoriasis can involve both fingernails and toenails. It presents clinically with nail pitting, onycholysis (separation of nail plate from nail bed), and "oil spots" (**Figure 12**). Other less common subtypes include guttate psoriasis (commonly seen in pediatric patients), palmoplantar psoriasis (frequently with pustules as the primary lesion), and inverse psoriasis (often seen without scale in the intertriginous areas). Inverse psoriasis is frequently misdiagnosed because of lack of scale, location (flexural), and resemblance to other common dermatologic conditions such as tinea, intertrigo, and allergic contact dermatitis.

Psoriasis is a systemic disease, not just a skin problem. Approximately 30% of patients have concurrent psoriatic arthritis. Patients with severe psoriasis also have a greater risk of cardiovascular disease, which is the leading cause of death

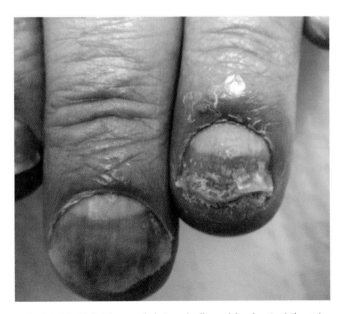

FIGURE 12. Nail pitting, onycholysis, and yellow-red discoloration (oil spots) are often present when the nails are involved in psoriasis.

among these patients, and chronic kidney disease. Psoriasis is associated with multiple cardiovascular risk factors including obesity, hypertension, diabetes, dyslipidemia, and the metabolic syndrome. The proposed link between psoriasis and cardiovascular disease is thought to be inflammation with similar cytokines involved in both psoriatic and atherosclerotic plaques.

Smoking tobacco may worsen psoriasis, and all patients should be counseled against smoking especially because of the elevated risk of cardiovascular disease. The pharmacologic treatment of psoriasis depends on the severity of the disease. Topical glucocorticoids are the mainstay of treatment for localized disease. Topical vitamin D analogues are also used as monotherapy or in combination with topical glucocorticoids. In patients with skin involvement of greater than 10% body surface area (severe psoriasis), psoriatic arthritis, psoriasis recalcitrant to topical treatments, or psoriasis in locations such as scalp or groin, systemic therapies, including phototherapy and traditional treatments such as methotrexate, acitretin, and cyclosporine, should be considered. Newer systemic therapies are the phosphodiesterase-4 inhibitor (apremilast) and biologic agents (tumor necrosis factor α inhibitors, interleukin-12/interleukin-23 inhibitors, and interleukin-17 inhibitors). These treatments target the cytokines involved in the pathogenesis of psoriasis.

KEY POINTS

- Psoriasis typically presents as thick, well-demarcated erythematous plaques with overlying silvery scale.
- Cardiovascular disease is the leading cause of death among patients with severe psoriasis.
- Topical glucocorticoids are the mainstay of treatment for localized disease; however, in patients with extensive involvement, psoriatic arthritis, psoriasis recalcitrant to topical treatments, or psoriasis in locations such as scalp or groin, phototherapy, methotrexate, acitretin, and cyclosporine should be considered.

Lichen Planus

Lichen planus is a T-cell–mediated disease classically presenting as pruritic, flat-topped, violaceous papules, often on the flexural surfaces of the extremities (wrists and ankles) and mucous membranes (**Figure 13**). This disease is fairly common with an incidence of 0.2% to 1% in adults. Other variants include mucosal, genital, bullous, atrophic, and hypertrophic lichen planus. Mucosal lesions have lacy white streaks (Wickham striae) or erosions and ulcerations. There can also be nail thickening and onycholysis, which can lead to scarring around the cuticle (dorsal pterygium).

Lichen planus tends to resolve over 1 to 2 years, although oral and nail lichen planus are more persistent. Some but not all studies have shown an increased prevalence of hepatitis C infection in patients with lichen planus. Squamous cell carcinoma transformation has been reported most

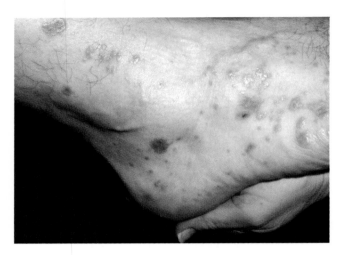

FIGURE 13. Lichen planus presents as purple, flat-topped papules most commonly on the ankles and wrists.

commonly in erosive oral lichen planus and hypertrophic lichen planus.

Potent topical glucocorticoids are effective in most patients. Systemic glucocorticoids, oral retinoids, sulfasalazine, and phototherapy are reserved for severe cutaneous or persistent oral disease.

KEY POINTS

- Lichen planus appears as pruritic, flat-topped, violaceous papules, often on the flexural surfaces of the extremities and mucous membranes.
- Lichen planus is treated with potent topical glucocorticoids; however, systemic glucocorticoids, oral retinoids, sulfasalazine, and phototherapy are used for severe or persistent oral disease.

Pityriasis Rosea

Pityriasis rosea is a common rash that may be related to reactivation of human herpesvirus 6 or 7. Pityriasis rosea begins as a single annular patch or plaque with fine scaling (the herald patch), typically on the trunk, followed by numerous smaller skin-colored to pink papules and plaques erupting along skin cleavage lines (**Figure 14**). This distribution on the posterior thorax can resemble a "fir tree" pattern. The herald patch is absent in up to 50% of cases, but when present it usually precedes the smaller plaques by several days up to 2 weeks.

Most patients do not need treatment, as these lesions are often asymptomatic and resolve over a few weeks to months. For patients with pruritus, a topical glucocorticoid and/or oral antihistamine can be used for symptomatic relief. Macrolide antibiotics, acyclovir, and phototherapy have all been reported to speed up resolution, but these treatments are generally not recommended. It is important to rule out secondary syphilis, which can look similar, but typically also involves the palms and soles and is usually associated with generalized lymphadenopathy.

KEY POINT

- Secondary syphilis can be mistaken for pityriasis rosea but it typically involves the palms and soles and is usually associated with generalized lymphadenopathy. **HVC**

Seborrheic Dermatitis

Seborrheic dermatitis is a common condition characterized by greasy yellow, scaly, erythematous patches in seborrheic areas (the scalp, face, ears, upper chest, axillae, and inguinal folds) (**Figure 15**). Specific areas of involvement on the face are the eyebrows, medial aspects of the cheeks, inter-eyebrow region, and the nasal ala. Men are more frequently affected than women. This disease is believed to be caused by a heightened sensitivity to lipophilic yeasts such as *Malassezia*. It is more prevalent in patients who are immunocompromised, such as those with HIV/AIDS or organ transplant patients. In HIV/AIDS patients, the severity of seborrheic dermatitis is inversely

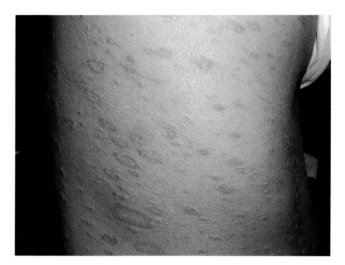

FIGURE 14. The oval-shaped patches of pityriasis rosea often follow along skin cleavage lines.

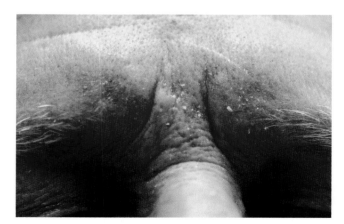

FIGURE 15. Seborrheic dermatitis, with fine, oily scale around the medial eyebrows.

correlated with the CD4 counts, may extend beyond typical locations, and may be difficult to control. Patients with Parkinson disease or Down syndrome also have a higher prevalence of seborrheic dermatitis. Diagnosis is made clinically based on the distribution and appearance. Factors contributing to flares include sleep deprivation and stress.

Treatment includes over-the-counter medications such as selenium sulfide or zinc pyrithione shampoos. Ketoconazole shampoo and cream are effective as well. Patients should be counseled to apply the shampoo on the skin and allow it to sit for 5 minutes before washing off. Weak or low-potency topical glucocorticoids can be used in combination with antifungal treatments when severely inflamed. Oral ketoconazole is not recommended owing to the risk of liver and adrenal gland toxicity, although other oral antifungal agents may be used for severe or refractory disease. If conventional therapies are not effective, other diagnoses must be considered including rosacea, lupus erythematosus, atopic dermatitis, and contact dermatitis.

KEY POINT

HVC
- Inexpensive treatment of seborrheic dermatitis includes over-the-counter medications such as selenium sulfide or zinc pyrithione shampoos.

Miliaria

Miliaria (prickly heat, heat rash) is caused by the occlusion and subsequent rupture of the eccrine sweat ducts at various levels. An overgrowth of *Staphylococcus epidermis* may contribute to the pathogenesis in miliaria. Clinically, it presents as numerous nonfollicular 1- to 3-mm papules or pustules that can arise with any condition causing sweating and skin occlusion. Miliaria can be subtyped by the level at which the eccrine sweat glands are occluded. Miliaria crystallina is caused by an occlusion at the stratum corneum and is characterized by asymptomatic clear subcorneal vesicles that can be easily ruptured (**Figure 16**). This tends to be more common in neonates.

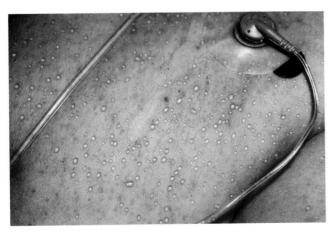

FIGURE 16. Miliaria crystallina with clear, fragile vesicles without inflammation.

Miliaria pustulosa describes the condition when vesicles have turbid fluid within them (**Figure 17**). Miliaria rubra is characterized by multiple small pink papules. It is the most common form and usually found on the trunk, particularly the back. It is the result of a deeper occlusion of the eccrine duct causing an intraepidermal-dermal vesicle.

Supportive therapy involves eliminating predisposing factors such as sweating and removal of occluding agents or conditions. Low-potency topical glucocorticoids can be used sparingly if symptomatic.

Transient Acantholytic Dermatosis

Transient acantholytic dermatosis, also known as Grover disease, is a relatively common benign eruption that is most often seen in middle-aged to elderly white men. The eruption presents as discrete papules, some of which may be scaly, and papulovesicles on the trunk (**Figure 18**). Symptomatically there are varying degrees of pruritus that may be associated with seasonal flares during the winter and spring. The cause is unknown, but there are specific conditions that are commonly

FIGURE 17. Miliaria pustulosa showing numerous 1-mm non-inflammatory pustules on the back of a hospitalized patient, seen in this image as small white dots.

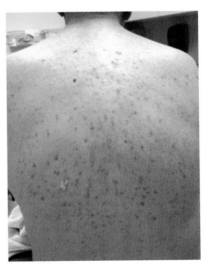

FIGURE 18. A patient with transient acantholytic dermatosis (Grover disease) showing recurrent outbreaks of pruritic, red papules, some of which are scaly, on the back. The image also shows numerous tan-colored seborrheic keratoses.

associated including chronic sun damage, eczema, and psoriasis. Transient acantholytic dermatosis can be triggered by dry skin, sweating, increased body temperature, acute sun exposure, certain medications, and internal neoplasms. The diagnosis can be confirmed by a skin biopsy that characteristically shows acantholysis of the epidermis with variable amounts of dyskeratosis.

Treatment includes moisturizers, emollients, and medium- to high-potency topical glucocorticoids. For severe and recalcitrant cases, oral retinoids, in particular isotretinoin, and psoralen with ultraviolet A (PUVA) can be used; neither is FDA approved for transient acantholytic dermatosis.

Disorders of Pigmentation
Vitiligo

Vitiligo is a common acquired autoimmune condition resulting in patchy depigmentation of the skin and is characterized by the loss of function or absence of melanocytes. Its prevalence is between 0.5% and 1.0%. Affecting both sexes equally, vitiligo can occur at any age, and it can be psychologically distressing. Clinically, it appears as completely depigmented, well-demarcated symmetric macules or patches with no scale. Its onset is insidious and asymptomatic, starting as smaller macules that gradually enlarge (**Figure 19**). It tends to be more visible in darker skin types (**Figure 20**) or in sun-exposed areas as the surrounding skin will become darker with sun exposure. The hair in the patches of vitiligo can become depigmented as well. The most commonly affected areas involve the extensor surfaces such as the dorsal hands and feet, elbows, and knees, and the periorificial areas such as around the mouth, eyes, rectum, and genitals. It can be associated with other autoimmune conditions such as diabetes and thyroid disease.

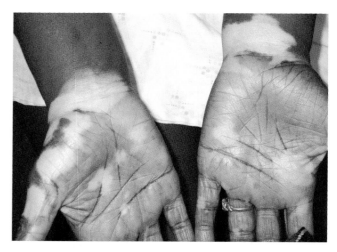

FIGURE 20. Classic vitiligo with well-demarcated symmetric patches of depigmented skin with no scale in a darkly pigmented person.

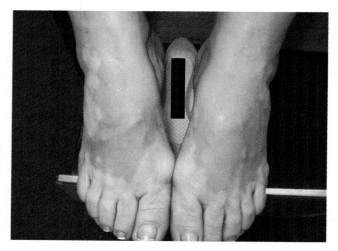

FIGURE 19. Well-demarcated symmetric patches of depigmented skin with no scale and accentuation of normal, sun-exposed skin typical of vitiligo.

Occasionally, it can be challenging to distinguish vitiligo from other conditions that cause depigmentation such as postinflammatory hyperpigmentation, tinea versicolor, pityriasis alba, and leprosy.

Postinflammatory hypopigmentation is a loss of skin pigmentation following resolution of inflammatory or infectious dermatoses. Topical or intralesional glucocorticoids can also cause hypopigmentation, which can be difficult to distinguish from postinflammatory hypopigmentation. Upon cessation of the glucocorticoid, the pigmentation will typically return. Other causes of postinflammatory hypopigmentation may include chemical irritants and destructive therapeutic procedures such as cryosurgery or laser therapy. The diagnosis of postinflammatory hypopigmentation is based upon recognition of hypomelanotic or amelanotic macules or patches that correspond to previous inflammatory lesions. If the diagnosis is in doubt, a skin biopsy may assist in identifying the responsible inflammatory lesion. Postinflammatory hypopigmentation typically resolves without specific therapy over weeks to months.

The diagnosis of tinea versicolor can be verified with a potassium hydroxide preparation showing hyphae and yeast cells. In addition, Wood lamp examination may disclose yellow to yellow-green fluorescence.

Pityriasis alba occurs in children and adolescents. Defining characteristics include patches of hypopigmentation on face, neck, upper trunk, and proximal extremities. Lesions typically manifest some border irregularity and are associated with a fine scale.

Tuberculoid leprosy presents with a small number of hypopigmented anesthetic lesions with raised margins.

Partial or complete depigmentation is also seen in idiopathic guttate hypomelanosis, a very common hypopigmentation disorder. Guttate hypomelanosis manifests as 2- to 6-mm hypopigmented round or oval macules on the trunk and extremities of middle-aged and older persons (**Figure 21**). Idiopathic guttate hypomelanosis may be the results of chronic ultraviolet (UV) exposure, trauma, and normal aging.

Other causes of depigmentation include drug-induced leukoderma and melanoma-associated leukoderma. Leukoderma has been reported in patients with advanced melanoma treated with immunotherapy such as high-dose interleukin-2, interferon alfa, ipilimumab (anti-CTLA-4), and granulocyte-macrophage colony-stimulating factor. Some genodermatoses such as tuberous sclerosis, piebaldism, and Waardenburg syndrome also cause depigmentation.

History and physical examination including a Wood lamp examination to help accentuate the depigmentation and the distribution of the lesions will help confirm the diagnosis. Lesions due to complete absence of melanin, such as vitiligo, will appear bright white and sharply delineated when examined with a Wood light. This is most helpful to identify hypopigmented or depigmented lesions in fair-skinned persons that otherwise may not be visible. Vitiligo can be associated with other autoimmune conditions such as diabetes mellitus and thyroid disease. Those conditions should be screened for,

but otherwise treatment involves methods to normalize the pigmentary discrepancies.

Treatment for depigmented skin can be challenging, prolonged, and suboptimal. Topical therapies involve high-potency topical glucocorticoids or immunomodulators (tacrolimus, pimecrolimus). Phototherapy with UV light is also an option and can be the treatment of choice for widespread involvement. Repigmentation occurs first around hair follicles as they are thought to be the reservoirs for melanocytes. As a result, repigmented skin will initially have a speckled appearance. Depigmentation therapy can also be considered if the vitiligo is so widespread that there are only a few remaining islands of normal pigmented skin. Monobenzyl ether of hydroquinone can be applied to the remaining normal islands of skin to permanently destroy the melanocytes.

KEY POINTS

- Vitiligo is an acquired autoimmune condition that causes the loss of melanocytes and subsequent depigmentation of the skin and can be associated with other autoimmune conditions such as diabetes and thyroid disease.

- Postinflammatory hypopigmentation is a loss of skin pigmentation following resolution of inflammatory or infectious dermatoses.

- Partial or complete depigmentation is seen in idiopathic guttate hypomelanosis manifesting as hypopigmented round or oval macules on the trunk and extremities of middle-aged and older persons.

Melasma

Melasma, also known as chloasma or the mask of pregnancy, is a common acquired condition resulting in patchy hyperpigmentation of the skin on the face. It can also be seen on the upper extremities. In this condition, the melanocytes overproduce melanin due to a multitude of factors including ultraviolet radiation, genetic predisposition, and hormonal influence (pregnancy, oral contraceptives). Women and those with darker skin types are more commonly predisposed. Clinically, it presents as ill-defined, tan to dark brown, reticulated patches mostly on the sun-exposed areas of the face (malar, mandibular, and centrofacial regions) (**Figure 22**). It worsens with sun exposure. The main differential diagnoses include postinflammatory hyperpigmentation, freckles, and lentigines. Melasma will fade during the postpartum period with sun protection and discontinuation of oral contraceptives. It will take months to years for pigmentation to normalize.

Treatment can be challenging and prolonged. The mainstay of treatment is strict sun protection, avoidance or discontinuation of the causative factors, and bleaching agents. Hydroquinone is typically used with concentrations ranging from 2% (over the counter) to 4% (prescription). The use of

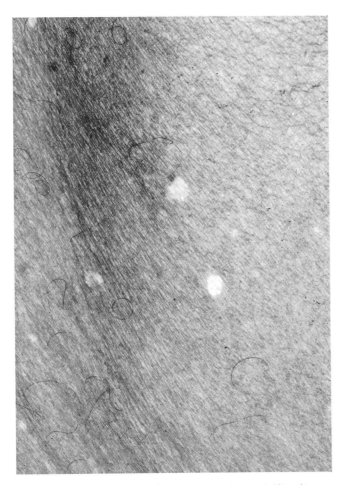

FIGURE 21. Partial or complete depigmentation is also seen in idiopathic guttate hypomelanosis, which manifests as 2- to 6-mm hypopigmented macules on the trunk and extremities.

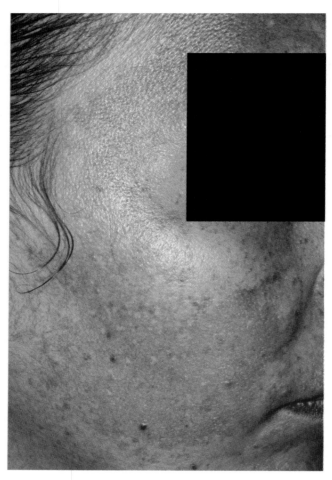

FIGURE 22. Ill-defined, reticulated hyperpigmented patches on malar cheeks typical for melasma.

hydroquinone should be monitored as it can cause drug-induced ochronosis, a bluish-gray discoloration. There are combinations of hydroquinone, tretinoin, and glucocorticoid topical creams that can be used nightly. Chemical peels can also help improve appearance. Laser and light-based therapies are another option for patients with refractory melasma, although they are used with caution as they can flare melasma as well. Caution must be used for darker skin types as irritating topical agents can result in inflammation and worsen pigmentation with postinflammatory hyperpigmentation.

Postinflammatory hyper- or hypopigmentation can occur after any cause of natural or iatrogenic-related inflammation (acne, dermatitis, folliculitis). Postinflammatory hyperpigmentation is most common in those with skin of color. It presents as hyperpigmented macules or patches at sites of previous inflammation. Postinflammatory hyperpigmentation can cause significant psychological stress and can take months to years to resolve. The first step in treatment is to treat the underlying skin condition causing the inflammation. Hydroquinone can be used and when used in combination

with tretinoin, it can augment its effect. Lasers and chemical peels can also be used with caution as any therapy that is irritating can be counterproductive.

KEY POINTS

- Melasma, which results in patchy hyperpigmentation on the face during pregnancy or with oral contraceptive use, is treated with strict sun protection, avoidance or discontinuation of causative factors, and bleaching agents such as hydroquinone.
- Postinflammatory hyperpigmentation presents as hyperpigmented macules or patches at sites of previous inflammation and is most common in those with skin of color.

Drug Reactions

Drug reactions are an important consideration when weighing a differential diagnosis for any rash, as medications can produce almost any pattern of skin disease. The most common types of cutaneous adverse reactions are exanthematous/morbilliform, urticarial, fixed drug, photosensitivity, hypersensitivity vasculitis, and the severe cutaneous adverse reactions (see Dermatologic Emergencies). Medications can also induce an array of specific diseases including psoriasis, bullous pemphigoid, and cutaneous lupus erythematosus (**Table 7**). Discontinuing the causative drug is the first step in treating drug reactions.

A morbilliform (measles-like) or exanthematous drug eruption consists of symmetrically arranged erythematous macules and papules, some discrete and others confluent. Morbilliform reactions are the most common drug reactions and are most likely a type IV delayed hypersensitivity reaction. As such, the rash appears in the first or second week after drug exposure, although subsequent exposures can produce a reaction much more quickly. Patients develop pink papules and macules that coalesce symmetrically to form plaques. The papules are often dense and monomorphic and are accompanied by varying degrees of pruritus beginning on the trunk and progressing distally across the limbs (**Figure 23**). Palms and soles are usually spared. This type of reaction is classically induced with amoxicillin use in acute Epstein-Barr virus infection. Treatment involves cessation of the causative agent, systemic and/or topical glucocorticoids, and oral H_1 antihistamines. Patients should be counseled to contact their clinician if they develop fevers, skin pain, blisters, pustules, or mucous membrane involvement indicating a more serious and potentially life-threating condition.

Urticarial reactions are the second most common type of cutaneous drug reaction and represent a type I hypersensitivity with IgE-mediated release of histamine. Wheals, pink-to-red effervescent edematous plaques with a surrounding flare, appear within minutes to a few hours after exposure to the

TABLE 7. Drug Reaction Patterns

Reaction Type	Classic Agents	Time to Onset	Additional Features
Exanthematous/Morbilliform	Antibiotics (penicillins, sulfonamides, cephalosporins), NSAIDs, allopurinol, antiepileptic agents	4-14 days	No effective test for causation, gold standard to determine causation is rechallenge (not recommended)
Urticarial			
Immunologic	Penicillin, anesthetic agents, ACE inhibitors	Minutes to a few hours	Most chronic urticaria are not drug related, but aspirin may cause or exacerbate chronic cases of urticaria
Non-immunologic	Vancomycin, rifampicin, acetylcysteine, opiates, radiocontrast agents	Minutes to a few hours	Red person syndrome is related to infusion rate of vancomycin
Photosensitivity			
Phototoxic	Voriconazole, demeclocycline, doxycycline, NSAIDs, fluoroquinolones, amiodarone, celery, limes	Hours	Voriconazole phototoxicity can cause skin cancer within a few years of treatment May result in fingernail shedding
Photoallergic	Hydrochlorothiazide, sulfonamide antibiotics, sulfonylureas, tricyclic antidepressants, sunscreens, fragrances containing 6-methylcoumarin, musk ambrette, or sandalwood oil	7-10 days for first exposure, hours for subsequent	May persist after ultraviolet light exposure (fall or winter months)
Neutrophilic			
Acneiform eruptions	EGFR inhibitors, glucocorticoids, androgens, lithium, iodinated cold medications	Variable	Acneiform eruptions with EGFR inhibitors portend a favorable treatment prognosis of the cancer
Sweet syndrome	GM-CSF, All-trans-retinoic acid, SMX-TMP	Variable	
Neutrophilic eccrine hidradenitis	Cytarabine	Variable	
Pigmentation	Minocycline, amiodarone, hydroxychloroquine, antiretroviral therapy, bleomycin, gold salts	Variable	Most appear on sun-exposed areas Bleomycin may cause flagellate pigmented macules on the back Zidovudine may cause pigmentation or pigmented streaking of the fingernails Minocycline may cause hyperpigmentation on sun-exposed areas and on acne scars
Fixed drug	Sulfonamides, NSAIDs, antiepileptic agents, tetracyclines	1-2 weeks after initial exposure, 24 hours for subsequent	Pseudoephedrine-related reactions may not pigment
Vasculitis	NSAIDs, antibiotics, hydrochlorothiazide, furosemide, minocycline, TNF inhibitors, propylthiouracil, GM-CSF, levamisole	1-3 weeks, within 3 days of rechallenge	Levamisole is used to add bulk and weight to cocaine. Drug-induced vasculitis is often ANCA positive, with both p- and c-ANCA patterns

EGFR = epidermal growth factor receptor; GM-CSF = granulocyte-macrophage colony-stimulating factor; SMX-TMP = sulfamethoxazole and trimethoprim; TNF = tumor necrosis factor.

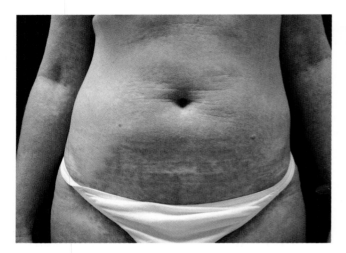

FIGURE 23. A morbilliform drug eruption consists of symmetrically arranged erythematous macules and papules, some discrete and others confluent.

 CONT.

causative agent (**Figure 24**). Patients may experience a spectrum of severity, from a few isolated wheals, to angioedema if the cutaneous edema becomes deep and confluent. In the most severe cases, anaphylaxis can occur, causing airway compromise and cardiovascular collapse. Nonimmunologic histamine release secondary to medications results in redness or flushing of the skin and variable pruritus without urticaria. Treatment of urticarial reactions is dependent on severity, with minor cases treated as described for exanthematous reactions, whereas anaphylaxis may require epinephrine, fluid resuscitation, and airway protection (for more information, see Urticaria). H

Fixed drug reactions recur in the same site (or sites) on the skin with each exposure. Pink-to-purple circinate plaques with central dusky discoloration or vesiculation appear most commonly on the lips, face, fingers, and genitals (**Figure 25**). The first exposure typically generates one plaque that recurs in the same location with each repeat encounter. Additional plaques may develop with subsequent exposures. Lesions typically resolve with muddy brown postinflammatory hyperpigmentation.

Photosensitivity disorders are a collection of conditions that have in common an abnormal skin response following exposure to ultraviolet radiation. Conceptually, it is useful to consider photosensitivity disorders that are idiopathic and those that are associated with application or ingestion of a drug or agent that causes cellular damage when exposed to ultraviolet radiation. Photosensitivity reactions related to exogenous agents are either phototoxic or photoallergic.

Polymorphous light eruption is the most common idiopathic photosensitivity disorder. It typically manifests before the age of 30 and is most common in fair-skinned women, first appearing in the spring and early summer. The rash will persist for weeks and resolve without scarring even with continued exposure to the sun. Lesions appear within hours of sun exposure and are found on the sun-exposed body parts. While many different types of eruptions may occur, the most

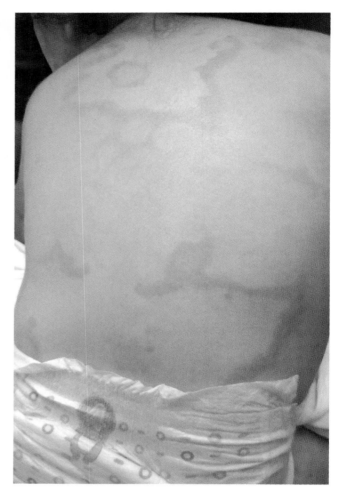

FIGURE 24. Urticarial drug reaction to amoxicillin with puffy pink plaques and an annular configuration.

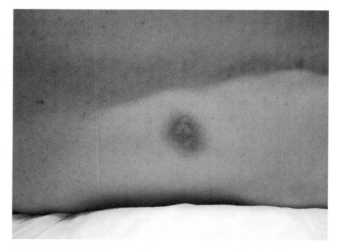

FIGURE 25. A fixed drug reaction causing an intense, dark red, oval patch. The patch will gradually fade, leaving postinflammatory hyperpigmentation.

common are pruritic skin-colored or pink papules. Other variants include vesicles, bullae, and plaques. The type of lesion will remain consistent in an individual with each occurrence.

Phototoxicity can occur in anyone with a threshold concentration of the responsible chemical or drug and is more common than photoallergy. Photoallergy is a cell-mediated immune response found in previously sensitized individuals that can be elicited by small amounts of offending agent. Phototoxic reactions present as an exaggerated sunburn within minutes to hours of sun exposure. Photoallergic reactions occur more commonly after topical exposure of a sensitizing agent and present as pruritic, eczematous eruptions within 24 to 48 hours after sun exposure on sun-exposed body parts (**Figure 26**). Treatment of photosensitivity disorders includes avoidance of allergens and photosensitizing drugs and broad-spectrum sunscreens if testing has ruled out sunscreen sensitivity.

Drugs are the most common cause of hypersensitivity vasculitis, a small vessel vasculitis. The American College of Rheumatology proposed criteria for the diagnosis of hypersensitivity vasculitis in a patient with vasculitis that are moderately sensitive and specific. Suggestive findings include palpable purpura and/or petechiae, which may be associated with fever, urticaria, arthralgia, and lymphadenopathy. These findings are typically associated with a low complement level and elevated erythrocyte sedimentation rate. The mainstay of treatment is drug discontinuation and avoidance. Severe or persistent symptoms may require systemic glucocorticoids. Medications can also cause a small/medium vessel ANCA-associated vasculitis (see Cutaneous Manifestations of Systemic Disease). **H**

KEY POINTS

- Morbilliform and urticarial reactions are the first and second most common drug reactions, respectively.
- Fixed drug reactions recur in the same site (or sites) with each exposure and consist of pink-to-purple circinate plaques with central dusky discoloration or vesiculation most commonly on the lips, face, fingers, and genitals.
- Photosensitivity disorders are a collection of conditions that have in common an abnormal skin response following exposure to ultraviolet radiation.
- Hypersensitivity vasculitis presents as palpable purpura and/or petechiae and may be associated with fever, urticaria, arthralgia, and lymphadenopathy.
- Discontinuation of the causative drug is the first step in treating drug reactions.   **HVC**

Acneiform Eruptions

Acne

Acne is a chronic inflammatory condition affecting the pilosebaceous unit (hair follicle and sebaceous gland). Although it is most common during adolescence, acne can affect people at any age. The clinical features of acne are open comedones (blackheads), closed comedones (whiteheads), inflammatory papules and pustules, and nodulocystic lesions on the face, neck, chest, shoulders, and back (**Figure 27** and **Figure 28**).

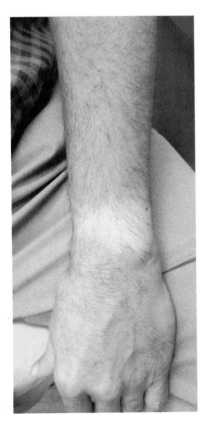

FIGURE 26. A photoallergic drug reaction from hydrochlorothiazide. The patient is experiencing pink, scaly, eczematous plaques on the arms. Note sparing of the area that was photo-protected by wristwatch. Phototoxic reactions (not pictured) result in pink edematous macules or blistering, much like a sunburn.

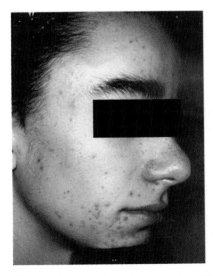

FIGURE 27. Note conspicuous papules and pustules (<5 mm), large open comedones on the nose, and one nodule (5 mm) at the lateral eyebrow area.

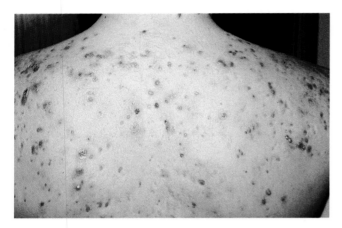

FIGURE 28. Extensive acne involvement of upper and mid-back with papules, pustules, nodules, granulation tissue, postinflammatory erythema, hyperpigmentation, and scarring.

TABLE 8.	Types of Acneiform Eruptions
Acneiform Eruption	**Distinguishing Characteristics**
Perioral/ periorificial dermatitis	Papules and pustules around mouth, eyelids, or nose; more common in women; possibly induced by topical glucocorticoids
Rosacea	Flushing, telangiectasias; lack of comedones; pustules common on nose, cheeks, forehead, and chin
Folliculitis	Follicular-based papules and pustules; often on scalp or trunk; most commonly caused by *Staphylococcus aureus*
Drug induced	Monomorphic pustules and papules; common inciting medications are glucocorticoids, lithium, anticonvulsants, and epidermal growth factor receptor inhibitors
Chloracne	Appears in scrotal region, postauricular scalp; history of exposure to halogenated aromatic compounds (dioxin)
Pseudofolliculitis barbae	Common in beard area; skin-colored or erythematous papules at hair-bearing sites; more common in black men

Acneiform lesions are common, and the differential diagnosis is broad. Variations in distribution and primary lesions may provide clues to help differentiate acne from other diagnoses (**Table 8**). Finally, rapid onset of acne combined with other signs of hyperandrogenism such as hirsutism and oligomenorrhea warrants consideration of polycystic ovary syndrome, congenital adrenal hyperplasia, or an underlying adrenal or ovarian tumor.

The pathogenesis is attributed to abnormal keratinization within the hair follicle, excess sebum production (stimulated by androgens), colonization of the follicle by *Propionibacterium acnes*, and the release of inflammatory cytokines. Treatments are directed at all four mechanisms (**Figure 29**).

There are numerous classification and grading scales used for the assessment of acne. These systems are typically based on factors such as the number and severity of the acne lesions. There is no universally agreed upon system. A common grading system is to classify acne as mild, moderate, and severe. Mild acne consists of primarily comedones with few inflammatory papules and no nodules or cysts. Moderate acne involves

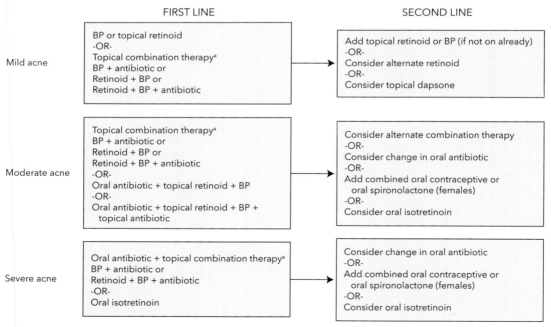

FIRST LINE / SECOND LINE

Mild acne

FIRST LINE:
BP or topical retinoid
-OR-
Topical combination therapy[a]
BP + antibiotic or
Retinoid + BP or
Retinoid + BP + antibiotic

SECOND LINE:
Add topical retinoid or BP (if not on already)
-OR-
Consider alternate retinoid
-OR-
Consider topical dapsone

Moderate acne

FIRST LINE:
Topical combination therapy[a]
BP + antibiotic or
Retinoid + BP or
Retinoid + BP + antibiotic
-OR-
Oral antibiotic + topical retinoid + BP
-OR-
Oral antibiotic + topical retinoid + BP + topical antibiotic

SECOND LINE:
Consider alternate combination therapy
-OR-
Consider change in oral antibiotic
-OR-
Add combined oral contraceptive or oral spironolactone (females)
-OR-
Consider oral isotretinoin

Severe acne

FIRST LINE:
Oral antibiotic + topical combination therapy[a]
BP + antibiotic or
Retinoid + BP + antibiotic
-OR-
Oral isotretinoin

SECOND LINE:
Consider change in oral antibiotic
-OR-
Add combined oral contraceptive or oral spironolactone (females)
-OR-
Consider oral isotretinoin

FIGURE 29. Treatment algorithm for the management of acne vulgaris in adolescents and young adults. BP = benzoyl peroxide.

[a]The drug may be prescribed as a fixed combination product or as a separate component.

Reprinted with permission from Zaenglein AL, Pathy AL, Schlosser BJ, et al. Guidelines of care for the management of acne vulgaris. J Am Acad Dermatol. 2016 May;74(5):945-73.e33. [PMID: 26897386] doi: 10.1016/j.jaad.2015.12.037. Epub 2016 Feb 17..

several comedones and inflammatory papules. A few nodules may be present as well. Severe acne is characterized by large lesion counts involving comedones and inflammatory pustules along with several cysts.

Topical retinoids (tretinoin, adapalene, tazarotene) are first-line treatments for all types of acne as they are effective for both comedonal and inflammatory acne. Retinoids help normalize the keratinization of the hair follicle and are comedolytic, thus reducing follicular plugging. They also decrease inflammatory cytokines that are activated by *P. acnes* and reduce postinflammatory hyperpigmentation. Topical retinoids may cause erythema, burning, and dryness. All topical retinoids are contraindicated in pregnancy. Adapalene and tretinoin are classified by the FDA as pregnancy category C whereas tazarotene is pregnancy category X.

Topical antibiotics are helpful in inflammatory acne as they target *P. acnes* and exhibit anti-inflammatory effects. Because of increased antibiotic resistance, topical antibiotics should not be used as monotherapy. It is recommended that topical antibiotics be combined with topical benzoyl peroxide in treatment for mild, moderate, or severe acne. Topical benzoyl peroxide has bactericidal properties and is not known to promote the development of resistant bacteria. Benzoyl peroxide may cause irritation and allergic contact dermatitis in some patients. The common topical antibiotics clindamycin and erythromycin are pregnancy category B while topical benzoyl peroxide is pregnancy category C.

Oral antibiotics are frequently used for moderate to severe inflammatory acne and acne resistant to topical treatment alone. Oral antibiotics inhibit *P. acnes* and can also decrease inflammation. Tetracycline-based antibiotics are often used as they exhibit both of these desirable properties. Oral antibiotics should be limited to 3 months, when possible, to decrease the risk of antibiotic resistance. Tetracycline-based antibiotics are pregnancy category D.

In severe nodulocystic or recalcitrant acne, oral isotretinoin should be considered. The iPLEDGE program is an FDA-approved regulatory program to prevent birth defects from isotretinoin. Isotretinoin is pregnancy category X.

Adult acne is more common in women and is related to androgenic hormones. It typically presents along the jawline and often flares with the menstrual cycle. Combined estrogen and progesterone oral contraceptives are effective acne treatments for inflammatory acne in women and girls older than age 14 years without evidence of hyperandrogenism. The use of spironolactone, an aldosterone receptor antagonist with antiandrogen activity, can also be effective in the treatment of acne. Oral contraceptives or spironolactone should be considered as second-line therapy that can to be added to other treatments in women with moderate to severe acne. Oral contraceptives are pregnancy category X whereas spironolactone is pregnancy category D.

When counseling patients with acne, it is important to stress the importance of adherence to treatment and the time course for improvement, often several weeks to months. In addition to prescribed medications, only products labeled as non-comedogenic should be used for cosmetics and moisturizers.

KEY POINTS

- The clinical features of acne are open comedones (blackheads), closed comedones (whiteheads), inflammatory papules and pustules, and nodulocystic lesions on the face, neck, chest, shoulders, and back.

- Treatment of comedonal and inflammatory acne includes topical retinoids, benzoyl peroxide, and topical antibiotics; because of increased antibiotic resistance, topical antibiotics should not be used as monotherapy. **HVC**

- Oral antibiotics are frequently used for moderate to severe inflammatory acne and acne resistant to topical treatment alone.

- Isotretinoin is indicated for severe nodulocystic and recalcitrant acne; it is associated with severe birth defects and must be administered through the federal regulatory program iPLEDGE.

Rosacea

Rosacea is an inflammatory condition that produces small pink papules and pustules on the central face in the third to sixth decades of life. Rosacea is most common among patients with light complexions from Irish and English decent. There are a variety of clinical presentations of rosacea including erythrotelangiectatic, papulopustular, phymatous, and ocular rosacea. This condition is defined by chronic inflammation of the pilosebaceous units with increased vascular reactivity. The pathogenesis of rosacea is still undetermined.

The papulopustular variant of rosacea can be confused with acne, but rosacea does not present with comedonal lesions (**Figure 30**). Telangiectasias are seen in the erythrotelangiectatic subtype (**Figure 31**). Most patients also have

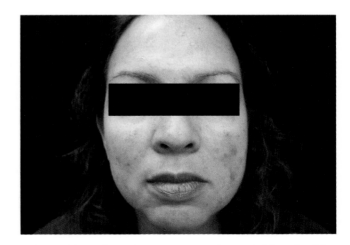

FIGURE 30. Papulopustular rosacea causes erythema and pink papules of the convexities of the face, namely, the forehead, nose, cheeks, and chin.

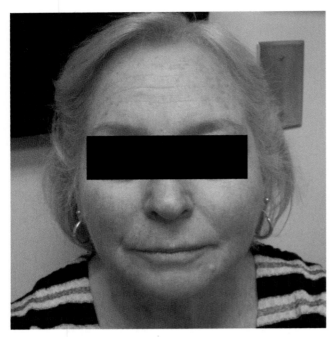

FIGURE 31. Erythrotelangiectatic rosacea presents predominantly with patches of erythema and telangiectasia.

frequent flushing in response to triggers such as stress, alcohol consumption, heat, and excessive sunlight. The erythema of the cheeks can mimic the malar rash of systemic lupus erythematosus. Unlike lupus, however, the erythema of rosacea includes the nasolabial folds. Ocular rosacea may present in isolation or with associated skin findings. In ocular rosacea, the conjunctiva appears injected, and patients often describe a "gritty sensation." In phymatous rosacea, severe sebaceous hyperplasia and chronic inflammation lead to fibrous overgrowth of the skin creating a nodular, tumor-like deformation of the facial structures. Rhinophyma is the form most frequently encountered, and it is almost exclusively found in men (**Figure 32**).

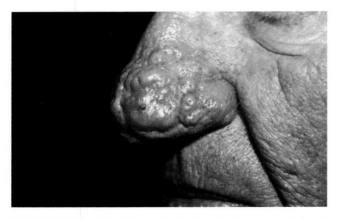

FIGURE 32. Rhinophyma, characterized by hyperplastic sebaceous glands and enlargement of the nose, in a patient with long-standing, uncontrolled rosacea.

Treatment for rosacea is targeted toward the most prominent signs and symptoms in each patient (**Table 9**). Treatment of erythrotelangiectatic rosacea focuses primarily on behavioral modifications such as: avoidance of identified triggers of flushing, proper use of sun protection, and use of gentle skin cleansers. Treatment for papulopustular rosacea includes topical metronidazole, azelaic acid, and topical ivermectin. Topical glucocorticoids should be avoided. Oral antibiotics, such as low-dose doxycycline, have been shown to help control inflammation in ocular and papulopustular rosacea. This low dose decreases side effects and reduces the prevalence of bacterial resistance. Topical brimonidine and oxymetazoline are alpha-2 agonists, which can be used for temporarily reducing erythema in rosacea. Laser therapy (pulsed dye laser) is also effective for erythema and telangiectasias. In severe cases, isotretinoin may be used. In the case of severe rhinophyma, surgery is the treatment of choice.

TABLE 9.	Management of Rosacea	
	Interventions	**FDA Pregnancy Category[a,b]**
Avoidance	Sun-protection (sunscreen or sun-protective clothing)	N/A
	Triggers: Foods (spicy, warm), alcohol, warm environments	N/A
Topical	Metronidazole, 0.75% or 1%	B
	Sodium sulfacetamide/sulfur	C
	Azelaic acid, 15%-20%	B
	Topical calcineurin inhibitors (pimecrolimus, tacrolimus)	C
	Permethrin	B
Systemic	Tetracycline antibiotics (doxycycline, 40 mg)	D
	Macrolide antibiotics	B
	Erythromycin, azithromycin, clarithromycin	C
Laser, light, and surgical	Lasers (PDL, Nd:YAG, CO_2, and others)	Avoid
	Intense pulsed light	
	Electrosurgery	

Nd:YAG = neodymium-doped yttrium aluminium garnet; PDL = pulsed dye laser.

[a]FDA categories: (A) Studies on pregnant humans show no risk (safe); (B) No clinical data of human risk but uncertain; (C) Risk cannot be ruled out; (D) Evidence of risk; (X) Contraindicated during pregnancy. See MKSAP 18 General Internal Medicine.

[b]The FDA has published changes in pregnancy and lactation labeling for prescription drugs, effective June 30, 2015 (see www.fda.gov/Drugs/DevelopmentApprovalProcess/DevelopmentResources/Labeling/ucm093307.htm). The pregnancy letter categories will be removed with the new labeling requirements; however, for prescription drugs that were previously approved, these changes will be phased in gradually. Labeling will include information relevant to the use of the drug in pregnant women (such as dosing and potential risks to the developing fetus), information about using the drug while breastfeeding (such as the amount of drug in breast milk and potential effects on the breastfed infant), and information regarding potential risks to females and males of reproductive potential who take the drug. Prescribing information for individual preparations should be consulted for more specific information.

KEY POINTS

- Rosacea is an inflammatory condition that produces small pink papules and pustules on the central face in the third to sixth decades of life.

- Most patients with rosacea have frequent flushing in response to triggers such as stress, alcohol consumption, heat, and excessive sunlight.

- Treatment for papulopustular rosacea includes topical metronidazole, azelaic acid, and topical ivermectin; oral antibiotics, such as low-dose doxycycline, have been shown to help control inflammation in ocular and papulopustular rosacea.

Hidradenitis Suppurativa

Hidradenitis suppurativa is an inflammatory skin disorder of the apocrine glands. This disease tends to occur more commonly in women and typically begins after puberty. Areas frequently affected are intertriginous areas such as the axilla, groin, and under the breasts. The condition is characterized by comedones, painful nodules, abscesses, draining sinuses, and scarring (**Figure 33**). Risk factors include obesity, family history, and cigarette smoking. For this reason, weight loss and smoking cessation are encouraged.

Hidradenitis suppurativa is extremely difficult to treat. No single treatment has been effective for all patients; however, there are several options available, depending on the patient's presentation and circumstances (**Table 10**). Decolonization with dilute bleach baths and chlorhexidine washes may be used in addition to topical clindamycin. Common systemic treatments are oral antibiotics, such as tetracyclines or the combination of clindamycin and rifampin. Systemic retinoids and oral zinc gluconate have been used as well with limited evidence of effectiveness. Recently, the tumor necrosis factor α

TABLE 10.	Treatment Options for Hidradenitis Suppurativa
Disease Severity	**Treatment Options/ Considerations**
Mild	
Predominantly comedones, small papules or pustules, solitary nodules	Antibacterial washes, topical antibiotics, analgesics, warm compresses Smoking cessation and weight loss recommended for all disease severity categories
Moderate	
Multiple nodules, abscesses or cysts; scarring	Oral antibiotics with antibacterial washes and/or topical antibiotics, analgesics, wide local excision Women: Oral contraceptives, spironolactone
Severe	
Multiple nodules, sinus tracts, scarring	Referral to dermatologist or surgeon for consideration of wide local excision, tumor necrosis factor α inhibitors, or clinical trial

inhibitor adalimumab became the first FDA-approved treatment for moderate to severe hidradenitis suppurativa.

Surgery may be required for chronic hidradenitis suppurativa. This may involve incision and drainage or deroofing of painful abscesses and sinus tracts. Radical wide excision may also be used for refractory cases after other therapeutic options have been exhausted. Even after successful surgical treatment, recurrence is common.

Common Skin Infections
Bacterial Skin Infections
Folliculitis

Folliculitis results from inflammation of the hair follicles. It typically presents as perifollicular erythematous papules and pustules on the face, scalp, trunk, and thigh; however, it can appear on any hair-bearing area of skin (**Figure 34**). Pruritus is a common symptom. Risk factors for folliculitis are occlusive dressings or clothing, increased sweating, obesity, and long-term topical glucocorticoid use.

Folliculitis can be noninfectious (HIV-associated eosinophilic folliculitis) or infectious. The most frequent cause of infectious folliculitis is *Staphylococcus aureus*. Other common infectious causes are gram-negative bacteria (*Klebsiella* species, *Enterobacter* species) from prolonged antibiotic treatment for acne and from *Pseudomonas aeruginosa*, which is associated with hot tubs (**Figure 35**). Other causes of infectious folliculitis are the yeast *Malassezia*; viral folliculitis from

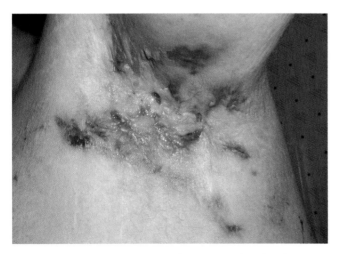

FIGURE 33. Hidradenitis suppurativa often presents with tender subcutaneous nodules. The nodules may spontaneously rupture or coalesce, forming painful, deep dermal abscesses.

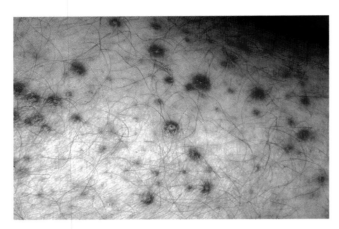

FIGURE 34. Pink papules and pustules centered on hair follicles, characteristic of folliculitis.

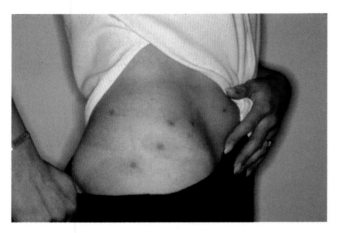

FIGURE 35. Erythematous papules with flare seen in hot tub folliculitis. The skin under the bathing suit is characteristically involved.

herpes simplex or varicella zoster; and *Demodex* folliculitis, which is caused by a mite found in the pilosebaceous unit of normal skin, causing a rosacea-like rash. The diagnosis of folliculitis can be made from history and clinical presentation. Bacterial cultures can be performed from pustules but are usually not necessary. Skin biopsies can be performed when causes other than bacterial infection, such as fungal or herpetic infections, are suspected.

Treatment for bacterial folliculitis is antibacterial soaps or antibacterial washes such as chlorhexidine, but topical antibiotics also can be used. Systemic antibiotics, with coverage against *S. aureus*, may be required for refractory or recurrent folliculitis. *Pseudomonas* folliculitis is usually self-limited, although oral ciprofloxacin may be effective. Gram-negative folliculitis is usually treated with ampicillin or ciprofloxacin. Refractory cases require oral isotretinoin therapy. *Malassezia* folliculitis often responds to topical antifungal agents, although oral fluconazole might be more effective. Systemic antiviral agents should be used for herpetic folliculitis, whereas topical permethrin or oral ivermectin is effective treatment for *Demodex* folliculitis.

- The diagnosis of folliculitis can be made from history and clinical presentation; however, skin biopsies can be performed when causes other than bacterial infection, such as fungal or herpetic infections, are suspected.

HVC

Abscesses/Furuncles/Carbuncles

Abscesses are soft tissue infections comprising collections of pus and bacteria within the dermis and subcutaneous tissue. They present as painful, fluctuant, erythematous nodules (**Figure 36**). Furuncles (or boils) are deeper infections of the hair follicle involving the dermis and subcutaneous tissue. Furuncles present as erythematous nodules with an overlying pustule. Multiple furuncles can coalesce into carbuncles, characterized by larger erythematous nodules with pus draining from multiple follicles. Carbuncles are typically located on the posterior neck, back, and the thighs. Fever and malaise can accompany carbuncles. *S. aureus* is the most common cause of abscesses, furuncles, and carbuncles, and there is an increasing prevalence of soft tissue infections caused by community-acquired methicillin-resistant *S. aureus* (MRSA).

Primary treatment for abscesses, furuncles, and carbuncles is incision and drainage. Gram stain and culture should be obtained from the purulent drainage when antibiotics are going to be administered (moderate and severe infections). Adjunctive oral antibiotic therapy is indicated for patients with moderate infections who have systemic signs of infection. Empiric treatment with an oral antibiotic active against MRSA such as trimethoprim-sulfamethoxazole or doxycycline is recommended. Empiric treatment with agents such as vancomycin, daptomycin, or linezolid is recommended in immunocompromised patients, patients who fail incision and drainage plus oral antibiotics, or patients with hypotension and systemic inflammatory response syndrome (severe infection). Treatment is then adjusted based on sensitivities from the culture of the purulent drainage.

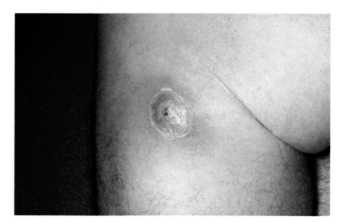

FIGURE 36. A staphylococcal abscess on the posterior thigh presenting as a tender, erythematous, fluctuant nodule topped by a central pustule.

CONT.

In the case of recurrent abscesses, other diagnoses should be considered, such as hidradenitis suppurativa, pilonidal cysts, or underlying conditions such as diabetes or HIV infection. Although MRSA decolonization in the community is controversial, the use of dilute bleach baths or chlorhexidine and topical mupirocin to the nares also may be considered for recurrent infections. **H**

> **KEY POINT**
>
> - Primary treatment for abscesses, furuncles, and carbuncles is incision and drainage; moderate infections should also be treated with trimethoprim-sulfamethoxazole or doxycycline.

Methicillin-Resistant *Staphylococcus aureus* in Hospitalized Patients

There has been a significant increase in hospital admissions for skin and soft tissue infections. MRSA infections have contributed to this increase and are associated with higher costs, longer hospitalizations, and higher morbidity and mortality rates.

Hospitalized patients are a common source of MRSA, but there is no consensus on effective screening measures. Active surveillance by performing screening cultures for MRSA is performed in many hospitals. Screening is usually performed by swabbing the nares, the most frequent site of colonization, although detection rates increase when screening of the nares is combined with cultures from the oropharynx and perineum. Screening policies also vary among hospitals. Some hospitals screen all admissions, whereas others screen only admissions to the ICU.

In patients who screen positive for MRSA, contact precautions using gown and gloves are effective in reducing transmission. Hand hygiene with soap and water or alcohol cleansers significantly reduces transmission and can decrease health care-associated infections. Decolonization of MRSA with daily chlorhexidine baths and the application of mupirocin to the nares twice a day for 5 days has shown to be effective in decreasing infections in the ICU.

In hospitalized patients with complicated skin and soft tissue infections, including purulent cellulitis, traumatic wound infections, and those who fail initial antibiotic therapy, therapy for MRSA should be considered pending culture data. Options include intravenous administration of vancomycin, daptomycin, telavancin, clindamycin, and linezolid. Oral linezolid is also an option. **H**

Impetigo

Impetigo is a superficial infection of the epidermis most commonly caused by *S. aureus* or group A streptococci. Impetigo is classified as bullous or nonbullous impetigo. It is most commonly seen in children but can present in adults as well.

Bullous impetigo is usually caused by *S. aureus*, which produces exfoliative toxins targeting the adhesion molecule desmoglein-1 between keratinocytes. This results in a localized blister formation (**Figure 37**). This same toxin is responsible for the more extensive exfoliation seen in staphylococcal scalded skin syndrome. Bullous impetigo presents as small vesicles that evolve into flaccid blisters. These blisters often rupture, leaving a collarette of scale and honey-colored crusted erosions. Nonbullous impetigo is more common and can be caused by either *S. aureus*, group A streptococci, or both. Nonbullous impetigo is characterized by erythematous papules or plaques with honey-colored crust (**Figure 38**). Satellite lesions are common. Nonbullous impetigo occurs on normal skin but can appear at areas of inflammatory conditions such as atopic dermatitis. Ecthyma is a variant of impetigo characterized by an ulcerative lesion with an overlying eschar that extends into the dermis and may be associated with lymphadenitis (**Figure 39**).

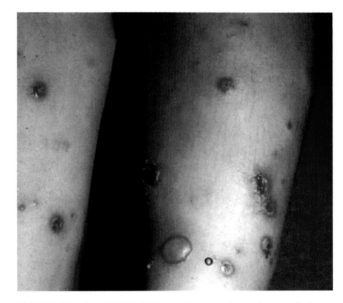

FIGURE 37. Clear, fluid-filled blisters with surrounding erythema on the legs of a patient with bullous impetigo.

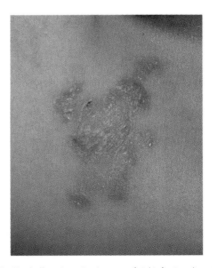

FIGURE 38. Nonbullous impetigo is a superficial infection characterized by a yellowish, crusted surface that may be caused by staphylococci or streptococci.

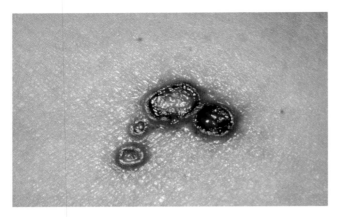

FIGURE 39. Superficial, saucer-shaped ulcers with overlying crusts are the classic findings of ecthyma. They almost always occur on the legs or feet and are usually caused by streptococci.

Diagnosis is typically made based on clinical appearance, but bacterial culture can be obtained from the blister fluid or exudative crust to identify the pathogen. Treatment consists of washing with soap and water and removal of the crust. Topical antibiotic treatment with mupirocin or retapamulin is effective in most cases of impetigo. Oral antibiotics are recommended for patients with widespread infection if outbreaks occur involving multiple people as well as in cases of ecthyma. Recommended antibiotics are cephalexin or dicloxacillin, unless MRSA is suspected or confirmed.

Cellulitis/Erysipelas

Cellulitis and erysipelas are both nonpurulent, superficial, spreading skin infections. Cellulitis typically refers to an infection involving the deeper dermis and subcutaneous tissue. Although erysipelas can be considered synonymous with cellulitis, it is often used to describe an infection limited to the upper dermis and superficial lymphatics. Erysipelas is also a term used when cellulitis only involves the face. Both cellulitis and erysipelas result from compromise in the skin barrier (trauma, ulcers, lymphedema, peripheral vascular disease, or previous cellulitis) allowing bacterial entry. The clinical presentation of cellulitis includes spreading patches of erythema with associated tenderness, warmth, and edema. It is usually found unilaterally on a lower extremity (**Figure 40**). Erysipelas classically has a more demarcated erythematous border than cellulitis. Systemic symptoms such as fever, tachycardia, and leukocytosis can be present in both. There are several conditions that can mimic cellulitis (**Table 11**). The

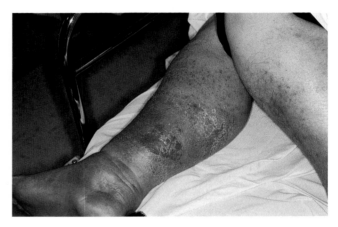

FIGURE 40. Cellulitis, a rapidly spreading, deep, subcutaneous-based infection, is characterized by well-demarcated area of warmth, swelling, tenderness, and erythema that may be accompanied by lymphatic streaking.

TABLE 11.	Differential Diagnosis of Cellulitis
Disease	**Clinical Characteristics**
Cellulitis	Well-demarcated erythematous plaque with erythema, pain, warmth, and swelling; associated lymphadenopathy can occur. Systemic symptoms include fever, chills, and malaise. Bilateral lower extremity cellulitis suggests an alternative diagnosis.
Stasis dermatitis	Erythematous, scaly, and eczematous patches most common on the lower extremities and usually affecting both legs with associated hyperpigmentation. Findings can persist for months to years. The medial ankle can be more severely involved, and ulcerations are common in this area. The erythema also can be striking, involving the ankle and extending to below the knee. Sharp demarcation often is less common in stasis dermatitis. Overlying cellulitis can develop in the setting of stasis dermatitis.
Contact dermatitis	Pruritic, geometric, and erythematous patches with superficial scale; differentiated from cellulitis by pruritus as opposed to pain.
Panniculitis (erythema nodosum)	Painful, erythematous, subcutaneous, ill-defined nodules present bilaterally. Many panniculitides will resolve with hyperpigmentation. The acute onset of pain and erythema may be concerning for cellulitis, although distinct subcutaneous nodules would be unusual.
Deep venous thrombosis	Pain, swelling, and associated erythema and warmth in one leg, with changes often more prominent in the calf. A brightly erythematous, well-demarcated plaque is not often seen, although red, blue, or violaceous surface changes can be seen.
Herpes zoster	Grouped vesiculopustules on an erythematous patch or plaque localized to one area (dermatome). The erythema can be well defined. The presence of grouped, crusted vesiculopustules or punched out erosions is uncommon in cellulitis. Bacterial superinfection can occur.

For a complete list of potential entities in the differential diagnosis of cellulitis, please see the bibliography.

CONT.

most common cause of cellulitis is group A streptococci followed by *S. aureus*. Blood cultures and skin biopsies are not usually needed.

For immunocompetent patients with mild cellulitis/erysipelas (no systemic signs of infection), empiric oral therapy directed against streptococci is recommended with penicillin, amoxicillin, cephalexin, dicloxacillin, or clindamycin. In patients with systemic signs of infection, intravenous treatment with penicillin, ceftriaxone, cefazolin, or clindamycin is recommended. In patients who have failed oral antibiotic therapy, who are immunocompromised, who have systemic inflammatory response syndrome and hypotension, or who have evidence of deeper necrotizing infection with findings such as bullae and desquamation, surgical evaluation for debridement and empiric broad spectrum antibiotic therapy with vancomycin plus either imipenem, meropenem, or piperacillin-tazobactam are recommended. Treatment is then adjusted based on culture and sensitivity results from lesion-associated specimens.

Patients with cellulitis have annual recurrence rates of 8% to 20%. Treating predisposing factors such as edema, obesity, diabetes, and venous insufficiency might decrease recurrence. Examination and treatment of the interdigital toe spaces for tinea infection, maceration, and fissuring can also prevent recurrence. The prophylactic use of antibiotics is effective in preventing recurrence of cellulitis and should be considered in patients with more than three episodes of cellulitis per year.

KEY POINTS

- For immunocompetent patients with mild cellulitis, begin empiric therapy with penicillin, amoxicillin, cephalexin, dicloxacillin, or clindamycin.

HVC
- Treating predisposing factors such as edema, obesity, tinea pedis, and venous insufficiency may decrease recurrent episodes of cellulitis.

Pitted Keratolysis

Pitted keratolysis is a bacterial infection of the soles of the feet, or (less commonly) the palms of the hand, with characteristic appearance and odor. As the name suggests, the infection manifests as scale and pitting of the skin surface. These pits may coalesce into larger erosions (**Figure 41**). In the United States, the infection is most common among patients with hyperhidrosis and prolonged occlusion of the feet (athletes, military personnel, laborers). Other than appearance and odor, symptoms are usually minimal and limited to mild pruritus or slight discomfort. Treatment is with topical antibacterial therapy such as clindamycin, erythromycin, or over-the-counter benzoyl peroxide preparations. In addition, the use of topical antiperspirants (aluminum hydroxide) and frequent changing and washing of socks should be used to keep the feet (or hands) dry and clean. The most common causative organisms are *Kytococcus*

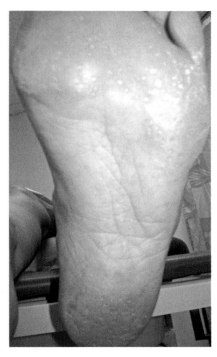

FIGURE 41. Pitted keratolysis presents with small indented pits on a background of hyperkeratosis and results from increased sweating of the feet. It is a superficial bacterial infection most commonly due to *Kytococcus sedentarius*, *Dermatophilus congolensis*, *Corynebacterium* or *Actinomyces* species.

sedentarius, *Dermatophilus congolensis*, *Corynebacterium* species, and *Actinomyces* species.

Erythrasma

Erythrasma is a benign superficial bacterial infection of the skin. Afflicted patients report red-brown plaques in the groin, crural folds, gluteal folds, axillae, or less commonly in the interdigital or inframammary regions (**Figure 42**). The skin often has a thin, wrinkled appearance similar to cigarette paper, and patients are often misdiagnosed with a dermatophyte infection. Symptoms, limited to mild pruritus, are minimal in most patients. In the immunocompromised patient, severe invasive disease has been described. The causative organism is most commonly *Corynebacterium minutissimum*. This organism produces porphyrins that fluoresce a soft, coral red under a Wood lamp. Clinical appearance and fluorescence are the best means of diagnosis, as histopathology may be unremarkable and skin scrapings are not helpful. Treatment is best accomplished with oral erythromycin, clarithromycin, or tetracyclines, but cure with topical antibiotics is reported.

Superficial Fungal Infections

Tinea

Tinea (dermatophytosis) is classified based on body site that is involved: tinea pedis ("athlete's foot") (**Figure 43**), tinea manuum

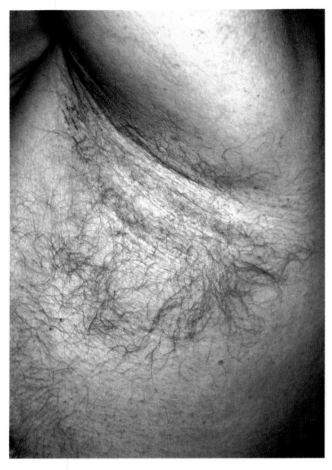

FIGURE 42. Erythrasma presents with sharply demarcated fine, pink-to-brown scaling patches that are typically found in skin-fold areas. The rash will fluoresce a coral red with Wood lamp illumination.

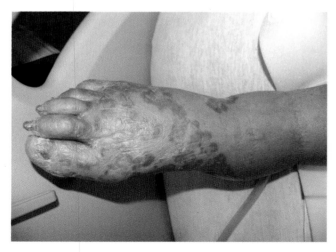

FIGURE 43. Erythematous patches with peripheral scale and associated onychomycosis (onychodystrophy with subungual debris of nails) in tinea pedis.

(hand), tinea cruris ("jock itch") (**Figure 44**), tinea capitis (scalp) (**Figure 45**), tinea faciei (face), and tinea corporis (body excluding the genital area or inguinal folds) (**Figure 46**). There are three species from the genera *Epidermophyton*, *Microsporum*, and *Trichophyton* that cause superficial fungal infections in humans, *Trichophyton rubrum* being the most common.

Dermatophytosis can also be classified as anthropophilic, zoophilic, and geophilic, based on host and mode of transmission. Anthropophilic dermatophytes are found in humans, cause little inflammation, and are transmitted from human to human or through fomites. Zoophilic dermatophytes are

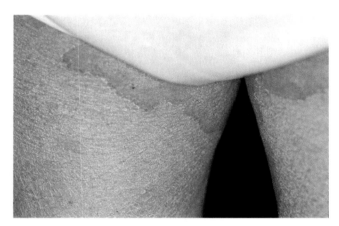

FIGURE 44. Tinea cruris, a dermatophyte infection of the groin, pubic region, and thighs, presents as erythematous annular to serpiginous lesions with peripheral scale and central clearing.

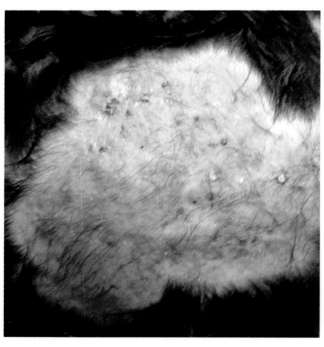

FIGURE 45. Kerion can be a result of tinea capitis infection and presents as painful boggy erythematous plaques with folliculitis and abscess formation.

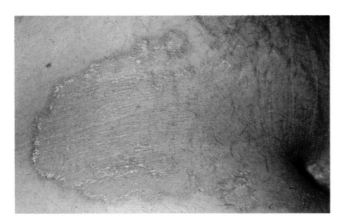

FIGURE 46. Tinea corporis presents with a characteristic erythematous annular centrifugally growing patches with a raised rim of peripheral scale.

transmitted from animals to humans from direct or indirect contact and cause inflammation and occasionally cause suppurative dermatophytosis. Geophilic dermatophytes only occasionally infect humans through direct contact but also cause inflammatory dermatophytosis. Infection is more prevalent in hot and humid climates and in patients who are immunocompromised, particularly those taking chronic glucocorticoid therapy.

The characteristic clinical presentation of tinea corporis, cruris, and faciei is annular scaly patches with central clearing and varying degrees of inflammation. Tinea cruris spares the scrotum in contrast to candida intertrigo, which is in the differential diagnoses. Concomitant tinea pedis and cruris are not uncommon. In tinea capitis, the invasion of the hair follicle leads to small broken hairs with the surrounding scalp showing erythematous scaly patches with varying degrees of crust and numbers of pustules. Occipital adenopathy is frequently seen. The chronic form of tinea pedis and tinea manuum presents as mildly pruritic scaly patches involving most of the palms and soles in a "moccasin" or "glove" distribution (**Figure 47**). One hand and two feet tinea is a characteristic pattern of

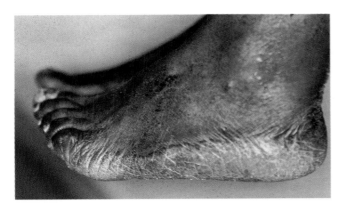

FIGURE 47. Mildly erythematous patches with fine scale that are well demarcated and are confined to the lateral foot, heel, and sole characteristic of "moccasin" type tinea pedis.

involvement. Tinea pedis can have a more acute form with 1- to 2-mm vesicles and can be extremely pruritic. The interdigital variant of tinea pedis shows fissures and maceration in the folds. Tinea incognito refers to tinea that has been erroneously treated with topical glucocorticoids, which initially decreases pruritus, but leads to a clinical presentation that is less inflammatory and can result in invasion of the follicular epithelium.

Tinea can be suspected based on clinical presentation and pruritus; however, diagnosis is based on visualization by microscopic examination of branching hyphae in the keratin (scale) using a potassium hydroxide preparation. To confirm the diagnosis, a fungal culture can be performed, which provides species identification, and is the preferred method for diagnosing tinea capitis. Hair shafts should be included in the specimen.

Dermatophytosis of non–hair–bearing skin with limited involvement can be treated topically with imidazole creams, such as miconazole, clotrimazole, and ketoconazole, applied once to twice daily for 2 to 4 weeks, ensuring that the application extends a few centimeters beyond the advancing border. Other topical agents including terbinafine 1% and ciclopiroxolamine 0.77% can also be used. Unlike superficial fungal infections caused by *Candida*, dermatophytes do not respond to topical nystatin. Combined antifungal agents and topical glucocorticoids should be avoided as they can lead to increased recurrences and treatment failures. Dermatophytosis of hair-bearing skin, including tinea capitis, or those with recurrent or extensive skin involvement, should be treated with oral antifungal agents such as terbinafine or itraconazole. Tinea should be treated to prevent skin breakdown, which can be an entry port for bacterial infection.

KEY POINTS

- The characteristic clinical presentation of tinea infection is annular scaly patches with central clearing and varying degrees of inflammation.

- Diagnosis of tinea is made by microscopic examination of branching hyphae in the keratin (scale) using a potassium hydroxide preparation.

- Dermatophytosis of non–hair–bearing skin with limited involvement can be treated topically with imidazole creams (miconazole, clotrimazole, ketoconazole); however, treatment of infections on hair-bearing skin or extensive or recurrent involvement should be treated with oral terbinafine or itraconazole.

Pityriasis Versicolor

Pityriasis versicolor or tinea versicolor is caused by commensal lipophilic fungi that live in the hair follicles and stratum corneum. Pityriasis versicolor is one of the most common, chronic, superficial fungal infections and is typically found in young adults. Caused by *Malassezia furfur*, pityriasis versicolor is most common in warm, humid environments. It presents as asymptomatic, oval-to-round, minimally scaly, hyperpigmented or hypopigmented macules that can coalesce into patches on the trunk and upper extremities (**Figure 48**).

The diagnosis of pityriasis versicolor can often be made by clinical presentation but may be confirmed by visualization of short rod-shaped hyphae and round yeast ("spaghetti and meatballs") on microscopic examination of skin scrapings using a potassium hydroxide preparation. Topical treatment using ketoconazole 2% shampoo or selenium sulfide suspension is effective. Either treatment should be applied from the upper neck to the thighs and used to wash the scalp. Oral itraconazole can be used for those with extensive disease or frequent recurrences. Because recurrences are high, weekly use of topical treatments can be preventive.

Candidiasis

Candida species, in particular *C. albicans*, can cause superficial infections in moist occluded skin such as the intertriginous areas, oropharynx mucosa, and genitals, as well as disseminated disease in immunocompromised, hospitalized patients (see MKSAP 18 Infectious Disease). Antibiotic therapy increases the number of colonizing organisms present in skin and mucous membranes leading to an increased risk of infection.

Intertrigo is an inflammatory skin disease that involves the axillae, inframammary, and inguinal folds (**Figure 49**). *Candida* is the most common secondary infection in intertrigo with obesity being an important risk factor. It presents as erythematous patches with satellite pustules that are often macerated. Diagnosis is frequently made on clinical grounds alone, but a potassium hydroxide preparation can show spores and pseudohyphae. For successful treatment, the area should be

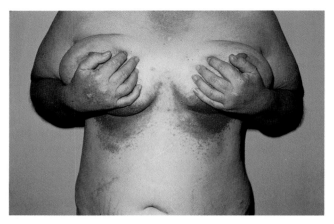

FIGURE 49. Bright red patches and plaques with satellite papules and pustules in the intertriginous area beneath the breasts characteristic of candidiasis.

dry, and use of absorbent powers and zinc oxide paste can be helpful. Topical imidazoles and nystatin are generally effective, but recurrences are common. For widespread infection, oral fluconazole can be added.

Chronic paronychia is associated with irritants or allergens and is caused by frequent exposure to water. Exacerbations can be caused by *Candida*, and successful treatment includes treating the underlying irritant or allergic contact dermatitis, as well as treatment with topical or oral antifungal agents, depending on the severity of the infection (see Nail Disorders).

Viral Skin Infections

Herpes Simplex Virus

For both herpes simplex virus types 1 (HSV1) and 2 (HSV2), transmission usually occurs by direct contact with infected secretions, skin lesions, or asymptomatic shedding. Both HSV1 and HSV2 can cause oral and genital lesions; however, infections with HSV1 are usually above the waist (oral, facial), whereas HSV2 infections are usually below the waist (genital). The seroprevalence of HSV increases with age, with HSV1 IgG antibodies being present in most adults. HSV2 seroprevalence increases with the number of sexual partners and high-risk sexual behaviors.

HSV causes a clinically unapparent primary infection through skin and mucous membranes where it replicates locally. This is followed by a short viremia, and the virus subsequently establishes latency through retrograde axonal transport in sensory nerve ganglions. Characteristically, HSV1 is found in the trigeminal ganglion and HSV2 in the sacral ganglion. Recurrent lesions are caused by reactivation of the virus. Symptomatic primary and recurrent infections typically remain localized and are named according to the site of infection, regardless of the HSV subtype responsible: herpetic gingivostomatitis, herpes labialis ("cold sore"), herpes facialis, and herpes genitalis.

The classic presentation is a group of painful, small vesicles on an erythematous base, transitioning to pustules and subsequent crusting of the lesions over time (**Figure 50**). Erosions or ulcers may also develop. HSV is the most common

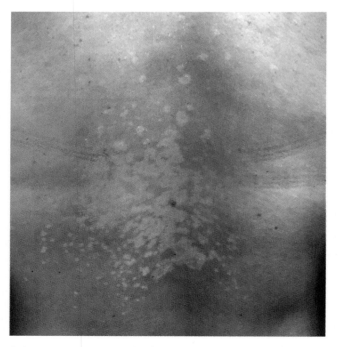

FIGURE 48. Hypopigmented scaly macules coalescing into patches on the back characteristic of pityriasis versicolor.

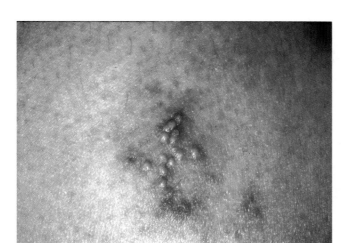

FIGURE 50. Herpes simplex virus infection with characteristic grouped vesicles on an erythematous base that recur in the same location.

CONT.

cause of painful genital ulcers, although chancroid also causes painful ulcers. Other infections (syphilis, granuloma inguinale, lymphogranuloma venereum) often cause nonpainful ulcerations (see MKSAP 18 Infectious Disease). However, a diagnosis based on the presence or absence of pain may be misleading.

With any sexually transmitted infection, HIV testing also is important. Symptomatic primary infections are usually more severe and of longer duration than recurrences. There is associated burning, tingling, and pain, which can be a prodrome in recurrences. Reactivation is higher in persons who are immunocompromised, and it can be triggered by trauma, ultraviolet light exposure, psychosocial stress, and fever. In herpes genitalis, recurrences are more frequent with HSV2 and in women, and asymptomatic shedding occurs in most patients with HSV2 but not HSV1.

The diagnosis is typically made on clinical grounds; however, for distinction between subtypes of HSV or from varicella zoster virus, other methods can be used (**Table 12**). Oral antiviral agents (acyclovir, valacyclovir, or famciclovir) can be used to treat primary infections, episodic or secondary recurrences, and as suppression or prophylaxis for patients with six or more recurrences per year. Oral antiviral agents are most effective when started during the prodrome of recurrences. Dosing varies for primary, secondary, and prophylaxis, as well as by site of infection and for immunocompromised patients. Topical therapies are less effective in improving symptoms and reducing disease duration. **H**

KEY POINTS

- The classic presentation of herpes simplex virus infection is a group of painful, small vesicles on an erythematous base, transitioning to pustules with subsequent crusting of the lesions over time.
- Oral antiviral agents (acyclovir, valacyclovir, or famciclovir) can be used to treat primary infections, episodic or secondary recurrences, and as suppression or prophylaxis for patients with six or more recurrences per year.

Varicella/Herpes Zoster

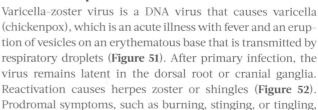

Varicella-zoster virus is a DNA virus that causes varicella (chickenpox), which is an acute illness with fever and an eruption of vesicles on an erythematous base that is transmitted by respiratory droplets (**Figure 51**). After primary infection, the virus remains latent in the dorsal root or cranial ganglia. Reactivation causes herpes zoster or shingles (**Figure 52**). Prodromal symptoms, such as burning, stinging, or tingling,

TABLE 12. Methods for Detecting Herpes Virus

Method	Sample	Utility
Hematoxylin and eosin staining	Skin biopsy	Characteristic histologic findings with immunohistochemistry to differentiate HSV from VZV
Direct fluorescence antibody	Unroofed vesicle	Discriminates between HSV1, HSV2, and VZV
Polymerase chain reaction	Unroofed vesicle	Discriminates between HSV1, HSV2, and VZV
Serologies	Peripheral blood	Diagnosis of primary infection with seroconversion of virus-specific IgG antibodies
Tzanck preparation	Unroofed vesicle	Multinucleated keratinocytes and cytopathic effect does not differentiate HSV from VZV. Technically difficult.
Viral culture	Unroofed vesicle	Delay of 48-72 hours but can discriminate HSV1, HSV2, and VZV; useful for antiviral sensitivities

HSV1 = herpes simplex virus 1; HSV2 = herpes simplex virus 2; VZV = varicella zoster virus.

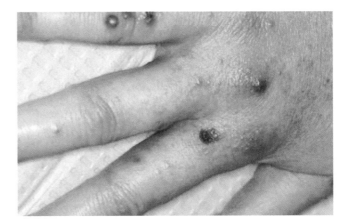

FIGURE 51. This patient has chickenpox (primary varicella zoster virus infection), which is characterized by the simultaneous onset of fever and a cutaneous eruption. Chickenpox lesions develop in crops such that lesions in different stages of development (macules, papules, vesicles, pustules, crusted erosions) are present at the same time on any one part of the body. Also, lesions are most prominent on the trunk rather than the extremities.

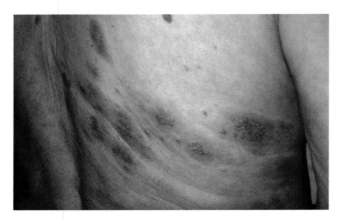

FIGURE 52. Typical herpes zoster of the trunk, characterized by painful grouped vesicles on an erythematous base in a dermatomal distribution.

CONT.

often occur in a localized region, followed by a dermatomal eruption of grouped vesicles or pustules on an erythematous base. The most common dermatomes affected are in the thoracic region. With involvement of the first division of the trigeminal nerve (forehead extending over upper eyelid, or nasal tip involvement), ophthalmologic evaluation is mandatory as herpes zoster ophthalmicus and possible blindness can result. If vesicles are noted in the external ear canal, evaluation by an otolaryngologist may be required as peripheral facial paralysis and auditory/vestibular symptoms can occur (Ramsay Hunt syndrome).

Herpes zoster can be complicated by postherpetic neuralgia and has been associated with an increased risk of cerebrovascular disease. Postherpetic neuralgia is defined as chronic neuropathic pain that persists for 3 months or more after the initial onset of herpes zoster. The risk, severity, and complications of herpes zoster, in particular postherpetic neuralgia, are increased in older patients, those with greater initial pain and more severe infection, and possibly in patients that are immunosuppressed or on immunosuppressive or immunomodulating medications.

Diagnosis of herpes zoster can usually be made by characteristic dermatomal presentation. For unusual cases or when the distinction between herpes simplex virus and herpes zoster is required, ancillary studies are available (see Table 12). Oral acyclovir, valacyclovir, or famciclovir is effective for treating herpes zoster if initiated within 72 hours of presentation and can shorten the disease course as well as help prevent postherpetic neuralgia. Current evidence is insufficient to support the addition of glucocorticoids with acyclovir to improve quality of life or the incidence of postherpetic neuralgia.

A recombinant zoster vaccine is now preferred to the live attenuated zoster vaccine in adults 60 years and older to prevent or attenuate illness caused by herpes zoster infection and to reduce the risk of postherpetic neuralgia. For individuals previously immunized with the live attenuated

vaccine, revaccination with the recombinant vaccine is recommended.

KEY POINTS

- After primary infection with the varicella zoster virus, the virus remains latent in the dorsal root or cranial ganglia, and reactivation causes herpes zoster or shingles, which presents as a painful dermatomal vesicular eruption.

- Oral acyclovir, valacyclovir, or famciclovir is effective for treating herpes zoster if initiated within 72 hours of presentation; it can shorten the disease course as well as help prevent postherpetic neuralgia.

Warts

Warts (verruca and condyloma) are caused by a human papillomavirus (HPV), which is ubiquitous. There are numerous HPV subtypes, but certain ones are associated with specific clinical lesions and are more common at certain sites (**Table 13**). Verruca vulgaris (common warts) are skin-colored digitate papules with thrombosed capillaries. Verruca plana (flat warts) are skin-colored, flat-topped papules (**Figure 53**). Condyloma acuminata (genital warts) are smooth to digitate papules that are skin-colored to tan (**Figure 54**). Verruca plantaris/palmaris (plantar/palmar warts) are exo-/endophytic papules with thrombosed capillaries manifesting as black dots when the top of the wart is pared down. HPV

TABLE 13.	Human Papillomavirus Subtypes
Subtype	**Clinical Lesion (Location)**
1	Verruca plantaris/palmaris (soles/palms)
2, 4	Verruca vulgaris (fingers, knees, and elbows)
3, 10	Verruca plana (face and legs; associated with shaving)
6, 11	Condyloma acuminata
16, 18, 31, 33	Condyloma acuminata (associated with high risk for cervical, anal, and penile cancer)

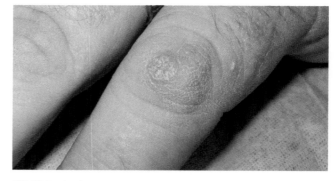

FIGURE 53. The common wart is a verrucous papule that is keratotic and exophytic.

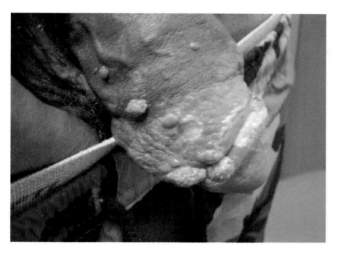

FIGURE 54. Anogenital warts (condyloma acuminatum) present as verrucous papules over the penile shaft and foreskin with adjacent erosions after imiquimod therapy.

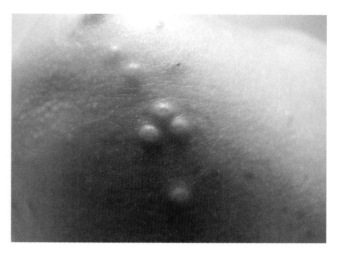

FIGURE 55. Molluscum contagiosum is a common cutaneous infection resulting from poxvirus infection. It occurs in young children and sexually active adults. It presents as firm, umbilicated yellow papules with varying degrees of surrounding erythema.

infection can occur at any age but is typically seen in children and young adults. Larger, more numerous lesions that are recalcitrant to treatment can be seen in immunocompromised persons.

Diagnosis is clinical. Warts are usually self-limited; however, in severe cases, including those with a protracted course or in immunocompromised persons, destructive treatments can be used. Location of the lesions has to be taken into account when selecting treatment, and can be associated with pigment change or scarring. Numerous treatments (salicylic acid, cryotherapy, tricarboxylic acid, cantharidin, and podophyllin) geared at destroying infected keratinocytes are available. All of these treatments should be repeated every 3 to 4 weeks until resolution. Larger lesions should be pared prior to treatment.

HPV vaccination is recommended for young persons to prevent cervical and anal carcinoma. Anogenital warts may also be prevented if the vaccine is effective against HPV 6 and 11 (see MKSAP 18 General Internal Medicine).

Molluscum Contagiosum

Molluscum contagiosum is caused by a poxvirus. Infection occurs in children, in adults as a sexually transmitted disease, and in patients with AIDS. The lesions are white-to-yellow smooth papules with an umbilicated center (**Figure 55**). Many patients develop a surrounding eczematous host response. They can be located anywhere on the skin, but in adults the genital area is typically involved, whereas in patients with AIDS the face is the most common area of infection and the lesions tend to be larger. Transmission is by direct contact or by fomites.

Diagnosis is based on clinical appearance, but skin biopsy on equivocal cases shows eosinophilic intracytoplasmic inclusions within keratinocytes. Molluscum contagiosum is usually self-limited, but in severe cases, those with a protracted course,

or in immunocompromised persons, destructive modalities or topical medications can be used. Any of these treatments can be associated with scarring and pigment change. Destructive treatments include cryotherapy, curettage, tricarboxylic acid, cantharidin, and podophyllin. Medical treatments consist of topical tretinoin and topical imiquimod.

Infestations

Scabies

Scabies (*Sarcoptes scabiei*) infestation is characterized by intensely pruritic, crusted papules, nodules, and burrows that develop in the interdigital spaces, wrists, ankles, breasts, periumbilical area, and genitals (**Figure 56**). In older adults, the immunocompromised, or Down syndrome patients, highly contagious crusted (Norwegian) scabies occurs with extensive thick concrete-like scale. Scabies is transmitted by close personal contact, and diagnosis is performed by microscopic identification of the mites, eggs, or feces from skin scrapings prepared with mineral oil (**Figure 57**). See **Table 14** for treatment. Pruritus may persist for weeks after eradication of scabies and does not necessarily represent resistance or reinfection. "Postscabetic pruritus" can be treated with antihistamines, topical glucocorticoids, and, if severe, oral glucocorticoids can be used.

KEY POINT

- Pruritus may persist for weeks after eradication of scabies and does not necessarily represent resistance or reinfection.

HVC

Lice

There are three types of lice that infest humans: head (*Pediculus humanus capitis*), body (*Pediculus humanus*

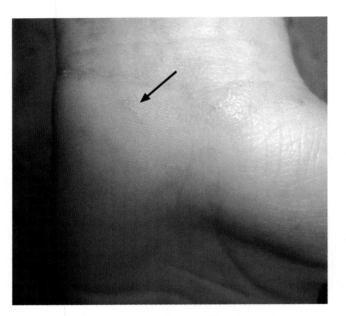

FIGURE 56. A burrow is present on the proximal hypothenar eminence. Scrapings of the black dot at the lower end of the burrow revealed the mite pictured in Figure 57.

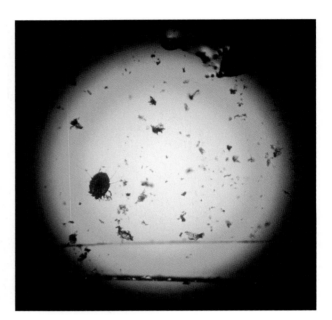

FIGURE 57. *Sarcoptes scabiei* mite seen on mineral oil preparation of skin scrapings.

TABLE 14. Treatment of Infestations	
Infestation	**Treatment**
Scabies (including pregnant women)	1. Treat all members of the household
	2. Wash and dry bedding, linens, clothing, towels in high heat; repeat in 1 week
	3. Topical 5% permethrin cream applied from neck down, repeat in 7 days; emphasize use under fingernails
Crusted scabies	1. In addition to 1 and 2 above, topical 5% permethrin applied daily for 7 days, then twice weekly until cure AND oral ivermectin on days 1, 2, 8, 9, and 15. Do not use ivermectin in pregnant women.
Pediculosis capitis (head lice) AND *Pthirus pubis* (pubic lice)	1. 1% permethrin cream rinse; 0.5% malathion for resistance
	2. Clear nits and eggs with fine tooth comb
	3. Wash and dry clothes and bedding in high heat
	4. Use petrolatum ointment for eyelash infestation
Pediculosis corporis (body lice)	1. Destroy or wash and dry clothing or bedding in high heat
Bed Bugs	1. Professional extermination
	2. Wash and dry clothing and bedding in high heat; repeat in 1 week

corporis), and pubic lice (*Pthirus pubis*). Head lice live on the scalp and attach eggs (nits) to the proximal hair shaft (**Figure 58**). Transmission occurs by close personal contact or by fomites such as bedding, clothing, or hairbrushes.

Body lice live in the seams of clothing and not on the skin. Excoriations result in crusted papules or linear petechiae on the trunk, neck, and proximal arms. Maculae ceruleae are blue-brown macules from subcutaneous hemorrhage at sites of feeding.

Pubic lice (crab louse) are typically spread by sexual contact but may attach to other sites such as eyebrows or eyelashes (*Pediculosis ciliaris*). Symptoms include itching in affected area and maculae ceruleae. See Table 14 for treatment.

Bed Bugs

Relaxed international travel and pesticide regulations have led to the resurgence of the bed bug (*Cimex lectularius*). Bed bugs live in floorboards, walls, vents, or furniture and crawl to the host to feed overnight. They do not live on the human body. Bites are characteristically linearly arranged urticarial papules ("breakfast, lunch, and dinner" bites) on exposed skin (**Figure 59**). See Table 14 for treatment.

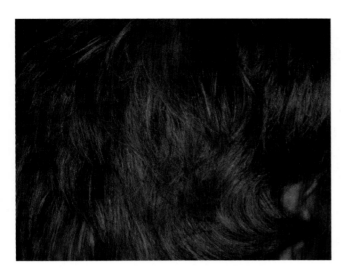

FIGURE 58. Multiple nits appearing as white adhesions to the black hair.

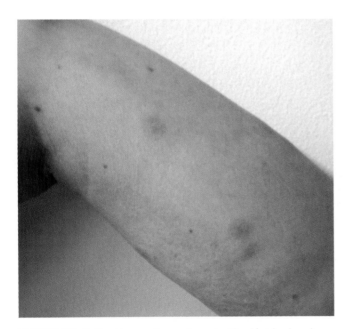

FIGURE 59. Bedbug bites usually occur in a series ("breakfast, lunch, and dinner"). The lesions are painless, pruritic, urticaria-like papules.

Bites and Stings

Spiders

There is often confusion in diagnosing spider bites. Most "spider bites" described by patients are actually folliculitis or furuncles; most spider bites are characterized by wheals, papules, or pustules. It is rare to see a punctum. Bites may itch or burn with most symptoms resolving in about 1 week. Bites may become secondarily infected from scratching.

Spider bites causing severe systemic symptoms are rare and are inflicted by a limited number of spiders. Each spider has a specific geographic distribution. For example, the brown recluse spider, *Loxosceles reclusa*, is found in the southern and central United States (**Figure 60**). Its bite can occasionally cause severe skin necrosis with significant pain and systemic symptoms.

KEY POINT

- Most "spider bites" described by patients are actually folliculitis or furuncles; most spider bites are characterized by wheals, papules, or pustules.

HVC

Hymenoptera

Bees, wasps, and ants belong to the order Hymenoptera. Following a sting, the stinger should be removed to prevent continuing envenomation. Small local reactions are treated with cold compresses, whereas large symptomatic local reactions (~10 cm) may require systemic glucocorticoids to reduce swelling and pruritus. In sensitized persons, systemic reactions such as hives, flushing, or even anaphylaxis may occur. These patients should carry an injectable epinephrine pen and be referred to an allergist for possible venom immunotherapy.

Fire ants (*Solenopsis invicta*), which are mostly found in the southern United States, have sharp jaws and a posterior stinger. The ants latch with their jaws and repeatedly sting while rotating around the bite site, which results in a central papule ringed with pustules. **H**

KEY POINT

- Persons sensitized to hymenoptera stings should carry an injectable epinephrine pen.

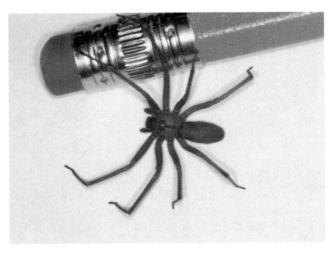

FIGURE 60. Brown recluse spiders are quite shy, and their bites are often misidentified and overdiagnosed.

Worms

Cutaneous larva migrans results from hookworm penetration of bare skin. As the worm migrates through the skin, it leaves elevated serpiginous pruritic lesions (**Figure 61**). Wearing shoes outdoors (especially on the beach) prevents transmission from animal feces. Treatment is ivermectin, albendazole, or cryotherapy at the advancing edge of the eruption.

Fleas

Fleas are the one of the most common causes of papular urticaria characterized by itchy papules on the legs and arms (**Figure 62**). The cat flea (*Ctenocephalides felis*) is the most common.

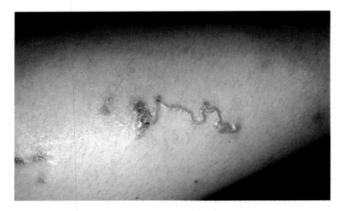

FIGURE 61. Serpiginous, linear red track marks that are pathognomonic for cutaneous larva migrans. Cutaneous larva migrans (creeping eruption) is a parasitic skin disease caused by migration of the hookworm larva within the superficial layers of the skin.

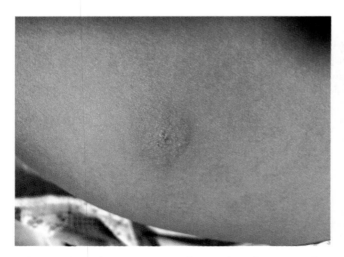

FIGURE 62. Papular urticaria reaction with surrounding inflammation on the leg characteristic of a flea bite.

Cuts, Scrapes, and Burns

Minor wounds can be cleaned gently with soap and water to remove any foreign materials and then properly bandaged. A thin layer of plain petrolatum can be applied to the damaged skin surface before applying a nonadherent bandage. Topical antibiotics can be used for wounds that are in locations that have increased risk for secondary infection such as the perineum or major skin folds. Topical antibiotics such as neomycin and bacitracin have activity against gram-positive and selected gram-negative organisms but may lead to contact allergy. Mupirocin is effective only against gram-positive organisms, with little risk of contact sensitivity, although bacterial resistance is increasing.

Cuts and Scrapes

Minor cuts and scrapes should be cleaned gently with soap and water, irrigated if necessary to remove any foreign material, and dressed with a bandage. If a cut extends into the dermis and is more than a puncture, it should be sutured together. Small cuts can be glued together with topical skin adhesive. Areas with increased tension (across the knee) are best sutured.

Burns

Burns may be caused by a multitude of agents including chemical, thermal, electrical, and ultraviolet light (**Figure 63**). Thermal burns are assessed based on the amount of surface area of involvement, depth of burn, and specific area involved. Grading of burns is seen in **Table 15**. Estimating the body surface area involved is based on the rule of 9s. The head and neck represent 9% body surface area, each arm is 9%, each leg 18%, the anterior trunk is 18%, the posterior trunk is 18%, and the genital region is 1% of body surface area. Minor burns in areas of low risk for infection with a small body surface area of involvement can be treated with gentle cleansing and application of a sterile dressing with petrolatum. Wounds prone to

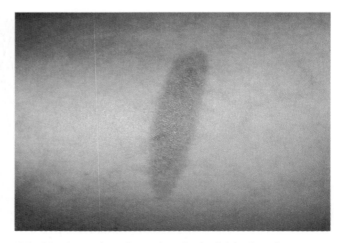

FIGURE 63. First-degree burn with small, red well-defined macule occurring after accidentally touching the skin with a hot curling iron.

TABLE 15.	Burn Grading	
Degree	**Structures Involved**	**Signs and Symptoms**
First	Epidermis	Red and tender skin
Second		
Partial thickness	Epidermis destroyed; partial dermis	Blisters, sloughed skin, red, painful
Full thickness	Epidermis and dermis destroyed	Dry, white, yellow, or red and painful
Third	Epidermis, dermis, and fat destroyed	Dry, black, minimal pain
Fourth	Same as third degree, but also involving muscle and or bone	Dry, black, minimal pain

developing infection may be best treated with a topical antibiotic in addition to the sterile dressing.

Common Neoplasms

Benign Neoplasms

Seborrheic Keratosis

Seborrheic keratoses are benign pigmented neoplasms of keratinocyte origin that are common in adults. They are "stuck-on" papules and plaques that occur anywhere on the body but are most common on the trunk and spare the palms, soles, and mucous membranes. Seborrheic keratoses range in size from a few millimeters to several centimeters. Usually they are brown, but they can range in color from tan to black (**Figure 64**). They can mimic melanoma and squamous cell carcinoma, but skin biopsy confirms the diagnosis. They may become irritated or excoriated. When seborrheic keratoses are symptomatic, they may be treated with cryotherapy or shave removal.

Melanocytic Nevi

Melanocytic nevi are benign neoplasms composed of melanocytes commonly referred to as "moles." They occur anywhere on the body including palms, soles, and mucous membranes. Melanocytic nevi can appear early in childhood and increase in number until middle age. They vary in clinical appearance depending on the location of melanocytes within the skin (**Table 16** and **Figure 65**). Clinically they can mimic melanoma, necessitating a biopsy for accurate diagnosis.

Dysplastic Nevi

Dysplastic nevi are melanocytic nevi that are often asymmetric, irregularly bordered, have more than one shade of brown, and may be quite large in diameter. Many have a "fried egg" appearance with an eccentric dark brown papular center and surrounding light brown ring. Dysplastic nevi can display one or more of the identifying characteristics of melanoma (see Malignant Melanoma), making an accurate clinical diagnosis impossible. In cases of uncertainty, a biopsy of the lesion can typically exclude melanoma; however, it is imperative to sample the entire lesion including a 1- to 2-mm border of normal surrounding skin.

TABLE 16.	Types of Melanocytic Nevi	
Type	**Location of Melanocyte Nests in Skin**	**Clinical Appearance**
Junctional melanocytic nevus	Dermal-epidermal junction	Brown-to-black macules
Compound melanocytic nevus	Dermal-epidermal junction and dermis	Tan-to-brown papules or nodules
Intradermal melanocytic nevus	Dermis	Tan-to-skin-colored papules

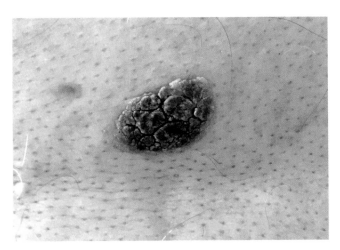

FIGURE 64. Seborrheic keratoses are brown, scaly, waxy papules/plaques that commonly occur in older persons. They frequently have a "stuck-on" appearance and often have verrucous (warty) surface changes as well. Seborrheic keratoses typically demonstrate horn cysts (epidermal cysts filled with keratin) on the surface that can best be visualized on dermoscopy.

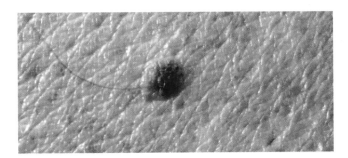

FIGURE 65. Compound melanocytic nevi are tan-to-brown papules with regular borders and even color.

CONT.

Although melanoma can arise within any melanocytic nevi, including dysplastic nevi, the risk of this occurring within any given lesion is quite small. Removal is reserved for those lesions that display particularly worrisome features, are changing in size and color, are symptomatic, or stand out from the patient's other nevi. Patients with multiple dysplastic nevi are at risk for developing melanoma and should be monitored closely (**Figure 66**). Some of these patients have dysplastic nevus syndrome. Criteria for this syndrome include a history of melanoma in one or more first- or second-degree relatives, the presence of a large number of nevi (>50), multiple nevi having atypical clinical features, and multiple nevi that have atypical histologic features. These patients are at increased risk of melanoma and should have yearly full-skin examinations. **H**

> **KEY POINTS**
>
> - Dysplastic nevi can display one or more of the identifying characteristics of melanoma; patients with multiple dysplastic nevi are at increased risk of melanoma and should have yearly full-skin examinations.
>
> **HVC**
>
> - Excision of dysplastic nevi is reserved for lesions that display particularly worrisome features, are changing in size and color, are symptomatic, or stand out from the patient's other nevi.

Halo Nevi

Halo nevi are melanocytic nevi with an admixed chronic lymphocytic infiltrate that signifies regression of the nevus. Halo nevi are central brown-to-tan macules or papules with a surrounding "halo" of hypopigmented or depigmented skin (**Figure 67**). They most frequently present on the back of teenagers or young adults. Multiple halo nevi have been associated with melanoma; therefore, these patients should have a complete skin examination.

Sebaceous Hyperplasia

Sebaceous hyperplasia is a common benign condition consisting of flesh-colored or yellow umbilicated papules found on the face of older patients, particularly the forehead (**Figure 68**). The lesions are often multiple and are more common in patients with rosacea. Histologically, there is enlargement of the sebaceous glands surrounding a hair follicle. Sebaceous hyperplasia can mimic basal cell carcinoma and may necessitate a biopsy for accurate diagnosis.

Callus/Corns

A callus is a collection of thickened, hardened stratum corneum that presents as a flat papule or plaque at the site of repetitive trauma, frequently under bones. Sometimes the term "corn" is used interchangeably with callus; however, corns have more distinct edges, are more rounded, and have a central core that can be soft or hard. Corns are typically seen on the sides or tops of toes. Treatment is by mechanical or chemical paring with salicylic acid, but removing the pressure from the site is necessary to prevent reformation.

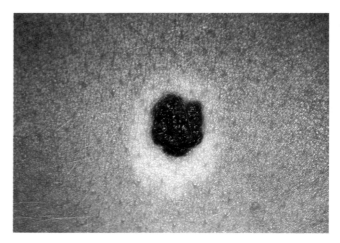

FIGURE 67. Halo nevus, with a depigmented halo surrounding a brown papule.

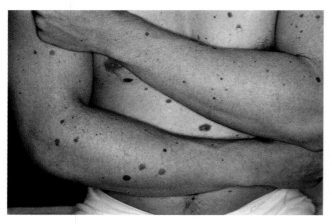

FIGURE 66. Dysplastic nevi are commonly larger than 6 mm and have irregular borders. This patient has numerous dysplastic nevi and is at increased risk for melanoma.

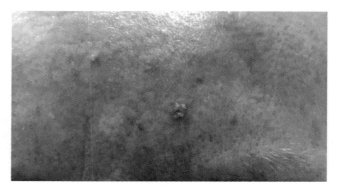

FIGURE 68. Sebaceous hyperplasia presenting as a yellow-to-pink papule with a central umbilication on the forehead.

Acrochordon (Skin Tags)

Acrochordons (skin tags) are skin colored, pedunculated papules (**Figure 69**). They are most commonly seen on the neck and skin folds in older adults. Skin tags appear with increased frequency during the second trimester of pregnancy and may regress postpartum. Skin tags are frequently seen in obese patients and in patients with diabetes mellitus. Perianal skin tags are common in patients with Crohn disease. If lesions become necrotic or crusted, they may require removal with cryotherapy or snip excision. They can be of cosmetic concern, especially when numerous. The presence of numerous lesions, particularly in the setting of obesity and acanthosis nigricans, is associated with insulin resistance.

Cherry Angiomas

Cherry angiomas are benign vascular lesions with a familial predisposition that present in adulthood and become more numerous with age. They are discrete red-to-violaceous papules that blanch with pressure, more common on the trunk but can be seen anywhere on the skin (**Figure 70**). Shave removal or electrocautery may be required for lesions that are traumatized or bleeding.

Dermatofibroma

Dermatofibromas are benign, fibrohistiocytic lesions that are common on the extremities, particularly the legs of young women, and are associated with trauma. Dermatofibromas are tan-to-brown discrete papules that often have a slightly darker brown ring encircling the main part of the lesion; they "dimple" when lateral pressure is applied to the lesion with the thumb and first finger (**Figure 71**). Treatment is not necessary, and recurrences are common after shave removal. Multiple dermatofibromas have been associated with HIV infection and systemic lupus erythematosus.

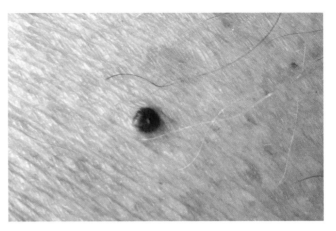

FIGURE 70. Cherry angioma is characterized by a blanchable, pink-to-red, small dome-shaped papule.

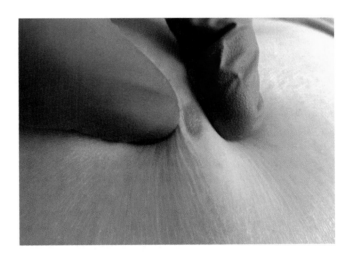

FIGURE 71. The "dimple sign" is a characteristic clinical feature of dermatofibromas which are firm tan papules.

Solar Lentigines and Ephelides

Solar lentigines are tan or light brown, 1- to 3-cm well-defined macules on sun-exposed areas of older adults, commonly referred to as "liver spots" (**Figure 72**). They are a marker of sun damage. Ephelides or "freckles" are 2- to 5-mm tan macules on sun-exposed areas that appear in childhood and darken with sun exposure. When solar lentigines or ephelides are larger than 1 cm or irregular in shape, melanoma is in the clinical differential diagnosis and a biopsy should be considered.

Hypertrophic Scars and Keloids

Hypertrophic scars are raised firm nodules or plaques at the site of an injury that can be tender or pruritic (**Figure 73**). They usually have a good response to intralesional glucocorticoids and may regress spontaneously.

Keloids are firm, rubbery papules, nodules, or plaques that extend beyond the site of injury, but can also form

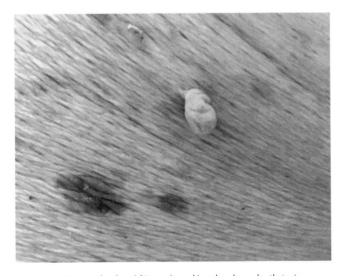

FIGURE 69. Acrochordons (skin tags) are skin-colored papules that arise on areas of friction, such as the neck, axillae, and groin.

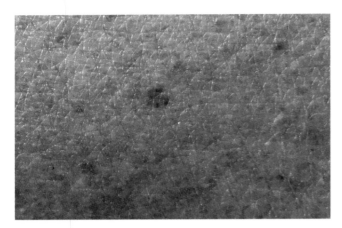

FIGURE 72. Solar lentigines (solar lentigo) are brown macules and patches that occur in middle aged to elderly fair-skinned persons in sun-damaged areas. Although benign, they may occasionally be difficult to distinguish from melanoma. Useful discriminating characteristics include more homogeneous pigmentation and lighter color.

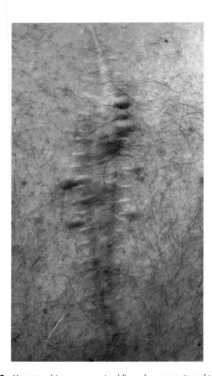

FIGURE 73. Hypertrophic scars are raised firm plaques at sites of injury. As opposed to keloids, they characteristically do not exceed the site of the original injury.

spontaneously, including from inflammatory lesions of acne. They are more common in people with pigmented skin and on the chest and ears. Treatment is difficult and is associated with high rates of recurrence. It requires excision with subsequent intralesional glucocorticoids.

Pyogenic Granulomas

Pyogenic granulomas or lobular capillary hemangiomas are friable red papules that grow quickly and bleed easily

(**Figure 74**). The name is misleading as they are neither pyogenic nor granulomatous. They are more common in women during pregnancy and with certain medications (antiretroviral agents and oral retinoids). Treatment for symptomatic lesions is shave removal or electrocautery.

Epidermal Inclusion Cysts

Epidermal inclusion cysts (sebaceous cysts) are subepidermal nodules with an epithelial lining and a core of accumulated keratin debris (**Figure 75**). They often have a central punctum by which foul-smelling material can be expressed. When epidermal inclusion cysts rupture, they may become tender, inflamed, and occasionally infected. Pilar cysts are similar

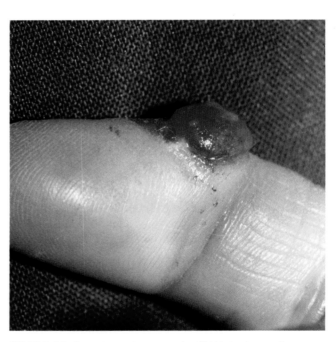

FIGURE 74. Pyogenic granulomas are red and friable benign vascular tumors that arise spontaneously or secondary to trauma and grow rapidly.

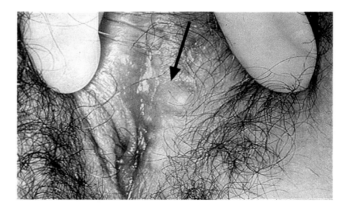

FIGURE 75. Epidermal inclusion cysts are either found incidentally or present as a firm non-tender lump. If they rupture, a local inflammatory response to the necrotic debris released can mimic infection. It is very common for women on the major or minor labia.

lesions that occur on the scalp. Treatment is by excision, but the epithelial lining must be removed to avoid recurrences.

Lipomas

Lipomas are benign neoplasms of mature adipocytes that present as mobile, subcutaneous nodules or tumors. Patients can have a single lesion or multiple, and they are most common on the trunk. Angiolipomas are a variant with a vascular component that is often painful and more common on the upper extremities. When symptomatic or larger, lipomas and angiolipomas can be excised.

Digital Myxoid Cysts

Digital myxoid (mucous) cysts are slow-growing, translucent papules most commonly seen in the distal interphalangeal joint or the proximal nail fold of the fingers, although the toes can also be affected. Nail deformity, pain, and discharge can be complications. Symptomatic treatment can be done by incision and drainage, but recurrences are common and there is a risk of infection and scarring.

Xanthoma

Xanthomas are characteristic skin conditions associated with primary or secondary hyperlipidemias. Xanthomas are yellow, orange, reddish, or yellow-brown papules, plaques, or nodules. The type of xanthoma closely correlates with the type of lipoprotein that is elevated. The most common xanthoma types include eruptive, plane, xanthelasma, tuberous, and tendinous.

Eruptive xanthomas present as clusters of erythematous papules typically on the extensor surfaces. They are most often associated with extremely high serum triglyceride levels. Plane xanthomas are yellow-to-red plaques found in skin folds of the neck and trunk. They can be associated with familial dyslipidemias and a variety of hematologic malignancies. Xanthelasma is a type of plane xanthoma localized to the periorbital area, most commonly on the upper medial eyelid (**Figure 76**), and is characterized by soft, nontender,

nonpruritic plaques. Xanthelasma can occur without hyperlipidemia, particularly in older persons, but is often associated with familial dyslipidemias when seen in a younger person. These lesions are a classic feature of primary biliary cirrhosis, a condition often associated with marked hypercholesterolemia. Tendon xanthomas are subcutaneous nodules occurring on the extensor tendons; they are associated with familial hypercholesterolemia.

Neurofibromas

Neurofibromas are benign nerve-sheath tumors that present as soft, skin-colored papules that show invagination of the papule with lateral pressure ("buttonhole" sign). Single lesions are common in adults, especially on the trunk. Multiple neurofibromas are seen in neurofibromatosis type 1 (von Recklinghausen disease) (**Figure 77**). Treatment of symptomatic lesions is by excisional biopsy.

Precancerous and Cancerous Neoplasms

Skin cancer is a major public health concern, and one in five people in the United States will develop it. Most cases are caused by excessive ultraviolet (UV) light exposure. People of all skin pigmentation can develop skin cancer, but fair skinned persons are more prone to the effects of UV light exposure.

Basal Cell Carcinoma

Basal cell carcinoma (BCC) is a malignant neoplasm arising from the basal layer of the epidermis. It is the most common type of skin cancer and cancer in general. Metastasis rarely occurs; however, without treatment, it can cause significant local tissue destruction. Vital structures, such as eyes, ears, and nose, may be damaged. The most common causative factor is UV light exposure. There are different histologic

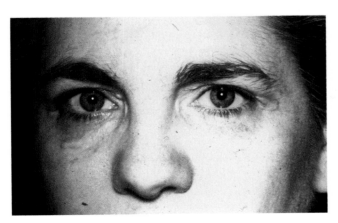

FIGURE 76. Xanthelasma is a type of plane xanthoma that presents as asymptomatic, flat, yellow-to-orange papules or plaques around eyelids that can be associated with familial dyslipidemia in young adults.

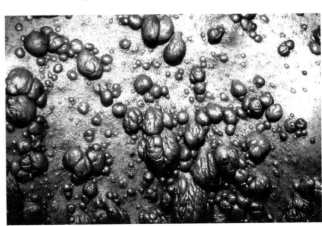

FIGURE 77. Neurofibromas present as soft, compressible, flesh-colored papules and nodules. Multiple neurofibromas are seen in neurofibromatosis type 1 (von Recklinghausen disease).

subtypes that result in varying clinical appearance including superficial, pigmented, sclerotic, and nodular. Patients usually present with a new growth that is bleeding or not healing. They often have other signs of photodamage, such as freckles, lentigines, and actinic keratoses.

Nodular basal cell carcinoma is the most common type of BCC. It presents as a pearly or translucent nodule or papule with arborizing telangiectasias. It may have a central depression or ulceration with a rolled waxy border (**Figure 78**). The term "rodent ulcer" is used to describe the ulceration. Nodular BCC is most commonly found on the face, especially the nose. Histologically, nodular BCC is a low-risk subtype, but its counterpart, micronodular BCCs, poses a higher risk. They can only be distinguished by histologic assessment.

The superficial type of basal cell carcinoma appears as a pink-red patch with or without scale. It may have a slight threadlike pearly rolled border. It can be confused for an actinic keratosis, squamous cell carcinoma in situ, or a patch of dermatitis such as psoriasis or nummular dermatitis. Superficial BCC tends to be a persistent solitary patch that does not respond to topical glucocorticoids. Biopsy provides definitive diagnosis.

Pigmented BCC presents as shiny blue-black papules, nodules, or plaques that can appear translucent with blue-black speckles with a rolled border. It is more common in patients with darker skin.

Sclerotic BCC, which includes morpheaform and infiltrative subtypes, presents as atrophic plaques or papules that can resemble a scar. Although it is the least common, it is a high-risk, aggressive histologic subtype.

The diagnosis of BCC should be confirmed histologically with a shave or punch biopsy. Treatment of BCC should be based on patient's preference and health status, the location of the lesion, histologic subtype, size, and primary versus recurrent nature. Therapeutic options include surgery (standard excision, Mohs micrographic surgery); electrodessication and curettage; cryosurgery; topical chemotherapy; radiation ther-

apy; and for metastatic or inoperable lesions, oral hedgehog pathway inhibitors (vismodegib, sonidegib). Surgical excision is the most commonly used intervention and results in the highest cure rate.

Mohs micrographic surgery is a highly specialized surgical technique that combines pathology and surgery for complete margin control and tissue conservation. It is appropriately used for cancers in the head and neck region, those that are large or recurrent, or in areas where tissue-sparing is critical for function (vital structures) (**Figure 79**). Radiation therapy is generally reserved for inoperable tumors or patients who refuse surgical treatment. Topical chemotherapy with 5-fluorouracil or imiquimod can be used for superficial BCC; however, its cure rate is user dependent.

Treatment course lasts for weeks and results in marked inflammation and irritation. Topical therapies are inappropriate for deep, recurrent, or sclerotic tumors. Curettage and electrodessication can be used for superficial or nodular BCCs on the trunk. It should not be used for tumors 2 cm or larger, those with poorly defined borders, recurrent or high-risk histologic subtypes, and those appearing in certain anatomic locations (face, scalp, eyelids). Cryosurgery for BCCs is different than that for actinic keratosis. The margin, depth, and temperature have to be monitored to achieve cure.

Follow-up skin examination every 6 to 12 months is recommended as the risk of developing another BCC is increased. Prevention with sun protection is highly recommended including routine use of sunscreens with sun protection factor greater than 35, protective clothing (wide brim hats, long sleeves), and avoidance of midday sun (10 AM to 2 PM).

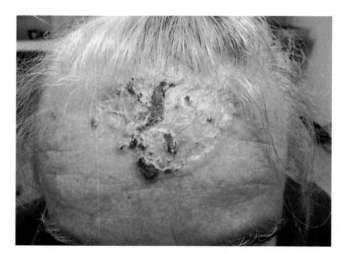

FIGURE 79. Untreated basal cell carcinomas (BCC) over time can become large and cause significant local tissue damage. BCC occurring in the mask area of the face and BCC with certain histology expand not only in the skin, but can invade deeper tissues including fascia, muscle, bone and nerves. These tumors are at high risk of recurrence after treatment along with structural damage. Biopsy of the tumor is needed to ascertain tumor histology, which directs appropriate management, which will likely include Mohs micrographic surgery.

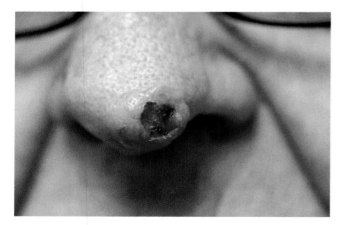

FIGURE 78. Pearly nodule with arborizing telangiectasias (bottom left) and ulceration characteristic of nodular basal cell carcinoma.

- Nodular basal cell carcinoma is the most common type of basal cell carcinoma, typically presenting as a pearly or translucent nodule or papule with arborizing telangiectasias; it may often have a central depression or ulceration with a rolled waxy border.

- The diagnosis of basal cell carcinoma should be confirmed histologically with a shave or punch biopsy.

- Surgical excision is the most commonly used treatment for basal cell carcinoma and results in the highest cure rate; Mohs micrographic surgery is used for cancers in the head and neck region, those that are large or recurrent, or in areas where tissue-sparing is critical for function.

Actinic Keratosis

Actinic keratoses are precancerous lesions of the epidermis. Approximately 1% to 5% of actinic keratoses will develop into squamous cell skin cancers. They present as ill-defined pink scaly ("sandpaper") thin papules or plaques mostly in sun-exposed areas (**Figure 80**). Individual lesions can be treated with cryotherapy. In patients with diffuse actinic damage, field treatment with topical chemotherapy creams (such as 5-fluorouracil or imiquimod) or photodynamic therapy can be used. Lesions that do not resolve with cryotherapy or are more indurated will require a biopsy to rule out an invasive neoplasm.

Squamous Cell Carcinoma

Squamous cell carcinoma (SCC), the second most common skin cancer, is a malignant neoplasm of keratinocytes. It presents as pink, scaly indurated plaques, papules, or nodules that can ulcerate, bleed, or become crusty (**Figure 81** and **Figure 82**). It can be painful. Risk factors are UV light, ionizing radiation, chemical carcinogens (coal tar, soot, and arsenic), viruses

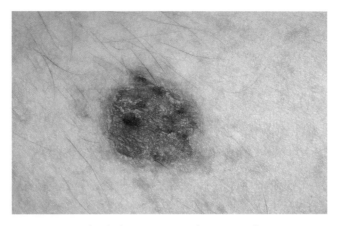

FIGURE 81. Pink scaly plaque consistent with squamous cell carcinoma.

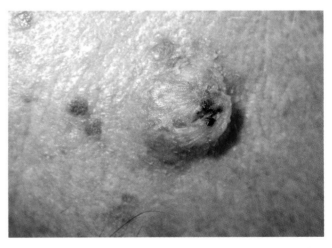

FIGURE 82. Pink hyperkeratotic nodule on sun exposed skin consistent with squamous cell carcinoma.

(human papillomavirus), and immunosuppression (organ transplant, hematologic malignancies, HIV infection). SCC occurs in areas of sun exposure and areas of chronic injury (burn scars, irradiated sites, erosive discoid lupus erythematosus). In comparison to lightly pigmented patients, those patients with darker pigment more often develop SCC in regions with chronic inflammation or scarring and more frequently on the lower extremities. SCC can be locally invasive and has the potential to metastasize. Histologically, it can range from well-differentiated SCC to poorly differentiated SCC, which is the more aggressive subtype. High-risk factors for SCC are tumor diameter greater than 2 cm, tumor thickness greater than 2 mm, poorly differentiated subtypes, perineural invasion, and tumor location of the ear or nonglabrous lip (**Figure 83**).

With SCC in situ (Bowen disease), malignant keratinocytes are confined to the epidermis. It appears as larger scaly pink and tan plaques with well-defined borders (**Figure 84**). Skin biopsy can distinguish SCC in situ from actinic keratoses.

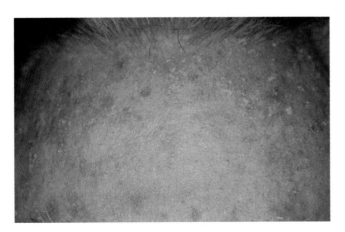

FIGURE 80. Actinic keratoses are typically pink thin papules that occur on sun-exposed areas, particularly the face and dorsal arms. Actinic keratoses result from chronic sun exposure, and their presence identifies persons who are at increased risk of developing invasive squamous cell carcinomas. Actinic keratoses are a precancerous condition.

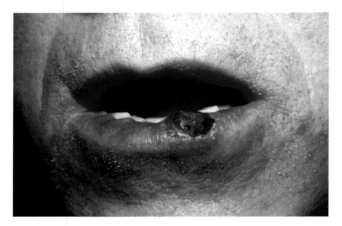

FIGURE 83. Squamous cell carcinoma lesions on the lower lip most commonly arise from sun damage, often in the setting of actinic cheilitis.

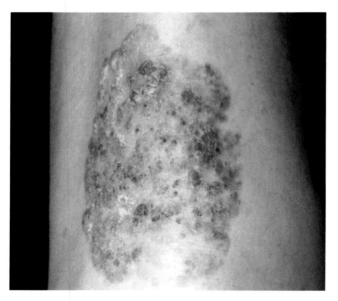

FIGURE 84. Bowen disease (squamous cell carcinoma in situ) typically presents as a gradually enlarging, well-demarcated erythematous plaque with an irregular border and surface crusting or scaling.

Surgical excision including Mohs micrographic surgery for high-risk SCC tends to be the first-line treatment given its potentially aggressive behavior and risk of metastasis. Radiation is an option if surgery is contraindicated. In cases of metastasis, chemotherapy can also be considered.

KEY POINTS

- Squamous cell carcinoma presents as pink, scaly indurated plaque, papules, or nodules that can ulcerate, bleed, or become crusty.
- Surgical excision, including Mohs micrographic surgery, is first-line treatment for squamous cell carcinoma on the head and neck, given its potentially aggressive behavior and risk of metastasis; in cases of metastasis, chemotherapy can also be considered.

Keratoacanthoma

Keratoacanthoma is considered to be a variant of SCC by some and a benign tumor by others. Histologically, it can resemble an SCC. It has a distinct appearance and clinical course. It appears rapidly (within 4 to 6 weeks) as a round pink nodule with a central, keratin-filled crater, giving it a "volcaniform" appearance (**Figure 85**). After its rapid growth, some keratoacanthomas tend to involute in 6 months. Because it is difficult to differentiate from SCC, they are often treated with surgical excision. **H**

Malignant Melanoma

Melanoma is a malignant neoplasm of the melanocytes. Although it is less common than BCC and SCC, it is histologically aggressive and has a much higher rate of metastasis. It is responsible for most skin cancer deaths. In the United States, the incidence of melanoma is increasing faster than any other cancer. The estimated lifetime risk of developing melanoma is 1 in 50. It tends to affect a younger population. There are four clinical subtypes: superficial spreading, lentigo maligna, acral lentiginous, and nodular melanoma. Risk factors include UV light (both chronic and intermittent blistering sunburns), genetics (family history, and *CDKN2A* and *CDK4* gene mutations), large number of nevi, dysplastic nevi, and fair skin.

In general, the ABCDEs of identifying characteristics can help diagnose melanoma where "A" stands for Asymmetry, "B" for irregular Border, "C" for multiple Colors, "D" for Diameter greater than 6 mm, and "E" for Evolution or change over time. Not all melanomas follow all of these characteristics, so if there is a lesion that is different from the patient's other nevi, a biopsy should be considered.

Superficial spreading melanoma is the most common type (**Figure 86**). It can occur anywhere on the body; however, in men, the most common location is the back, whereas in women, it is more often found on the legs.

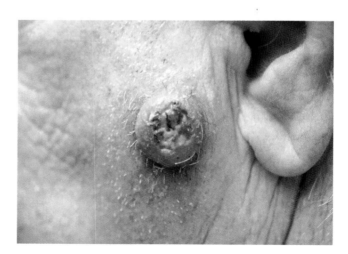

FIGURE 85. Rapidly growing, pink "volcaniform" nodule with central crust that is characteristic of a keratoacanthoma.

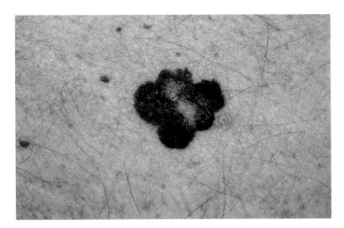

FIGURE 86. A superficial spreading melanoma with prominent Asymmetry, irregular Borders, Color variation, and large size (Diameter)—ABCD.

CONT.

Lentigo maligna is more often found on the head and neck region. It is associated with frequent chronic UV light exposure. It is usually found in older patients, peaking in the seventh and eighth decades of life. It presents as ill-defined, asymmetric brown or black macules or patches, often reaching a diameter of 5 to 7 cm prior to invasion (**Figure 87**). The change and darkening of the lesion can be very insidious and can be mistaken for a solar lentigo or seborrheic keratoses.

Acral lentiginous melanoma occurs on the palms, soles, and distal fingers and toes. It is an ill-defined, black macule plaque, and it more frequently occurs in patients with darker skin (**Figure 88**). The average time to diagnosis is 2 years. The 5-year survival rate for melanoma in blacks and Hispanics, even after adjusting for age, stage, site, and socioeconomic status, is lower compared with white patients.

Nodular melanoma begins in the vertical growth phase and is more aggressive. It is rapid growing and presents as blue-black, smooth, or eroded nodules occurring anywhere on the body (**Figure 89**).

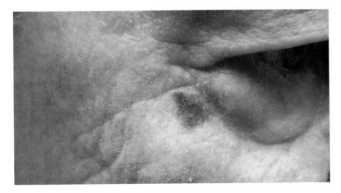

FIGURE 87. Ill-defined asymmetric brown patch consistent with a lentigo maligna which presents as a slowly enlarging, variegated, pigmented patch on sun-damaged skin.

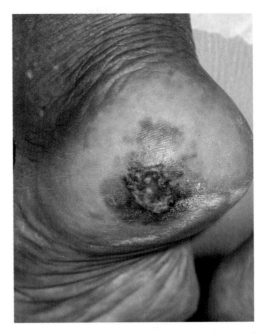

FIGURE 88. Ill-defined, asymmetric black gray ulcerated plaque on the heel typical of acral lentiginous melanoma.

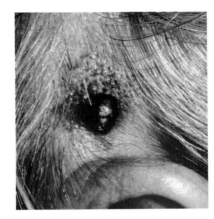

FIGURE 89. Nodular melanomas typically present as uniformly dark blue or black "berry-like" lesions that most commonly originate from normal skin. They can also arise from preexisting nevi, as did this melanoma. Nodular melanomas grow vertically rather than horizontally.

All suspicious pigmented lesions must be biopsied. The preferred method to biopsy a pigmented lesion is an excisional biopsy with 1- to 2-mm margin to obtain the entire lesion and to prevent sampling error. Shave biopsies should be avoided in most pigmented lesions as there is risk of transecting a melanoma and preventing true staging of the lesion. A modified technique that can be helpful is the "scoop" biopsy where the deep dermis or subcutaneous tissue is removed to get underneath the lesion. In wide, ill-defined lesions, it may be prohibitive to remove the entire lesion, so an incisional biopsy is acceptable. Definitive treatment cannot be determined until histologic confirmation and final staging of the tumor is completed.

Poor prognostic factors include male gender, increasing age, increased tumor thickness (Breslow depth), ulceration, increased tumor mitotic rate, and head/neck/trunk locations. Melanomas are staged with the tumor, nodal, and metastasis (TNM) system (https://cancerstaging.org/references-tools/quickreferences/Documents/MelanomaLarge.pdf).

Survival is dependent on early diagnosis. Treatment is based on the stage of melanoma. In the first and second stage, surgical treatment is used to remove the lesion and a margin of clinically normal skin (wide local excision). The size of the margin is based on the depth of the lesion. Melanomas that are stage IB or higher are often considered for sentinel node biopsy for assessing prognosis. Stage III melanoma is treated with wide local excision, lymph node dissection, and possible adjuvant interferon. Immunotherapy has emerged as the primary systemic treatment for stage IV melanoma. Combination treatment with an anti-PD1 antibody (pembrolizumab, nivolumab) with ipilimumab, an anti-CTLA4 antibody, is most often selected for patients with metastatic melanoma (see MKSAP 18 Hematology and Oncology). Survival data suggest that up to 80% of patients receiving this combination will be alive at 2 years. Chemotherapy is typically reserved for patients who have progressed despite optimal systemic therapy. Radiation is usually reserved for palliative therapy for metastasis to the brain and bones. Thorough follow up including a full-body skin examination at routine intervals is crucial for patients with a history of melanoma.

KEY POINTS

- Identifying characteristics of melanoma are Asymmetry, irregular Border, multiple Colors, Diameter greater than 6 mm, and Evolution or change over time (ABCDEs).

- All suspicious pigmented lesions must be biopsied; the preferred method to biopsy is an excisional biopsy with 1- to 2-mm margin.

- For stage I and stage II, treatment of melanoma is surgical excision with the size of the margin based on the depth of the lesion; stage III is treated with wide local excision, lymph node dissection, and possible adjuvant interferon; and stage IV is treated with immunotherapy; chemotherapy is reserved for patients who progress despite optimal immunotherapy.

Pruritus

Pruritus, or itching, is one of the most common symptoms in dermatology. Itch sensation is transmitted to the central nervous system by C-fibers (which are distinct from C-fibers that transmit pain signals) and can be very disruptive to a patient's quality of life. Pruritus is commonly associated with a variety of skin diseases, yet it may also be seen independent of skin pathology. When first evaluating pruritus, it is important to establish if the itch is secondary to an inflammatory skin condition or present without a primary rash.

Several inflammatory skin diseases are associated with pruritus, including atopic dermatitis, contact dermatitis, lichen planus, and urticaria. Significant pruritus is also associated with burns and healing skin, and in xerotic, or dry skin, especially in older patients.

When pruritus occurs in the absence of skin findings, a variety of systemic diseases should be considered. Uremic pruritus is common in patients with chronic or end-stage kidney disease. It typically presents within 3 months of starting hemodialysis. Pruritus can also be associated with cholestatic hepatobiliary diseases (**Figure 90**). Pruritus associated with cirrhosis from alcoholic liver disease or hepatitis C infection can occur in the absence of cholestasis. Thyroid disease and polycythemia vera are other systemic diseases that might present with itching. Generalized pruritus may also be the presenting symptom in malignancies such as lymphocytic leukemia and Hodgkin lymphoma. Certain infections, such as HIV, may present with generalized itching as well.

Various psychiatric or somatization conditions can also manifest as itching (psychogenic itch) (**Figure 91**). Pruritus typically worsens during stressful or traumatic events. Patients with chronic pruritus have increased depression and impaired quality of life. Neuropathic pruritus describes the itch that is caused by dysfunction of a peripheral or central nerve(s) due to surgery, trauma, arthritis, neuropathy, or infection (postherpetic neuralgia). Neuropathic itch is often localized to a small, well-circumscribed area; examples include the forearm (brachioradial pruritus), posterior shoulder, or mid to upper back (notalgia paresthetica) (**Figure 92**).

A review of systems, complete blood count, thyroid function studies, kidney function tests, liver chemistry tests, HIV

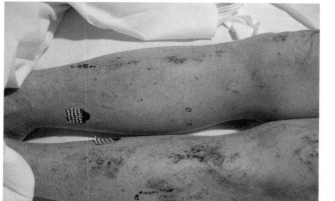

FIGURE 90. Linear excoriations in a patient with cholestatic liver.

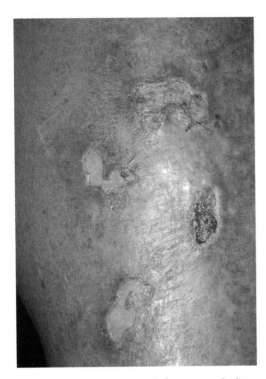

FIGURE 91. Patients with psychogenic itch often report nonhealing sores, such as those seen on this patient's arm. The lesions often have a linear or irregular shape from repeated manipulation. Scars from previous episodes are often seen among the active lesions.

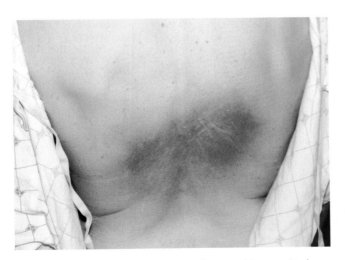

FIGURE 92. A localized and persistent area of pruritus without associated primary skin lesions, usually on the back or forearms, suggests neuropathic itch. This patient's area of hyperpigmentation is secondary to chronic scratching.

TABLE 17. Common Medications That May Cause Pruritus
Calcium channel blockers
Hydrochlorothiazide
Opioids
NSAIDs
ACE inhibitors
Anticoagulants
Antibiotics (trimethoprim/sulfamethoxazole)
Selective serotonin reuptake inhibitors

Patient education is critical to the management of any pruritic condition. The primary lesson for most patients is scratching causes skin damage that contributes to an "itch-scratch-itch" cycle. Treatment of pruritus is directed at addressing the underlying cause. The treatment of inflammatory skin conditions with topical glucocorticoids and emollients can help alleviate pruritus. Topical anti-itch medications containing menthol can also be helpful. First-generation oral antihistamines can be sedating and helpful for pruritus at night. For older patients with xerotic skin, comprehensive dry skin care should be reviewed. This includes bathing in warm water followed by immediate application of a thick emollient. Products that contain perfumes or dyes should be avoided as xerotic skin is at greater risk of irritation due to a compromised skin barrier.

Topical treatments may not be as effective for systemic causes of pruritus. Gabapentin can be effective in treating pruritus associated with burns, neuropathic itch, and uremic pruritus. Phototherapy can also be used for uremic pruritus. Ursodeoxycholic acid can be considered for cholestatic pruritus.

KEY POINTS

- When pruritus occurs in the absence of skin findings, a variety of systemic causes, including kidney or liver diseases, thyroid disease, or HIV, should be considered.
- Reactions to common medications, such as opiates, calcium channel blockers, hydrochlorothiazide, and NSAIDs, are frequent causes of pruritus.
- Topical glucocorticoids and emollients are appropriate treatment for pruritus associated with inflammatory skin conditions.

CONT. test, and chest radiograph are necessary to help guide further workup. In addition, a review of the patient's medications, including supplements and illicit drugs, should be performed. Common medications that can cause pruritus are opiates, calcium channel blockers, hydrochlorothiazide, and NSAIDs **(Table 17).**

Urticaria

Urticaria (hives) are localized areas of edema caused by mast cell degranulation and the release of inflammatory proteins, including histamine, leukotrienes, complement, and prostaglandins. Urticaria is characterized by well-demarcated

CONT.

erythematous plaques ranging in size from 1 to 8 cm that appear quickly and resolve in a matter of hours (**Figure 93**). Individual lesions may be erythematous or white, often surrounded by a red halo, and have a variety of shapes including round, oval, annular, arciform, and serpiginous. The center of a lesion is typically blanchable pink or clear skin. These lesions are extremely pruritic and tend to appear on body sites with repetitive pressure or rubbing, such as the waistline and posterior neck. Although individual urticarial lesions should resolve in less than 24 hours, recurrent crops of hives may last for weeks. Most cases of urticaria resolve spontaneously, and the cause is never determined. If the episodes last for longer than 6 weeks, the condition is classified as chronic urticaria. If the individual urticarial lesions do not resolve after 24 hours, or if they are accompanied by systemic symptoms (joint pain, fever), urticarial vasculitis must be considered.

The diagnosis of urticaria is clinical. Physical maneuvers that can help with diagnosis include circling lesions and seeing if they have resolved within 24 hours, and gently scratching uninvolved skin with the wooden end of tongue depressor to see if urticaria (not just redness) can be induced (dermatographism). The cause of urticaria is investigated primarily by history and physical examination; skin biopsies are not generally needed. Skin biopsy, however, is helpful in the diagnosis of urticarial vasculitis and should be considered in patients with painful lesions, systemic symptoms, or persistent individual lesions.

Viral infection and medication reaction are the most common causes of acute urticaria in adults. Food-induced allergic reactions can be severe, and the most commonly implicated foods are shellfish, peanuts, and tree nuts. Infrequent but important causes include autoimmune thyroid disease and malignancies, particularly lymphoma. Physical urticaria is induced by a physical stimulus such as sunlight, sweating, physical pressure, vibration, water, or cold temperature.

Angioedema is a transient, localized subcutaneous or submucosal form of urticaria caused by extravasation of fluid into interstitial tissues. Angioedema may occur with or without urticaria and can be a component of anaphylaxis. Angioedema involving the face and airway is an emergency, and its initial treatment involves systemic epinephrine and glucocorticoids.

Hereditary angioedema, distinct from the more typical mast-cell associated angioedema, is caused by activation of the complement cascade due to lack of or dysfunction of C1 esterase inhibitor. Hereditary angioedema may cause sporadic localized edema involving the head and neck and is differentiated from mast cell-associated angioedema by the lack of typical urticarial lesions. Diagnosis is by testing for quantitative and functional levels of C1 esterase inhibitor and C4 complement levels.

Diagnostic workup for urticaria is not recommended unless history suggests a specific cause. If symptoms persist, laboratory tests, including a complete blood count with differential, urinalysis, erythrocyte sedimentation rate or C-reactive protein, thyroid-stimulating hormone, and liver chemistry tests, can be considered. If associated with systemic symptoms or suspicion of urticarial vasculitis, testing directed by the findings should be considered. **H**

KEY POINTS

- Urticaria is characterized by well-demarcated erythematous pruritic plaques that appear quickly and resolve in a matter of hours; diagnostic workup for urticaria is not recommended unless history suggests a specific cause. **HVC**

- Hereditary angioedema is caused by activation of the complement cascade due to lack of or dysfunction of C1 esterase inhibitor.

- Nonsedating, long-acting antihistamines are the treatment of choice for urticaria; topical antihistamines have not been found to be effective and may lead to allergic contact dermatitis. **HVC**

Autoimmune Bullous Diseases

Bullous or blistering dermatoses can be acquired from an autoimmune process or from a genetic defect and are characterized by blistering or erosion of the skin. Autoimmune bullous diseases (ABDs) are caused by antibodies interfering with cohesion between keratinocytes of the epidermis (desmosomes) or between the epidermis and dermis (basement membrane zone) (**Table 18**). ABDs can be subdivided into intraepidermal and subepidermal disorders. Intraepidermal ABDs present with flaccid vesicles that rupture easily, whereas

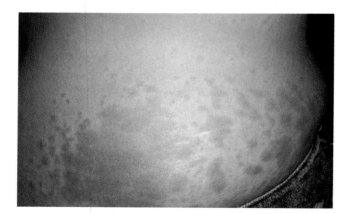

FIGURE 93. Urticarial lesions on the waist characterized by small and large edematous and erythematous plaques of various shapes.

TABLE 18. Characteristics of Autoimmune Blistering Diseases

Disease	Clinical Characteristics	Pathology	Comments
Pemphigus vulgaris	Tender, fragile blisters and erosions seen in oral mucosa and skin; mucous membrane lesions much more common than in bullous pemphigoid; Nikolsky sign (rubbing of the skin resulting in blister formation) is positive	Suprabasilar clefting compared with subepidermal clefting seen in bullous pemphigoid DIF/IIF: intercellular pattern within the epidermis	Incidence varies by country and ethnicity and is estimated to be 0.5 to 3.2 cases per 100,000 persons per year
Pemphigus foliaceus	Scaling and crusted lesions on face and upper trunk, and erythroderma with no mucosal involvement; Nikolsky sign is positive	High granular or subcorneal clefting compared with suprabasal clefting seen in pemphigus vulgaris DIF/IIF: intercellular pattern within the epidermis	Incidence varies by country with estimated occurrence of 0.5 to 6.6 cases per million persons per year Endemic pemphigus foliaceus (fogo selvagem) occurs in central and southwestern Brazil and Colombia and has a higher incidence with up to 50 cases per million persons per year and up to 3.4% of the population affected
Paraneoplastic pemphigus	Painful oral, conjunctival, esophageal, and laryngeal erosions occur more commonly than in pemphigus vulgaris; it is a polymorphous skin eruption marked by confluent erythema, bullae, erosions, and intractable stomatitis; patients also have respiratory problems that may be fatal	Mixed pattern of both suprabasal acantholysis and interface dermatitis DIF/IIF: IgG binds in an intercellular pattern within the epidermis; reactants at the dermal-epidermal junction. The combination of intercellular and subepidermal deposition of immunoreactants is a clue to the diagnosis.	High mortality rate (up to 90%) and association with underlying neoplasms: non-Hodgkin lymphoma (42%), chronic lymphocytic leukemia (29%), Castleman disease (10%)
IgA pemphigus	A vesicopustular eruption with clear blisters that rapidly transform into pustules; trunk and proximal extremities are most commonly involved, with relative sparing of the mucous membranes	Subcorneal collection of neutrophils DIF shows deposition of intercellular IgA at the epidermal surfaces	Newly described disease with unknown frequency
Bullous pemphigoid	Tense blisters preceded by intense pruritus or urticarial lesions most commonly seen in the elderly on the trunk, limbs, and flexures; does not usually present with oral lesions	Subepidermal bullae without acantholysis and with prominent eosinophils DIF shows linear IgG deposition at the basement membrane zone	One of most common autoimmune blistering diseases with up to 4.3 cases per 100,000 persons per year
Epidermolysis bullosa acquisita	Mechanically induced bullae and erosions mostly on extensor areas that heal with scarring and milia	Subepidermal cleavage without acantholysis DIF shows IgG deposition at the basement membrane zone that localizes to the base on salt-split skin	Rare disease with unknown frequency Can be associated with inflammatory bowel disease
Cicatricial pemphigoid	Presents with bullae, erosions, milia, and scarring seen on mucous membranes and conjunctivae of middle-aged to elderly persons; oral mucosa is almost always involved; conjunctival lesions are also common	Histology is similar to bullous pemphigoid DIF may reveal patterns similar to bullous pemphigoid, linear IgA bullous dermatosis, or epidermolysis bullosa acquisita	Rare disease with estimated incidence of 0.9 to 1.1 cases per million persons per year Increased risk for malignancy in some patients Prompt treatment should be initiated to avoid permanent ocular and oral scarring

(Continued on the next page)

TABLE 18. Characteristics of Autoimmune Blistering Diseases *(Continued)*

Disease	Clinical Characteristics	Pathology	Comments
Dermatitis herpetiformis	Severely pruritic grouped vesicles or erosions on elbows, knees, back, scalp, and buttocks; lesions occur in crops and are symmetrically distributed; often the vesicles are not seen because the process is so itchy that they are almost immediately broken	Histology shows neutrophilic infiltrate at the tips of the dermal papillae causing subepidermal separation DIF shows granular IgA deposition	Common blistering disease with 10 to 11 cases per 100,000 persons per year Nearly all patients with dermatitis herpetiformis will have celiac disease
Linear IgA bullous dermatosis	Pruritic, discrete, or clustered bullae in a herpetiform pattern ("cluster of jewels"); annular or polycyclic lesions with vesicles and bullae at the periphery are common	Subepidermal bullae with neutrophils Can be indistinguishable from dermatitis herpetiformis, epidermolysis bullosa acquisita, or bullous lupus DIF shows linear IgA deposition	In adults, the estimated incidence is 0.6 cases per 100,000 persons per year Ocular involvement can occur A variant can occur in children called chronic bullous dermatosis of childhood
Porphyria cutanea tarda (and pseudoporphyria)	Erosions and bullae on hands and forearms, and occasionally face and feet, that heal with milia, hyperpigmentation, and hypopigmented scars. Porphyria cutanea tarda (but not pseudoporphyria) can also present with hypertrichosis on the face	Subepidermal bullae with little inflammation; dermal papillae protrude upward into the blister cavity and thickened upper dermal capillary walls DIF: deposition of immunoglobulins and complement around the dermal capillaries and linear at the basement membrane zone	Common disorder with estimated incidence of 1 case per 25,000 persons per year Not a true autoimmune blistering disorder but should be included in the differential diagnosis Can be associated with hepatitis C infection

DIF = direct immunofluorescence; IIF = indirect immunofluorescence.

subepidermal ABDs show intact, tense bullae. Although most of the ABDs are idiopathic, medications can also cause variants of almost all the disorders, and a thorough medication review is essential (**Table 19**).

The most sensitive method for the diagnosis of ABD is a skin biopsy. A skin (shave or punch) biopsy of an intact, early vesicle or bullae with adjacent normal skin should be submitted in formalin and processed for hematoxylin and eosin staining. Each of the ABDs has characteristic histologic findings that suggest a differential diagnosis. In addition, a biopsy for direct immunofluorescence (DIF) in Michel transport medium should be performed. For optimal sensitivity, biopsies for DIF should be from noninvolved perilesional skin. The histologic findings together with the pattern on DIF can usually render a diagnosis.

 Bullous pemphigoid is the most common subepidermal ABD and overall the most common ABD. Onset is usually in adults 60 years of age and older and presents with urticarial and eczematous lesions that progress to tense bullae on an erythematous base (**Figure 94**). Oral involvement is present in approximately 20% of patients. There are varying degrees of pruritus with bullous pemphigoid. Bullae heal with pigment change but otherwise do not scar. It typically has a protracted course with exacerbations and remission. In the past, morbidity was high, but steroid-sparing agents result in successful management.

Pemphigus vulgaris is the most common intraepidermal ABD, and its incidence increases with age. It presents with oral or vaginal erosions and flaccid vesicles that rupture easily and leave erosions (**Figure 95**). Pemphigus vulgaris has a positive Nikolsky sign whereby light lateral friction on perilesional skin induces a blister. Lesions heal with pigment change but otherwise do not scar. Prior to the use of oral glucocorticoids and steroid-sparing agents, mortality was high owing to secondary infection and sepsis. **H**

Pemphigus foliaceus is a superficial intraepidermal ABD that is most common in middle-aged adults. It presents with crusted erosions on the scalp, head/neck, and trunk without mucous membrane involvement (**Figure 96**). It can be associated with autoimmune diseases, in particular lupus erythematosus.

Epidermolysis bullosa acquisita is a subepidermal ABD with a varied clinical presentation with onset in adulthood. Unlike bullous pemphigus, classic epidermolysis bullosa acquisita presents at sites of friction or trauma (hands, elbows, buttocks, axillae) with tense bullae that are not on an erythematous base. It heals with scarring (milia). Because of the generally noninflammatory nature of epidermolysis bullosa acquisita, treatment is difficult and avoidance of trauma is an important aspect of the regimen.

Dermatitis herpetiformis is a subepidermal ABD that is extremely pruritic. It is a lifelong condition with onset in

TABLE 19.	Drug-Induced Autoimmune Blistering Disorders
Condition	**Medications**
Pemphigus	Thiol group (D-penicillamine, captopril, gold, pyrithioxine)
	Amoxicillin
	Ampicillin
	Cephalosporins
	Rifampin
Pemphigoid	Furosemide
	Amoxicillin
	Ampicillin
	Phenacetin
	Penicillin
	Penicillamine
	Psoralen plus ultraviolet A (PUVA)
	β-Blockers
	Terbinafine
Cicatricial pemphigoid	Penicillamine
	Indomethacin
	Practolol
	Clonidine
	Topical pilocarpine
Linear IgA bullous dermatosis	Vancomycin
	Captopril
	Amoxicillin
	Ampicillin
	Diclofenac
	Lithium
Pseudoporphyria	Furosemide
	Naproxen
	Oxaprozin
	Tetracycline
	Voriconazole

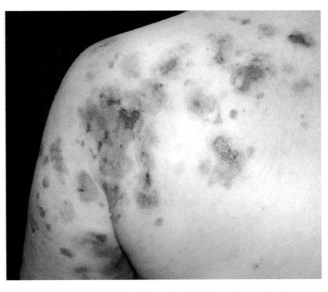

FIGURE 95. The flaccid, intraepidermal vesicle of pemphigus vulgaris are readily broken, leaving behind weeping erosions.

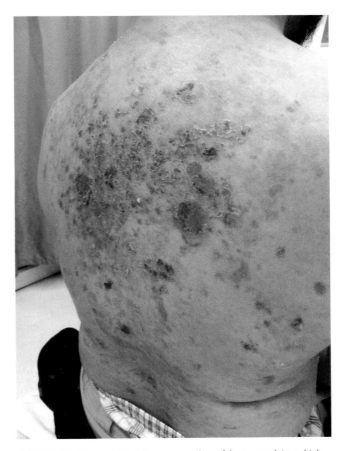

FIGURE 96. The superficial blisters in pemphigus foliaceus result in multiple erosions and crusting (similar to "corn flakes"). Intact vesicles are not seen regularly.

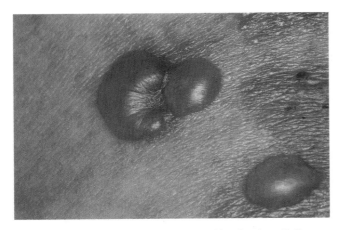

FIGURE 94. Bullous pemphigoid is characterized by subepidermal bullae blisters that are tense and do not rupture easily. It predominantly involves nonmucosal surfaces. Sites of predilection are the lower abdomen, inner thighs, groin, axillae, and flexural aspects of the arms and legs.

adulthood. There are small tense vesicles and papules, which are rarely intact, presenting as excoriations on the elbows, knees, and buttocks (**Figure 97**). Most patients have celiac disease. A gluten-free diet is first-line treatment for dermatitis herpetiformis, but additional therapy with dapsone is often is required. Before initiating therapy with dapsone, patients should be checked for glucose-6-phosphate dehydrogenase deficiency.

Management of ABDs depends on the symptoms, extent of disease, and associated comorbidities. For localized disease, topical or intralesional glucocorticoids may be sufficient. Because the epidermal barrier is disrupted in these conditions, secondary bacterial infection can lead to exacerbations. In general, treatments for ABD are not FDA approved and recommendations are based on expert opinion, consensus, and published evidence. The goal is to decrease circulating antibodies with the subsequent elimination of antibodies binding to skin antigens and the restoration of function. Initial treatment is with prednisone until no new vesicles or blisters are present. This is followed by a slow taper and the addition of a steroid-sparing agent. Recently rituximab has been shown to have high efficacy in pemphigus vulgaris.

KEY POINTS

- Autoimmune blistering diseases are characterized by persistent pruritic or painful vesicles or bullae with erosions of the skin.

- **HVC** A gluten-free diet is first-line treatment for dermatitis herpetiformis, but additional therapy with dapsone is often is required.

- Management of autoimmune bullous diseases depends on the symptoms, the extent of disease, and the associated comorbidities; immunosuppressive medications are often required.

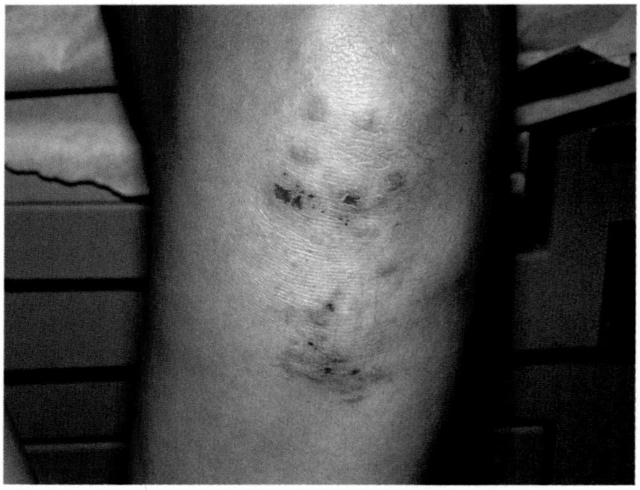

Cutaneous Manifestations of Internal Disease

Rheumatology

Lupus Erythematosus

Lupus erythematosus (LE) is a family of autoimmune conditions featuring autoantibodies directed against nuclear targets. Cutaneous lupus erythematosus (CLE) can exist with or without systemic disease; however, as many as 80% of systemic lupus erythematosus (SLE) patients have some degree of skin disease. CLE is divided into two broad categories: lupus-specific skin disease and lupus-nonspecific skin disease. Lupus-specific skin disease is further divided into three groups: acute cutaneous lupus erythematosus (ACLE), subacute cutaneous lupus erythematosus (SCLE), and chronic cutaneous lupus erythematosus (CCLE) (**Figure 98**). The lupus-specific skin diseases are defined by their clinicopathologic characteristics and are not found in other conditions. Nonspecific skin disease may appear in other unrelated disorders.

The classic malar "butterfly" rash (**Figure 99**) is characteristic of ACLE; however, ACLE can also manifest as a "maculopapular" variant that is photosensitive and distributed over the chest, upper back, and arms. Both rashes are pink-violet macules to scaly papules and plaques. In vibrant cases, severe inflammation can cause separation of the epidermis, which appears similar to Stevens-Johnson syndrome/toxic epidermal necrosis (SJS/TEN) and may involve oral ulcerations. This is sometimes referred to as apoptotic epidermolysis syndrome. Bullous lupus, a variant of ACLE, is a blistering disorder caused by antibodies to the anchoring fibrils of the epidermis. Essentially all patients with ACLE have SLE and as such tend to

FIGURE 97. Dermatitis herpetiformis is an autoimmune bullous disease that causes intensely pruritic small papulovesicles classically grouped on the scalp, elbows, knees, back, and buttocks. Due to intense pruritus, erosions and excoriations are the most common clinical finding.

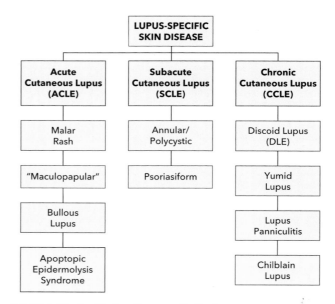

FIGURE 98. Classification of lupus-specific skin disease.

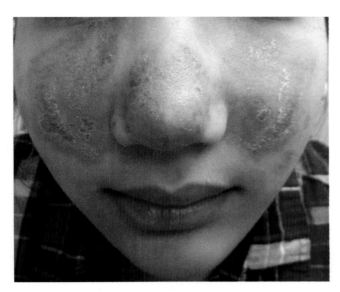

FIGURE 99. Malar butterfly rash in a patient with acute cutaneous lupus erythematosus showing pink-violet plaques with sparing of the nasolabial folds.

TABLE 20. Most Common Medications Causing Drug-Induced Cutaneous Lupus
ACE inhibitors
Griseofulvin
Hydralazine
Hydrochlorothiazide
NSAIDs
Proton pump inhibitors
Terbinafine
Tumor necrosis factor inhibitors

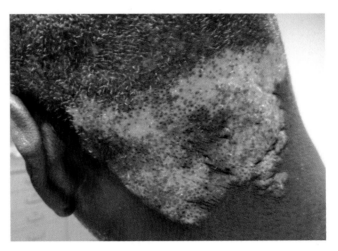

FIGURE 101. Chronic discoid lupus erythematosus on the occiput, with hyperpigmented borders, depigmented centers, dilated empty follicular ostia.

have systemic symptoms and positive serologies. The rash of ACLE does not scar.

SCLE appears as one of two variants: annular and polycyclic photosensitive plaques on the back, chest, and extremities, or psoriasiform scaly plaques in a similar distribution (**Figure 100**). SCLE does not scar, but may resolve with temporary pigmentary changes. Fewer than one in four SCLE patients have SLE, and as many as one in three are drug induced (**Table 20**). The latter may resolve with withdrawal of the causative agent. Up to 70% of patients with SCLE have an elevated antinuclear antibody titer, with anti-Ro and anti-La being overrepresented.

CCLE is another group of related skin diseases. Discoid lupus (DLE) is the most common. DLE lesions start as red-to-violet plaques that develop a hyperpigmented border and thick adherent scale in the center (**Figure 101**). Pulling back

the scale will reveal projections from the underside that resemble carpet tacks. Eventually the centers of lesions become atrophic and depigmented, causing permanent alopecia if occurring in hair-bearing areas (**Figure 102**). Plaques favor the head and neck, particularly the scalp and conchal bowls (the hollow of the auricle of the external ear). CCLE in general has a low association with SLE, and DLE of the head and neck has approximately a 10% risk of underlying systemic disease.

Lupus panniculitis appears as painful red indurated subcutaneous plaques that eventually cause atrophy and scarring depressions of the skin. DLE can often be seen overlying lupus panniculitis. The condition typically appears on the cheeks, lateral arms, breasts, and buttocks. Rarely lupus panniculitis transforms to a form of cutaneous T-cell lymphoma.

Chilblains or pernio are tender purple papulovesicles or plaques that appear on toes and fingers (**Figure 103**). They are triggered by exposure to cold or moisture and are unrelated to Raynaud phenomenon. They respond well to warming and calcium channel blockers.

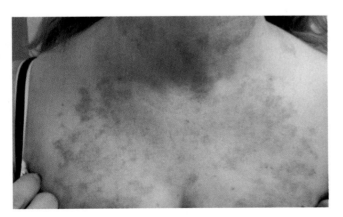

FIGURE 100. Subacute cutaneous lupus erythematosus presenting as pink nonscarring annual and polycyclic macules and plaques on the chest and neck.

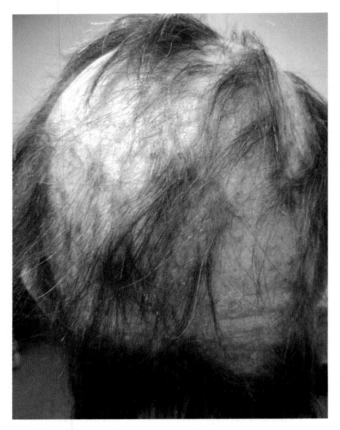

FIGURE 102. Active discoid lupus erythematosus of the scalp with scarring hair loss.

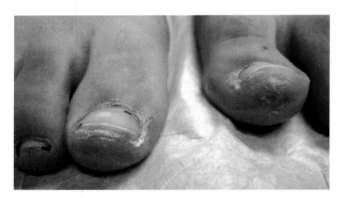

FIGURE 103. Chilblains/pernio in a patient with systemic lupus erythematosus appearing as tender purple plaques on the toes.

Tumid lupus presents with dermal macules or plaques on sun-exposed skin and is the most photosensitive of the lupus-specific skin diseases. It is uncommonly found in association with SLE (**Figure 104**).

Two lupus-nonspecific features are included in the Systemic Lupus International Collaborating Clinics criteria. First, oral or nasal ulcerations, a variant of minor aphthae, appear as white tender erosions of the oro- or nasopharynx. Second, "lupus hair," which is a variant of nonscarring alopecia, is a form of telogen effluvium. It may be localized, patchy,

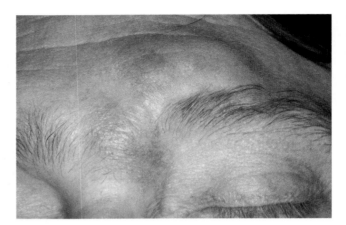

FIGURE 104. Tumid lupus showing reticulate pink dermal plaques on the forehead in typical photodistribution.

or diffuse. Most typical is a recession of the frontal hairline with sparse, short, wiry, and broken hairs left behind. Hair regrowth can be a sign of disease control.

Therapy for cutaneous lupus includes antimalarial agents such as hydroxychloroquine, methotrexate, mycophenolate mofetil, cyclosporine, dapsone, and combination therapy (**Table 21**). Thalidomide is effective for some patients with chronic cutaneous lupus.

The importance of photoprotection in the patient with lupus cannot be overstated. Patients should avoid peak sun hours and use barrier protection such as protective clothing and wide brim hats. Broad spectrum sunscreen (ultraviolet A and B filters) should be worn every day, with frequent reapplication. Sunlight and other sources of ultraviolet light drive disease activity, cause flares in stable patients, or even flare systemic disease.

KEY POINTS

- Lupus-specific skin disease is further divided into three groups: acute cutaneous lupus erythematosus (ACLE), subacute cutaneous lupus erythematosus (SCLE), and chronic cutaneous lupus erythematosus (CCLE)

(Continued)

TABLE 21. Treatment for Cutaneous Lupus Erythematosus
Antimalarial agents (hydroxychloroquine, may add quinacrine if not effective, or switch to chloroquine)
Cyclosporine, dapsone
Immunosuppressants (methotrexate, azathioprine, mycophenolate mofetil)
Rigorous solar protection and avoidance
Systemic retinoids (acitretin)
Thalidomide, leflunomide
Tobacco cessation
Topical anti-inflammatory agents (glucocorticoids or calcineurin inhibitors)

- Essentially all patients with ACLE have systemic lupus erythematosus (SLE), and the most common manifestation of ACLE is a malar rash; SLE is much less commonly associated with SCLE and CCLE.

- Therapy for cutaneous lupus is antimalarial agents such as hydroxychloroquine, methotrexate, mycophenolate mofetil, cyclosporine, dapsone, and combination therapy.

HVC
- Photoprotection, including avoiding peak sun hours, protective clothing, and the use of a broad-spectrum sunscreen, is an essential part of therapy for all forms of lupus.

Dermatomyositis

Dermatomyositis is an autoimmune disease that affects skin and proximal muscles in varying degrees of combination. Heliotrope rash (with pink-violet macules to edematous plaques on the eyelids) and Gottron papules (with lichenoid pink-violet papules on the knuckles, elbows, or knees) are pathognomonic signs of dermatomyositis. Patients commonly exhibit pink scaly plaques or macules on the scalp that extend onto the superior forehead, with varying degrees of nonscarring hair loss. The "shawl sign" refers to the pink-violet or poikilodermatous photodistributed macules with spotty hyper- and hypopigmentation ("salt and pepper") with telangiectasia and atrophy on the upper back, whereas the anterior V-sign references similar findings on the upper chest in a V shape (**Figure 105**). The Gottron sign manifests as pink macules over the knuckles, elbows, or knees without papules (**Figure 106**). The nailfold capillary beds of patients with dermatomyositis often demonstrate alternating areas of dilatation and dropout with periungual erythema. Cuticular overgrowth and hemorrhagic infarcts are also characteristic.

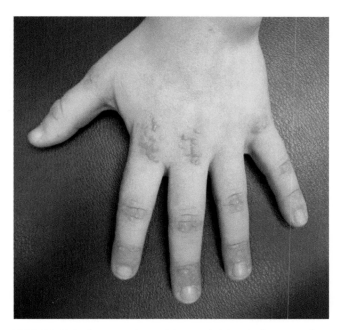

FIGURE 106. Gottron papules are violaceous, slightly scaly plaques over the bony prominences on the hands.

Dermatomyositis and cutaneous lupus erythematosus can appear clinically similar. These conditions can be distinguished by sparing of the knuckles and upper eyelids in cutaneous lupus erythematosus, whereas dermatomyositis favors these areas. Dermatomyositis and CLE are essentially indistinguishable on skin biopsy.

Amyopathic dermatomyositis refers to characteristic skin findings without clinical or laboratory evidence of muscle disease for 6 months without treatment. This variant of dermatomyositis is about as common as classical disease. Amyopathic dermatomyositis is important to recognize because it carries similar risks for malignancy and interstitial lung disease (see MKSAP 18 Rheumatology).

The antisynthetase syndrome is a constellation of findings including dermatomyositis, hyperkeratotic, fissured skin on the palmar and lateral aspects of fingers (mechanic's hands), fevers, Raynaud phenomenon, elevated titers of anti-synthetase antibodies, and often interstitial lung disease. Anti-Jo1 is the prototypical antisynthetase antibody (**Figure 107**).

The cutaneous manifestations of dermatomyositis typically improve with the treatment of the associated myositis. It is a photosensitive disease, so aggressive photoprotection is foundational. Topical glucocorticoids are recommended as initial therapy but are often inadequate to control the skin lesions. Antimalarial agents can be helpful but can also flare the disease or cause drug-induced myopathy. Methotrexate, azathioprine, mycophenolate mofetil, and cyclosporine can be helpful. There are several reports supporting the use of JAK/STAT inhibitors in resistant cases. Intravenous immunoglobulin is a valuable tool in cases of severe recalcitrant skin disease.

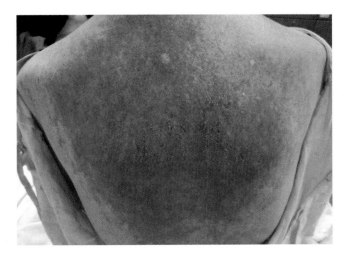

FIGURE 105. The shawl sign demonstrating a photodistributed erythematous patchy rash on the upper back in a patient with dermatomyositis.

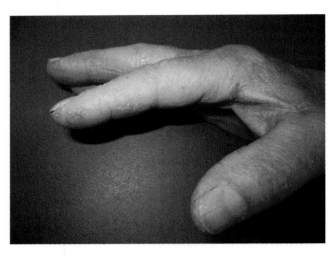

FIGURE 107. Mechanic hands with hyperkeratotic, fissured skin on the palmar and lateral aspects of fingers seen in a patient with antisynthetase syndrome.

KEY POINTS

HVC
- The heliotrope rash and Gottron papules are pathognomonic signs of dermatomyositis.

- Cutaneous lupus erythematosus can be distinguished from dermatomyositis by sparing of the knuckles and upper eyelids; dermatomyositis favors these areas.

- Photoprotection, topical glucocorticoids, antimalarials, and other systemic agents are typically needed to control the skin manifestations of dermatomyositis.

Sclerosing Disorders

The scleroderma family of disorders is discussed in the MKSAP 18 Rheumatology section. Patients with sclerosing disorders may exhibit skin findings that include "puffy hands" (early diffuse systemic sclerosis) and skin tightening (advanced diffuse systemic sclerosis) (**Table 22**). Raynaud phenomenon, especially with periungual capillary changes, is very common in systemic sclerosis and usually precedes skin disease (**Figure 108**).

Treatment with disease-modifying anti-inflammatory drugs such as methotrexate and mycophenolate are recommended to slow the progression of cutaneous sclerosis but

TABLE 22.	Cutaneous Features of Systemic Sclerosis
Digital infarction that may lead to autoamputation
Fingertip ulcers with rat bite appearance
Matte telangiectases (face and lips mostly, but also on body)
Periungual erythema, and tortuous dilated capillary loops
Rhagades (radial creases extending outward from lips)
Salt and pepper hyperpigmentation or depigmentation (typically in areas of sclerosis)
Sclerodactyly

result in only modest benefit. Patients with progressive sclerosis will progress to sclerodactyly or thick, hide-like skin of the fingers. This skin sclerosis will progress from distal to proximal (**Figure 109**). Both diffuse and limited sclerosis can affect the face resulting in restriction of the oral aperture, atrophied lips, and perioral creases radiating around the mouth (**Figure 110**). Sclerosis can result in acroosteolysis (resorption of the finger tips) and fixed contractures of the fingers, wrists, elbows, or feet.

Localized scleroderma (morphea) begins as red-violet plaques that progress to isolated sclerotic circumscribed plaques (**Figure 111**). The scarring sclerosis is permanent, and

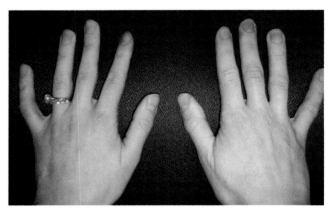

FIGURE 108. The hand is the most likely site for attacks of vasospasm that characterize Raynaud phenomenon. A typical episode is precipitated by cold exposure, which is soon followed by distinctive color changes of white (ischemic phase) or blue (cyanotic phase). With rewarming there is the onset of redness, which heralds reperfusion.

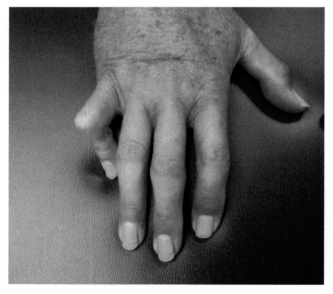

FIGURE 109. Sclerodactyly (skin thickening over the fingers) extending proximal to the metacarpophalangeal joints in a patient with diffuse systemic sclerosis. Flexion contractions of the digits are present, most notable in the fifth digit.

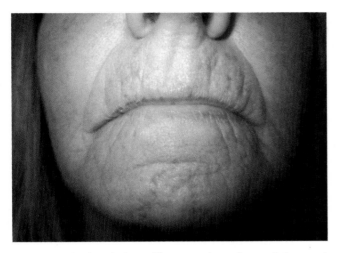

FIGURE 110. Rhagades (perioral fissures or a cluster of scars radiating around the mouth), lip atrophy and telangiectases in patient with limited systemic sclerosis.

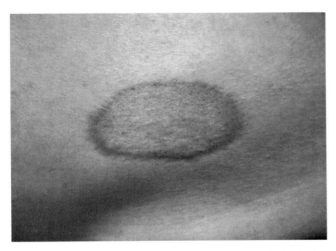

FIGURE 111. Plaque morphea with red-violet inflammation at the border that indicates continued inflammatory activity.

active lesions will have a violet-pink border that fades as disease activity burns out. Most commonly, patients will have one to a few plaques, but the disease can generalize. Morphea is not associated with sclerodactyly or systemic disease (esophageal dysmotility, interstitial lung disease, or kidney involvement). Raynaud phenomenon is uncommon in these patients. Treatment is best accomplished with topical and systemic glucocorticoids or calcineurin inhibitors, methotrexate, or UVA therapy.

Eosinophilic fasciitis is sclerosis of the deep dermis and subcutis. Patients report tightening of the skin, mostly on the arms, and the appearance of the "dry river bed sign." This sign alludes to the collapsed appearance veins in the arms. The condition has been described to appear after periods of intense physical activity. Treatment includes systemic glucocorticoids or methotrexate.

- Raynaud phenomenon, especially with periungual capillary changes, is very common in systemic scleroderma and usually precedes skin disease.

- Patients with sclerosing disorders may exhibit skin findings that include "puffy hands" (early diffuse systemic sclerosis) and skin tightening (advanced diffuse systemic sclerosis).

Rheumatoid Arthritis

Rheumatoid arthritis may feature several cutaneous features, most notably rheumatoid nodules and rheumatoid vasculitis.

Rheumatoid nodules are the most common cutaneous manifestations of rheumatoid arthritis and are recognized as firm, nontender, dermal-to-subcutaneous nodules that can be moveable or bound to underlying fascia or bone. They vary in size from 2 mm to 5 cm and appear most commonly over pressure points and on the extensor surfaces of joints or tendons (**Figure 112**); however, they have been described almost everywhere on and in the body, including lungs, lymph nodes, and other organs. About one third of rheumatoid arthritis patients develop rheumatoid nodules. During treatment with methotrexate, the nodules may rapidly proliferate (accelerated nodulosis).

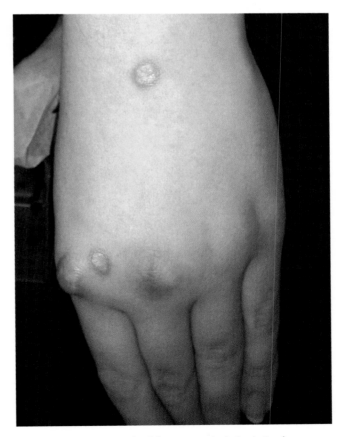

FIGURE 112. Rheumatoid nodules appear as slowly developing, firm, painless, subcutaneous nodules located at pressure points or over the extensor surfaces of joints and tendons.

Rheumatoid vasculitis is much less common and typically occurs in elderly male smokers with long-standing disease and high titers of rheumatoid factor. It can appear as a small or medium-sized vasculitis, with pigmented purpura, nodules, or stellate purpura and ulcers, and may affect nerves or organs.

Vasculitis

Vasculitis is discussed in detail in MKSAP 18 Rheumatology. This section focuses only on the cutaneous findings of vasculitis.

Small-vessel vasculitis affects the capillaries and venules. Patients develop palpable purpura, and/or petechiae, which are nonblanching hemorrhages, on dependent areas such as the shins, feet, hips, and buttocks, as well as pressure areas such as under the elastic band of clothing (**Figure 113**). Lesions may coalesce to form purpuric plaques or ulcerate.

Small-vessel vasculitis is a finding, not a diagnosis, and determining the cause is critical. Idiopathic small-vessel vasculitis involving only the skin is common, but the findings of small-vessel vasculitis can be seen in many systemic diseases such as granulomatosis with polyangiitis, eosinophilic granulomatosis with polyangiitis, microscopic polyangiitis, cryoglobulinemic vasculitis, immunoglobulin A (IgA) vasculitis, drug reactions, and infective endocarditis. Skin biopsy with direct immunofluorescence is important, as cases with IgA deposition (rather than IgG or IgM) are more likely to have systemic effects. An urticarial variant will deplete complement levels and is highly associated with systemic lupus erythematosus. Complement levels, rheumatoid factor, antinuclear antibody, cryoglobulin, and hepatitis testing can be helpful to narrow the differential diagnosis.

Treatment of idiopathic cutaneous small-vessel vasculitis includes elevation, compression, NSAIDs, and antihistamines. Complicated or chronic cases may require glucocorticoids, dapsone, colchicine, or immunosuppressants.

Medium-vessel vasculitis affects the arterioles, including those that travel through the subcutis to supply segments of the skin. Inflammation and destruction of the vessels results in tender nodules on the legs and livedo reticularis and may be associated with reticulate purpura (**Figure 114**) or stellate ulceration (see Dermatologic Emergencies). Severe cases can cause ischemia or infarction of the digits, nose, ears, or genitals. Examples of conditions that can cause medium-vessel vasculitis skin findings include polyarteritis nodosa, granulomatous polyangiitis, eosinophilic granulomatous polyangiitis, drug-induced vasculitis (particularly from cocaine cut with levamisole), and cryoglobulinemic vasculitis. Consider testing for hepatitis B and C in patients with medium-vessel vasculitis. There is a cutaneous-only variant of polyarteritis nodosa, which is treated in a similar fashion to idiopathic cutaneous small-vessel vasculitis.

Large-vessel vasculitis does not typically involve skin findings, except for a palpable temporal cord in giant cell arteritis or in severe cases of Takayasu arteritis where ischemia or necrosis may occur.

Cryoglobulinemia is a condition characterized by soluble antibodies that precipitate from serum when cooled below body temperature. The disease may manifest as a combination of small- and medium-vessel vasculitis (cryoglobulinemic vasculitis) and may exhibit symptoms from both or either category. Palpable purpura, subcutaneous nodules, reticulate purpura, or stellate ulceration may occur starting on the lower legs. Cryoglobulinemic vasculitis is usually secondary to another condition. Treatment is best directed at the underlying disease, but systemic glucocorticoids or rituximab can be helpful, particularly in cases associated with viral hepatitis.

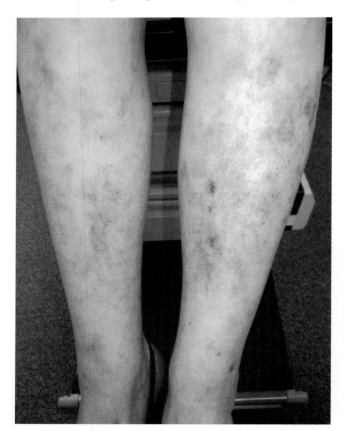

FIGURE 113. Small-vessel vasculitis manifesting as palpable purpura and petechiae in a patient with subacute lupus erythematosus.

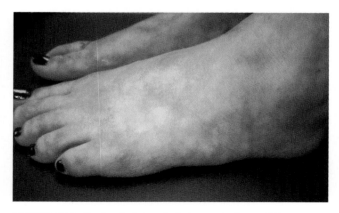

FIGURE 114. Livedo reticularis on the feet, recognized as a red-blue, reticulated vascular network in a patient with systemic lupus erythematosus.

- Small-vessel vasculitis, recognized by the presence of palpable purpura, and/or petechiae in dependent areas, may be idiopathic and limited to the skin, or secondary to systemic vasculitides, autoimmune diseases, cryoglobulinemia, drugs, and infective endocarditis.

- Medium-vessel vasculitis can present with tender nodules on the legs and livedo reticularis and may be associated with reticulate purpura or stellate ulceration.

- Cryoglobulinemia may manifest as a combination of small- and medium-vessel vasculitis with palpable purpura, subcutaneous nodules, reticulate purpura, or stellate ulceration starting on the lower legs.

Nephrology

Persons with end-stage kidney disease often have cutaneous findings. These findings have an insidious onset and can be quite subtle in the early stages. Xerosis and pruritus are most frequently seen. Pruritus may lead to chronic excoriations, lichenification, and prurigo-like changes. The exact mechanism of how end-stage kidney disease causes pruritus is still unknown. It is likely caused by diminished excretion of metabolites.

Dialysis is helpful in some patients, but not all. The itching can be treated with oatmeal baths, the liberal use of emollients, and over-the-counter antipruritics. Traditional soaps should be avoided and replaced with synthetic detergent cleansers (Dove, Cetaphil, and Olay). Topical glucocorticoids, antihistamines, and phototherapy have also been found to be helpful. There are three unique skin disease states seen predominately in persons with end-stage kidney disease: calciphylaxis, Kyrle disease, and nephrogenic systemic fibrosis.

Calciphylaxis

 Calciphylaxis is a rare disease seen most commonly in persons with chronic end-stage kidney disease, and those on dialysis with an elevated calcium-phosphorous product greater than 70 mg^2/dL^2. Parathyroid hormone levels are often dramatically elevated. Although the precise mechanism is not fully elucidated, those with end-stage kidney disease exhibit abnormalities in the endothelial cells, which allow for an abnormal deposition of calcium within the lumen of the dermal arterial and capillary vasculature. As the calcium deposition increases, small thromboses form that lead to ischemia and infarctions of the overlying tissue (**Figure 115**). The tissue becomes necrotic, painful, and a potential source for secondary infection that may lead to sepsis and death. Patients with calciphylaxis have a greater than 80% 1-year mortality rate. Body areas with high adipose tissue content are preferentially affected. The thighs and abdominal pannus are two of the most frequent areas involved.

The initial presentation may start as tender dusky red macules or a livedo reticularis pattern. It quickly progresses to

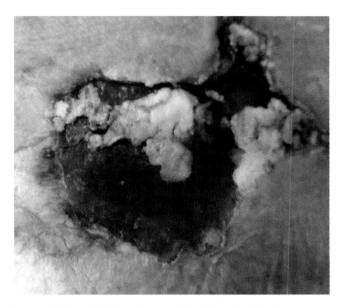

FIGURE 115. Calciphylaxis showing eschar with angulated border on a patient's thigh. Note the central necrosis with surrounding erythema.

develop tender subcutaneous plaques with an overlying dusky red discoloration. Surrounding purpura is often found. The area of involvement quickly expands in an angulated arrangement. As the skin infarcts, a black eschar forms. Because of poor underlying blood flow, the sores do not heal, which leads to chronic open ulcers and eschars that are highly susceptible to infections.

In those patients with hyperparathyroidism, parathyroidectomy may be helpful. Surgical debridement of dead tissue and prompt treatment of infection is important. Using a low-calcium dialysate during dialysis may help reduce the calcium-phosphorous product and slow down the deposition of calcium in the small vessels. The use of intravenous sodium thiosulfate has been reported to be beneficial because it works by increasing the solubility of the calcium deposits, thus clearing the blockages. Bisphosphonates may be beneficial in patients who have failed other forms of therapy.

- Calciphylaxis lesions are painful areas of necrotic tissues caused by dermal vascular calcification in patients with severe chronic end-stage kidney disease and a high calcium-phosphorus product.

- Sodium thiosulfate, along with meticulous wound care, may be beneficial in treating patients with calciphylaxis.

Kyrle Disease

Kyrle disease, a type of perforating dermatosis, is seen in patients with end-stage kidney disease and diabetes mellitus. Patients develop pruritic hyperkeratotic umbilicated papules or nodules with overlying hyperpigmentation. Within the umbilicated region is a firm central keratin plug or core (**Figure 116**). This plug contains collagen bundles that are

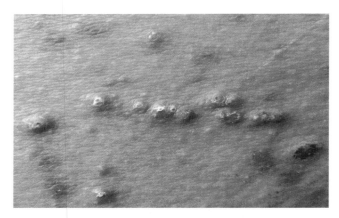

FIGURE 116. Kyrle disease showing hyperkeratotic hyperpigmented umbilicated papules with a central keratin plug. This is caused by extrusion of collagen from the dermis into and through the epidermis.

being extruded through the epidermis. Treatment is directed at the pruritus with the use of oatmeal baths, synthetic detergent cleansers, and liberal use of emollients and topical antipruritic agents. If only a few nodules are present, surgical removal is a treatment consideration.

KEY POINT

- Pruritic umbilicated papules or nodules with hyperkeratotic cores are characteristic of Kyrle disease.

Nephrogenic Systemic Fibrosis

Nephrogenic systemic fibrosis occurs in patients with end-stage kidney disease who have been exposed to gadolinium-containing contrast agents. Patients present with symmetrical, fibrotic indurated papules, plaques, or subcutaneous nodules most commonly located on the legs, the mid-thighs, and upper arms (**Figure 117**). The skin findings can occur weeks to years after exposure to gadolinium-containing contrast dyes. There are many anecdotal treatments including ultraviolet A phototherapy, extracorporeal photopheresis, kidney transplantation, and cyclophosphamide. Because of screening protocols that have been put in place before patients are given gadolinium-based contrasts, there has been a marked reduction in the number of new cases of nephrogenic systemic fibrosis.

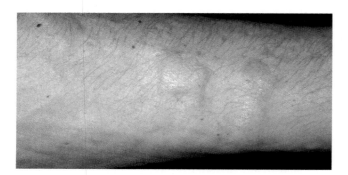

FIGURE 117. Indurated papules and plaques are characteristic of early nephrogenic systemic fibrosis. These will eventually coalesce into large plaques.

KEY POINTS

- Nephrogenic systemic fibrosis presents with symmetrical, fibrotic indurated papules, plaques, or subcutaneous nodules most commonly located on the legs, the mid-thighs, and upper arms.
- Gadolinium-based contrast dyes should be avoided in patients with severe end-stage kidney disease.

Gastroenterology

Inflammatory bowel disease has been found to have an association with the development of erythema nodosum and pyoderma gangrenosum. Although these skin conditions can be idiopathic, their presence should alert the clinician to look for an underlying inflammatory bowel disease.

Dermatitis herpetiformis is associated with celiac disease. Porphyria cutanea tarda is seen most frequently in association with alcoholic liver disease, hepatitis C infection, or hemochromatosis.

Patients with cirrhosis will often develop nonspecific skin findings such as palmar erythema, spider telangiectasia, xerosis, and pruritus. Terry nails, manifested by whitening of the nail bed caused by edema, are seen in end-stage liver disease (see Nail Disorders).

Pyoderma Gangrenosum

Approximately half the cases of pyoderma gangrenosum are associated with an underlying disease, such as inflammatory bowel disease, leukemia, or lymphoma. Pyoderma gangrenosum presents with an exquisitely tender papule, pustule, or nodule. The area quickly enlarges and begins to ulcerate in a cribriform pattern, with intervening strands of epithelium. There is a characteristic violaceous border with an overhanging epithelium (**Figure 118**) around the central exudative ulcer, which is often described as a "wet ulcer." The most frequent location is the lower leg. Pyoderma gangrenosum is also seen frequently in association with a stoma site (peristomal) after ostomy placement in a patient with inflammatory bowel disease. Pyoderma gangrenosum often occurs in the site of trauma (pathergy), and there are numerous reports of pyoderma becoming much worse after surgical debridement. Once the inflammation has been treated and the ulcer heals, patients are often left with a prominent atrophic scar.

Pyoderma gangrenosum is a diagnosis of exclusion and is made after ruling out other causes of ulcerations. For this reason, diagnosis can be challenging and delayed. Skin biopsies are nonspecific but will often show a neutrophilic-rich ulceration with marked tissue edema. Tissue cultures should be negative, but are frequently complicated by surface colonization.

Management of pyoderma gangrenosum is multidimensional. The underlying disease state must be evaluated and treated. Initial therapy directed at the ulcer is with glucocorticoids, and small areas can be treated with intralesional glucocorticoids or potent topical glucocorticoids; however, most patients will require systemic glucocorticoid treatment.

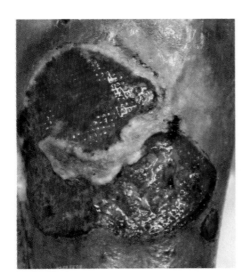

FIGURE 118. Pyoderma gangrenosum is an uncommon, neutrophilic, ulcerative skin lesion that begins as tender papules, pustules, or vesicles that spontaneously ulcerate and progress to painful ulcers with a purulent base and undermined, ragged, violaceous borders.

H CONT. Many treatment options are available and include cyclosporine, infliximab, dapsone, colchicine, mycophenolate mofetil, intravenous immunoglobulin, methotrexate, and thalidomide. Trauma and surgical debridement should be avoided to prevent pathergy. Local wound care is often best achieved with a wound care specialist to ensure proper care to avoid secondary infection and to minimize other complications. Recognition and treatment of secondary infection are difficult and require vigilance and frequent evaluations. **H**

KEY POINTS

- Pyoderma gangrenosum presents as a tender papule, pustule, or nodule that rapidly develops into an ulcer; there is often a characteristic violaceous rim with a rolled or overhanging border.

- Approximately half the cases of pyoderma gangrenosum are associated with an underlying disease, such as inflammatory bowel disease, leukemia, or lymphoma.

- Pyoderma gangrenosum usually responds well to systemic glucocorticoids; trauma and surgical debridement should be avoided to prevent pathergy.

H **Dermatitis Herpetiformis**

Dermatitis herpetiformis is a neutrophilic dermatoses caused by IgA antibodies against tissue and epidermal transglutaminase. Dermatitis herpetiformis typically presents with intensely pruritic papules and fragile vesicles that rapidly break leaving tiny erosions (see Autoimmune Bullous Diseases and MKSAP 18 Gastroenterology and Hepatology). The elbows, knees, scalp, and lower back are the most common sites of involvement. A skin biopsy will show numerous neutrophils stuffing the dermal papillae, and a granular pattern of IgA deposition will be seen on direct immunofluorescence.

Most patients with dermatitis herpetiformis will have an underlying gluten-sensitive enteropathy; however, they are usually free of gastrointestinal symptoms. Interestingly, only 20% of patients with celiac disease will go on to develop dermatitis herpetiformis; however, all patients with dermatitis herpetiformis should be evaluated for underlying bowel involvement. Treatment is usually initiated with dapsone and a gluten-free diet. Dapsone is quickly effective in inducing a clinical remission, but a gluten-free diet is the preferred long-term management of both the skin and bowel disease. **H**

KEY POINT

- Patients with dermatitis herpetiformis should be evaluated for celiac disease, and long-term treatment is best achieved with a gluten-free diet. **HVC**

Porphyria Cutanea Tarda

Porphyria cutanea tarda presents with increased skin fragility noted on sun-exposed areas, most frequently on the dorsal hands. Small vesicles rupture leaving erosions (**Figure 119**). On close examination, milia are often seen in the healed areas that were once vesicles. Milia represent small epidermal inclusion cysts that develop after subepidermal blister formation. As the disease progresses, hyperpigmentation of skin and hypertrichosis of the forehead/temples is commonly seen. Jaundice may be present.

Porphyria cutanea tarda is most commonly caused by an acquired defect of hepatic uroporphyrinogen decarboxylase (UPDC) enzyme. Reduced UPDC activity results in the accumulation of porphyrinogens that are oxidized to porphyrin. Accumulated porphyrins are photosensitizing and when they are transported to the skin cause phototoxicity on light

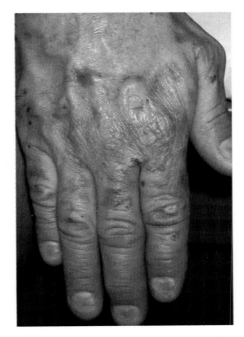

FIGURE 119. Porphyria cutanea tarda manifests as a chronic blistering disease with epidermal erosions on sun-exposed skin, especially on the backs of the hands.

CONT.

exposure. Chronic hepatitis C infection is the most likely cause, followed by alcohol-induced liver damage and hemochromatosis. A urine sample examined under Wood lamp illumination will fluoresce. The diagnosis can be confirmed by increased plasma or urine porphyrin level analysis.

The treatment is aimed at decreasing iron overload. In addition to treating the underlying condition, phlebotomy is the mainstay of therapy. Low-dose hydroxychloroquine is an effective second option for those who do not have significant iron overload. It is dosed at 200 mg once or twice weekly.

Hematology/Oncology

Cutaneous manifestations of malignancy include both malignancy-related cutaneous paraneoplastic syndromes and skin disorders (**Table 23**) and hereditary syndromes with an

TABLE 23.	Paraneoplastic Disorders: Conditions That Are Strongly Linked to Internal Malignancy	
Condition	**Clinical Findings**	**Associated Malignancy/Comments**
Acanthosis nigricans	Velvety or verrucous hyperpigmentation of intertriginous areas, weight loss, glossitis	Adenocarcinoma, usually GI or GU, most commonly of the stomach; also occurs in patients with endocrinopathy
Amyloidosis	"Pinch purpura" in sites of thin skin such as the periorbital area, usually accompanied by macroglossia and smoothing of the tongue	Seen in multiple myeloma or systemic amyloidosis
Bazex syndrome (also known as acrokeratosis paraneoplastica)	Psoriasiform, violaceous scaling on the acral surfaces (fingers, toes, nose, and ears); keratoderma may also be present	Squamous cell carcinoma of the upper respiratory tract or upper GI tract; effective therapy of an associated cancer is followed by resolution of the dermatosis
Carcinoid syndrome	Episodic flushing, often accompanied by diarrhea and bronchospasm; can eventually result in telangiectasia or permanent ruddiness	Primarily due to GI carcinoid tumors metastatic to the liver; tumor removal is followed by resolution of the skin and systemic findings
Dermatomyositis	Heliotrope rash, Gottron papules, shawl sign, photodistributed violaceous erythema; scaly erythema of the scalp with diffuse alopecia; periungual telangiectasias and cuticular overgrowth	20% to 25% of patients with dermatomyositis had, have, or will have a malignancy; ovarian cancer is overrepresented; paraneoplastic course is possible but unusual
Ectopic ACTH syndrome	Generalized hyperpigmentation	Small cell lung cancer; tumor removal can result in improvement of the pigmentation
Extramammary Paget disease	Erythematous scaly patch or plaque on the perineal skin, scrotum, or perianal area	Cancer of the GI or GU tract is present in 25% of patients; it is not contiguous with the dermatosis; the dermatosis is a malignancy and needs appropriate excision or ablation
Leser-Trélat sign	Rapid appearance or inflammation of multiple seborrheic keratoses; often occurs in conjunction with acanthosis nigricans	Same cancer association as acanthosis nigricans; seborrheic keratoses are common lesions; Leser-Trélat sign is very rare
Necrobiotic xanthogranuloma	Purple-orange nodules and plaques, often on the upper eyelids, which frequently ulcerate	90% of patients have an associated paraproteinemia (generally IgG κ) and may develop multiple myeloma
Necrolytic migratory erythema	Intertriginous erythema, scales, and erosions; glossitis and angular cheilitis are common	Glucagon-secreting tumor of the pancreas
Neutrophilic dermatoses	Sweet syndrome; atypical pyoderma gangrenosum (bullous lesions with a blue-gray border, often on the hands, arms, or face)	Myeloid leukemia, myelofibrosis, and refractory anemias; these disorders also occur without malignancy in 80% to 90% of patients
Paget disease of the breast	Erythematous, irregularly bordered plaque on the nipple	Represents an extension of a ductal adenocarcinoma of the breast
Paraneoplastic pemphigus	Severe mucosal erosions, tense and flaccid bullae that may be widespread	Non-Hodgkin B-cell lymphoma, Castleman disease, chronic lymphocytic leukemia
Scleromyxedema	Waxy fine papules over the face, neck, and upper trunk	Most patients have an associated paraproteinemia (generally IgG λ) and may develop overt multiple myeloma
Tripe palms	Rugose folds on the palms and soles; may occur with or without acanthosis nigricans	If occurring with acanthosis nigricans, same cancer association; if occurring without acanthosis nigricans, squamous cell carcinoma of the head and neck or lungs

ACTH = adrenocorticotropin hormone; GI = gastrointestinal; GU = genitourinary.

associated risk of malignancy with cutaneous findings as part of the syndrome (**Table 24**).

Sweet Syndrome

Sweet syndrome, or acute febrile neutrophilic dermatosis, is characterized by fever, neutrophilia, a dense dermal infiltrate on histology, and characteristic skin lesions. Skin lesions are painful, edematous, red-to-violaceous "juicy" papules and plaques, most common on the face, neck, and extremities (**Figure 120**). Additional diagnostic criteria include responsiveness to oral glucocorticoids and absence of infection. Most cases of Sweet syndrome typically develop after an upper respiratory or gastrointestinal infection or in the setting of hematologic abnormalities, particularly myelodysplastic syndrome and myelodysplastic syndrome evolving into acute myeloid leukemia (**Table 25**). Sweet syndrome has also been associated with solid malignancies and medications (particularly neutrophil-stimulating

medications such as granulocyte-colony stimulating factor and all-trans retinoic acid. In addition to the skin eruption, patients typically have high fevers, leukocytosis with a left shift, elevated inflammatory markers, and often muscle or joint pain.

Amyloidosis

The hallmark of systemic amyloidosis with cutaneous involvement and cutaneous amyloidosis is extracellular deposition of altered amyloid protein in the skin. In primary (systemic) immunoglobulin light-chain amyloidosis (AL), AL amyloid deposits in multiple organs including the skin. Skin manifestations are present in 30% to 40% of patients and include generalized waxy appearance, easy bruising with minor pressure (pinch purpura) (**Figure 121**), violaceous discoloration around the eyes ("raccoon eyes"), yellow waxy papules and plaques especially in a periorbital location (**Figure 122**), dystrophic nails, and macroglossia (**Figure 123**). When the

TABLE 24.	Genetic Diseases with Cancer Associations and Skin Findings[a]	
Condition	**Clinical Findings**	**Associated Malignancy/Comments**
Birt-Hogg-Dube syndrome	Fine white sclerotic facial papules (fibrofolliculomas or trichodiscomas); spontaneous pneumothoraces	Kidney cancer
Cowden syndrome	Tan facial papules (tricholemmomas) and oral papillomas or cobblestoning	Adenocarcinomas of the breast or thyroid and/or polyps of the gastrointestinal tract
Muir-Torre syndrome (Lynch syndrome)	Sebaceous neoplasms and keratoacanthomas (squamous cell carcinoma subtype)	Adenocarcinomas of the gastrointestinal tract or other tumors of the genitourinary tract. Lung, breast, and hematologic malignancies may occur.
Reed syndrome	Tender cutaneous papules (leiomyomas); uterine fibroids	Kidney cancer
Tuberous sclerosis complex	Multiple cutaneous lesions (facial angiofibromas, ash leaf spots, hypopigmented macules, subungual papules); cortical tubers and seizures; female patients may develop lymphangioleiomyomatosis	Kidney cancer

[a]This table is a brief review focused on genetic diseases that can present in adulthood; this is not a comprehensive list of genetic skin diseases with cancer associations.

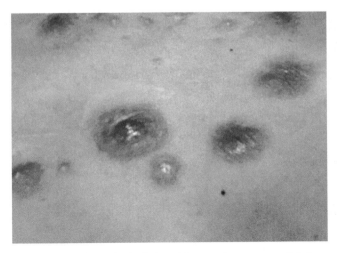

FIGURE 120. The tender skin lesions of Sweet syndrome appear as "juicy" indurated edematous red-purple plaques and nodules, sharply demarcated from the adjacent skin.

TABLE 25. Associations with Sweet Syndrome
Acute myelogenous leukemia
Behçet disease
Chronic leukemias
Inflammatory bowel disease
Multiple myeloma
Myelodysplastic syndrome
Myeloproliferative disorders
Relapsing polychondritis
Rheumatoid arthritis
Solid tumors (rare)
Thyroid disease

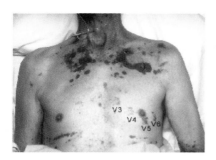

FIGURE 121. Extensive purpura in a 66-year-old man with amyloidosis. Only minor pressure will cause dermal bruising ("pinch purpura"). The ecchymoses labeled V3-V6 are from suction cup ECG chest leads used the day before this photo was taken.

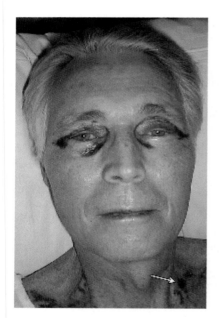

FIGURE 122. A 50-year-old man with prominent periorbital purpura. Easy bleeding leads to characteristic "pinch purpura" (arrow).

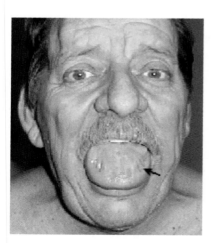

FIGURE 123. Massive infiltration by amyloid leading to macroglossia. Note the indentations from teeth pressing on the firm and enlarged tongue (arrow).

diagnosis is suspected, patients should be screened with immunofixation of serum and urine and serum free light chain assay. Skin biopsies for the diagnosis of AL are controversial, as even when amyloid protein is seen in the dermis, the biochemical composition must be established with immunofixation studies (see MKSAP 18 Hematology and Oncology).

Endocrinology

Many patients with endocrine disorders have associated dermatologic conditions. This section will focus on some conditions associated with thyroid disease and diabetes mellitus, since a high proportion of these patients have at least one dermatologic complication.

Eruptive Xanthomas

Eruptive xanthomas are characterized by a rapid onset of numerous yellow papules with surrounding erythema primarily on the extensor surfaces of the extremities and buttocks. Diagnosis is made by a skin biopsy that shows lipid-laden macrophages in the dermis. Eruptive xanthomas are pathognomonic of hypertriglyceridemia with a vast number of these patients also having a diagnosis of diabetes mellitus. Lesions typically resolve with control of carbohydrate and lipid metabolism.

Acanthosis Nigricans

Acanthosis nigricans presents as velvety-to-verrucous, gray-to-brown thickening with accentuation of skin marking and is seen in the intertriginous folds and neck (**Figure 124**).

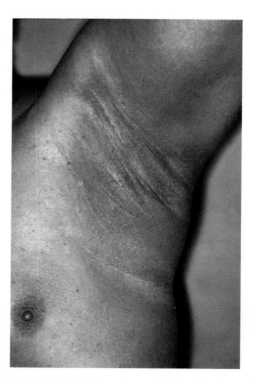

FIGURE 124. Acanthosis nigricans, characterized by a velvety brown plaque in a patient with insulin resistance.

CONT.

Histologically, the pigment change results from epidermal thickening. Acanthosis nigricans is more common in persons of color. It can be associated with diabetes or a malignant and paraneoplastic syndrome. Therefore, a diagnosis of acanthosis nigricans should prompt screening for diabetes and, if of acute onset, screening for malignancy. It is mainly of cosmetic concern and resolves when the underlying condition is treated. Topical salicylic acid, retinoids, and ammonium lactate have modest benefit.

Necrobiosis Lipoidica

Necrobiosis lipoidica is a chronic condition that is seen mainly in patients with diabetes mellitus, both type 1 (more commonly) and type 2. Necrobiosis lipoidica presents as well-demarcated, indurated, yellow-brown oval plaques with central atrophy and telangiectasias. Lesions are typically seen on the bilateral pretibial areas but can occur anywhere on the body.

The diagnosis is usually made on clinical findings, but a punch biopsy of skin to include subcutaneous tissue can be performed to confirm the diagnosis. Histology shows a necrobiotic granulomatous dermatitis. Only a small portion of patients with diabetes (0.3% to 1.6%) develop necrobiosis lipoidica, and in most patients the diabetes precedes necrobiosis lipoidica. Patients with necrobiosis lipoidica without diabetes should be monitored closely for diabetes. Glycemic control does not usually lead to resolution of necrobiosis lipoidica. Treatment is challenging, and relapses are common.

Pretibial Myxedema

Autoimmune thyroid disease, particularly Graves disease, may uncommonly be associated with pretibial myxedema, an accumulation of glycosaminoglycans in the dermis, usually over the lower legs. Pretibial myxedema presents with firm nodules and plaques with a "peau d' orange" appearance on the pretibial area (**Figure 125**). Diagnosis is based on clinical

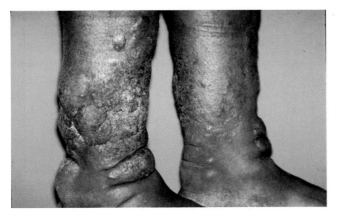

FIGURE 125. Pretibial myxedema is generally seen in patients with Graves disease. It is also termed thyroid dermopathy. It results from the accumulation of glycosaminoglycans in the dermis that leads to characteristic thickening and the development of firm, compressible plaques with a "peau d'orange" appearance.

findings, elevated thyroid-stimulating immunoglobins, and skin biopsy showing characteristic accumulation of mucin in the dermis. Control of the hyperthyroidism does not usually lead to resolution of pretibial myxedema.

Infectious Disease

Dermatologic conditions are very common in patients with HIV and AIDS, and in some this may be the first clue of infection. Cutaneous manifestations can be divided into three categories: immunologic (decreasing CD4 count), related to antiretroviral therapy, and increased prevalence or severity of endemic infections. Many of these conditions are also found in the general population; however, in patients with HIV, they tend to have increased severity, prevalence, atypical presentations, and be recalcitrant to treatment. Because of atypical presentations and the increased risk of infections, if the diagnosis cannot be made on clinical grounds, two skin biopsies should be performed: one for histologic evaluation and the second for bacterial, mycobacterial, and fungal culture.

Acute seroconversion syndrome (primary HIV infection) is an acute mononucleosis-like illness that occurs in many (90%) but not all patients 2 to 4 weeks after infection. Clinical presentation includes fever, sore throat, cervical adenopathy, and an exanthem. The exanthem is made up of asymptomatic erythematous macules and papules involving the face and trunk. The recommended algorithm for diagnosing HIV infection involves use of the fourth-generation HIV test. This test combines an immunoassay for HIV antibody with a test for HIV p24 antigen.

Many HIV-associated primary dermatologic disorders, including xerosis, atopic dermatitis, seborrheic dermatitis, and psoriasis, are related to the T-cell imbalances. Atopic dermatitis and xerosis are related and present with dry skin and eczematous patches. Both conditions are associated with pruritus, which is often severe and can be recalcitrant resulting in a high burden of morbidity for these patients. In seborrheic dermatitis, there are erythematous patches with greasy scale on the scalp, nasal labial folds, and chest. This condition is extremely common in patients with HIV, and most patients with AIDS have some compatible findings. The prevalence of psoriasis, which presents with plaques with overlying scale, and psoriatic arthritis, is increased in patients with AIDS but not those with HIV. New-onset pruritus, atopic dermatitis, seborrheic dermatitis, and psoriasis that is severe and recalcitrant to treatment should prompt testing for HIV/AIDS.

Eosinophilic folliculitis is a condition that is almost exclusively seen in AIDS, in particular in later stages. It presents as extremely pruritic, erythematous follicular-based papules and pustules on the upper trunk, neck, and face. Skin biopsy is diagnostic, showing numerous eosinophils within the follicular infundibulum with destruction of the sebaceous gland. Treatment is challenging with first-line therapy being medium- to high-potency topical glucocorticoids.

Pulmonary

Sarcoidosis is an inflammatory granulomatous disease commonly associated with skin manifestations, some of which predict specific internal organ involvement. Lupus pernio is sarcoidosis of the nose and central face, manifesting as violaceous subcutaneous plaques or nodules, often with some overlying scaling. Lupus pernio is more common in skin of color and is associated with an increased risk for extracutaneous disease, particularly intrathoracic sarcoidosis. Sarcoid lesions may also preferentially develop in sites of trauma, and these lesions are also associated with an increased risk of pulmonary disease. Other more common cutaneous manifestations of sarcoidosis include violaceous papules on the nose, periorbitally and around the oropharynx, and nasal openings.

Limited cutaneous sarcoidosis is treated with topical or intralesional glucocorticoids and more extensive disease is typically treated with hydroxychloroquine. Patients who fail to respond may be treated with thalidomide, methotrexate, or occasionally TNF-α inhibitors.

Erythema nodosum is the most common form of panniculitis, or inflammation of the fat. Erythema nodosum manifests as ill-defined, tender, bilateral dermal red or violaceous nodules, most commonly on the bilateral shins (**Figure 126**). Most resolve spontaneously over 4 to 6 weeks. Erythema nodosum is a nonspecific reaction to some systemic process.

The most common associations are streptococcal infection, hormones (including oral contraceptives, hormone replacement therapy, or pregnancy), inflammatory bowel disease, sarcoidosis, and other medication reactions. The appearance of erythema nodosum in patients with sarcoidosis usually signifies an acute presentation with a good long-term prognosis. The combination of erythema nodosum, arthritis, hilar lymphadenopathy, and fevers constitute Löfgren syndrome. This set of findings is so specific for sarcoidosis that a biopsy is not needed to confirm the diagnosis. Most cases of erythema nodosum resolve spontaneously, and therapy is supportive in nature with NSAIDs and compression stockings. **H**

Dermatologic Emergencies
Retiform Purpura

Retiform is a descriptive term for a net-like, branching, or stellate configuration, reflecting the vascular structure of the skin. Purpura refers to the nonblanching dark red or purple color resulting from extravasation of erythrocytes into the skin (**Figure 127**). Retiform purpura signifies total occlusion of cutaneous arterioles with downstream necrosis and hemorrhage in the watershed area of the vessel. Occlusion of several adjacent vessels may result in purpura and necrosis of body segments (**Figure 128**), particularly in acral regions (digits, ears, genitals).

Retiform purpura is a description, not a diagnosis, and the cause must be determined to preserve life and limb. Because of their devastating consequences, thrombotic and embolic causes should be considered first. Thrombotic causes can be due to unregulated coagulation such as disseminated intravascular coagulation, thrombotic thrombocytopenic purpura, or warfarin- or heparin-induced thrombosis. The heart and large vessels may be sources of emboli as seen with bacterial or marantic endocarditis, atrial myxoma, or cholesterol emboli following an intravascular procedure.

Diagnosis is made by history and examination (**Table 26**). The evaluation should be directed by the most likely associated disorder. A wide net of testing may be necessary in the critically ill patient without a clearly identified underlying condition. In a stable patient, skin biopsy can further direct the evaluation. Treatment is directed toward the underlying cause.

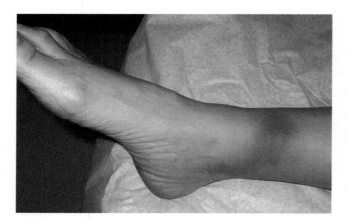

FIGURE 126. Erythema nodosum manifests as painful, red-brown nodules on the anterior shins.

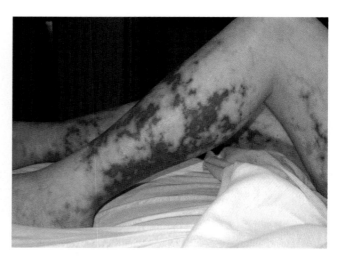

FIGURE 127. Retiform purpura on the lower legs due to vasculitis characterized by dark red or purple net-like, branching, or stellate configuration.

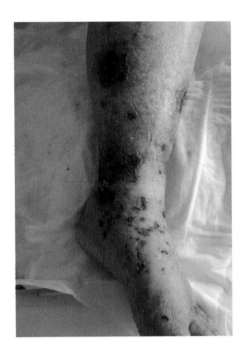

FIGURE 128. Retiform purpura resulting in ulceration and necrosis secondary to total occlusion of cutaneous arterioles.

TABLE 26.	Differential Diagnosis for Retiform Purpura
Category	**Examples**
Vasculitis	Rheumatoid vasculitis
	Polyarteritis nodosa
	Granulomatosis with polyangiitis
	Eosinophilic granulomatosis with polyangiitis
	Systemic lupus erythematosus
	Cryoglobulinemic vasculitis
	Scleroderma
Thrombotic	Disseminated intravascular coagulopathy
	Thrombotic thrombocytopenic purpura/ hemolytic uremic syndrome
	Antiphospholipid syndrome
	Inherited and acquired thrombophilias
	Myeloproliferative disorders
Embolic	Fat emboli
	Septic emboli
	Cholesterol emboli
	Infectious and marantic endocarditis
Arteriopathy	Calciphylaxis
Infectious	Meningococcemia
	Angioinvasive fungi
	Ecthyma gangrenosum
	Necrotizing fasciitis
Drug-related	Heparin
	Warfarin
	Levamisole-adulterated cocaine

Erythema Multiforme

CONT.

Erythema multiforme (EM) minor is an immune-mediated condition that can be recognized by its classic targetoid plaques with characteristic histopathologic features. The sharply defined circinate plaques feature two differently colored concentric rings (pale inner ring, red outer ring) surrounding a pale, dusky, vesiculated or crusted center (**Figure 129**). These plaques typically appear on the face and acral sites, such as the back of the hands, the arms, legs, or feet. The palms and soles may also be involved. Crops of lesions persist for approximately 7 days and resolve without scarring. Most cases of EM minor are caused by infections, herpes simplex virus 1 and 2 being the most common followed by *Mycoplasma pneumoniae*, particularly in children. Drug-induced cases of EM minor are less frequent and typically result from NSAIDs, antiepileptic agents, or sulfonamides. Mucosal involvement is rare, but if present, is trivial.

EM major has severe mucosal involvement and systemic symptoms in addition to typical skin findings found in EM minor. Lesions in the mouth blister and become painful erosions. They are often polycyclic and involve the buccal mucosa and lips, where the edges may suggest the concentric rings of EM. The eyes, nasopharynx, and genitals are less commonly affected. Fever and malaise may precede rash, and joint pain and swelling have been described. Internal organ involvement should prompt reconsideration of the diagnosis. Skin biopsy can be helpful when the diagnosis is unclear, and direct immunofluorescence can be used to exclude the possibility of autoimmune blistering disease. EM can recur, and in approximately 70% of patients this is associated with herpes simplex virus infection. These patients may benefit from suppressive antiviral therapy. Antimicrobial therapy is helpful if *M. pneumoniae* is the trigger of EM. If a drug is implicated, the immediate first step is stopping the drug. Systemic

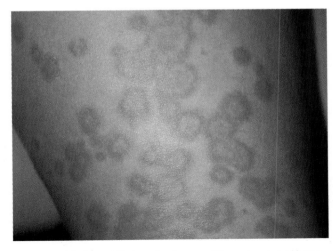

FIGURE 129. Targetoid lesions of erythema multiforme characterized by two concentric rings (pale inner ring, red outer ring) surrounding a pale or dusky center.

CONT.

glucocorticoids are highly effective for decreasing inflammation and pain, even when patients have an infectious trigger, and short courses (3-4 weeks) should be considered early in the disease. H

KEY POINTS

- Erythema multiforme can be recognized by classic targetoid plaques that appear on the face and acral sites, such as the back of the hands, the arms, legs, or feet.

- Most cases of erythema multiforme are caused by herpes simplex virus or *Mycoplasma pneumoniae*; drug-induced cases of erythema multiforme minor are less frequent and typically result from NSAIDs, antiepileptic agents, or sulfonamides.

HVC
- Erythema multiforme can recur, and in approximately 70% of patients this is associated with herpes simplex virus infection; these patients may benefit from suppressive antiviral therapy.

Stevens-Johnson Syndrome and Toxic Epidermal Necrolysis

Stevens-Johnson syndrome (SJS) and toxic epidermal necrolysis (TEN) represent a spectrum of severe mucocutaneous reactions defined by the extent of affected body surface area (BSA) involved with blisters and erosions. They are the most severe and deadly of the cutaneous adverse drug reactions. SJS refers to patients with less than 10% BSA affected. Greater than 30% BSA affected is the criterion for TEN. Patients with BSA between 10% and 30% are referred to as SJS/TEN overlap syndrome. Key features include full-thickness epidermal necrosis with involvement of mucous membranes. Essentially all cases of TEN are temporally correlated with medications (**Table 27**), whereas about 25% of SJS cases are caused by infection or vaccination. HIV infection, kidney disease, uncontrolled autoimmune disease, and human leukocyte antigen type (HLA-B*1502 and HLA-B*5801) also contribute to increased risk. Patients of Asian and South Asian ancestry who are positive for HLA-B*1502 have up to a 10% risk for SJS/TEN when exposed to aromatic anticonvulsants (carbamazepine, phenytoin, and

phenobarbital). HLA-B*5801 positivity predicts risk of SJS/TEN upon exposure to allopurinol. The role of genetic screening to prevent these reactions is unsettled.

Symptoms begin usually within 1 to 3 weeks of exposure to the inciting agent. Patients may notice fever, malaise, and symptoms of upper respiratory infections followed by skin pain, grittiness or sand-like irritation of the eyes, and odynophagia. Shortly thereafter, patients develop red or purple dusky macules on the trunk that progress to vesicles, erosion, and ulceration (**Figure 130**). Painful erosions develop in the mouth, eyes, or genitals in as many as 95% of patients. Unlike EM's predilection for the extremities, SJS and TEN favor the trunk and face. SJS/TEN patients may exhibit atypical targetoid macules demonstrating one or two colored rings, which can be distinguished from the three colored zones of EM. The presence of extensive epidermal sloughing and a positive Nikolsky sign further differentiate SJS/TEN from EM major (**Table 28**).

Systemic manifestations are common in SJS/TEN patients. All patients experience fever and malaise. Lymphadenopathy, elevated transaminase levels, and cytopenias are common. Pneumonitis, nephritis, hepatitis, and myocarditis are possible. Hypovolemia and electrolyte imbalances due to loss of the skin barrier are common.

The acute phase of the disease lasts 1 to 2 weeks, and skin reepithelization may take 2 to 4 weeks. Mortality is high with 5% to 10% of SJS cases being fatal and as many as one in three patients with TEN dying from complications related to the disease. Most deaths result from secondary infection, complications of transcutaneous fluid loss, or respiratory distress. Early identification and withdrawal of the causative medication improve outcomes. The SCORTEN scale is a validated, severity-of-illness tool for TEN and SJS that can be applied early in the course of the disease. The mortality rate is directly correlated with the number of SCORTEN variables that are fulfilled (**Table 29**).

Treatment of SJS/TEN is highly controversial. Intravenous glucocorticoids or intravenous immune globulins are probably the most commonly used treatments, but neither is supported by strong evidence. Supportive care in an ICU with experienced nursing staff is critical for wound care, and many

TABLE 27. Medications Most Commonly Leading to Stevens-Johnson Syndrome/Toxic Epidermal Necrolysis
Allopurinol
Aminopenicillins (ampicillin, amoxicillin)
Carbamazepine
Lamotrigine
Nevirapine
Phenytoin
Sulfamethoxazole-trimethoprim
Sulfasalazine

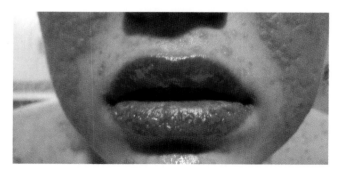

FIGURE 130. Swelling of the lips with vesicles on the lower lip and erosions and mucosal sloughing on the upper lip secondary to Steven-Johnson syndrome.

TABLE 28. Comparison of Erythema Multiforme, Stevens-Johnson Syndrome, and Toxic Epidermal Necrolysis

	Erythema Multiforme (EM)	Stevens-Johnson Syndrome (SJS)	Toxic Epidermal Necrolysis (TEN)
Morphology	Typical 3-zoned target	Atypical targets and confluent erythema with sloughing	Extensive, confluent erythema with sloughing
Distribution	Favors extremities	Trunk and extremities; up to 10% body surface area involvement[a]	Trunk and extremities; at least 30% body surface area involvement[a]
Mucosal disease (oral, eye, genitourinary)	1 or 2 sites	2 or more sites	2 or more sites
Constitutional symptoms	+	++/+++	+++
Etiology:			
Infection (%)	50	26	6
Drugs implicated in (%)	50	74	94
Mortality rate (%)	0	5-13	25-39

[a]SJS/TEN overlap: 10% to 30% body surface area involvement, remaining features the same as SJS.

TABLE 29. SCORTEN Tool Values

SCORTEN Features	Values Associated with Poor Prognosis
Age	>40 years
Malignancy	Present
Heart rate	>120/min
Body surface area	>10%
Plasma glucose	>252 mg/dL (13.98 mmol/L)
Blood urea nitrogen	>28 mg/dL (9.99 mmol/L)
Bicarbonate	<20 mEq/L (20 mmol/L)

The likelihood of death increases with each feature. Five or more features is associated with a 90% mortality rate.

Data from: Bastuji-Garin S, Fouchard N, Bertocchi M, Roujeau JC, Revuz J, Wolkenstein P. SCORTEN: a severity-of-illness score for toxic epidermal necrolysis. J Invest Dermatol. 2000 Aug;115(2):149-53. PubMed PMID: 10951229.

 CONT. patients are transferred to a burn center. Infection is a significant cause of mortality. A low threshold is recommended for performing cultures and initiation of empiric antibiotics, but use of prophylactic antibiotics is not recommended. Ophthalmologic and urologic consultations are mandatory if ocular or genital involvement is present, as destructive scarring may occur in these areas. **H**

KEY POINTS

- Key features of Stevens-Johnson syndrome and toxic epidermal necrolysis include full-thickness epidermal necrosis with involvement of mucous membranes, which is potentially lethal due to secondary infection, complications of transcutaneous fluid loss, or respiratory distress.
- Stevens-Johnson syndrome and toxic epidermal necrolysis are distinguished by the amount of skin detachment that is involved.

(Continued)

KEY POINTS *(continued)*

- Intravenous glucocorticoids or intravenous immune globulins are the most commonly used treatments for Stevens-Johnson syndrome and toxic epidermal necrolysis; supportive care in an ICU or burn unit is critical for wound care.
- The role of genetic screening for HLA-B*1502 and HLA-B*5801 to prevent Stevens-Johnson syndrome and toxic epidermal necrolysis is unsettled.

HVC

Drug Hypersensitivity Syndrome (or DRESS Syndrome)

Drug hypersensitivity syndrome (DHS) and drug reaction with eosinophilia and systemic symptoms (DRESS) are synonymous and represent another severe life-threatening medication reaction. The most common culprit medications include sulfonamide antibiotics, allopurinol, and anticonvulsants, but many more medications have been implicated (**Table 30**). Unlike other medication reactions, the onset of symptoms is delayed, often by 2 to 6 weeks, from the time of exposure. Patients begin with fever and flulike symptoms, which are quickly followed by burning skin pain and rash. Patients typically develop a morbilliform exanthem that starts on the face and upper trunk and spreads distally (**Figure 131**). Eventually

TABLE 30. Medications Most Commonly Causing DRESS Syndrome

Abacavir
Allopurinol
Aromatic antiepileptic drugs (carbamazepine, phenytoin, and phenobarbital)
Minocycline
Proton pump inhibitors
Sulfasalazine

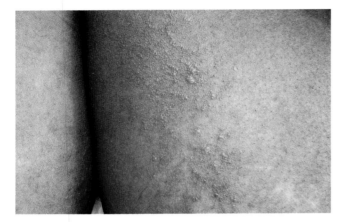

FIGURE 131. Generalized morbilliform eruption in a patient with drug reaction with eosinophilia and systemic symptoms (DRESS). Vesicles, blisters, and pustules may also be seen.

CONT.

the patients develop striking facial edema and redness, a hall-mark of this condition. Oral mucosal involvement is common but is less severe than SJS/TEN or EM major.

Systemic involvement is necessary for the diagnosis and most commonly features eosinophilia or an atypical lympho-cytosis and elevated transaminase levels. Hypotension, shock, and multisystem organ damage are possible, and death occurs in about 10% of patients. Immediate discontinuation of the causative agent is mandatory, and systemic glucocorticoids tapered over weeks to months can be helpful. DRESS caused by an aromatic antiepileptic agent can also pose a serious threat due to cross-reaction with other aromatic antiepilep-tics. For example, if phenytoin causes DHS but is appropriately stopped, neither phenobarbital nor carbamazepine should be substituted because of the risk of cross-reaction.

Acute Generalized Exanthematous Pustulosis

Acute generalized exanthematous pustulosis (AGEP) refers to the rapid onset of a pustular rash following a medication expo-sure in a patient without a history of pustular psoriasis. Onset may be as soon as 1 day after exposure to the medication or a few days at most. Patients present with fever, erythema, and eventually develop myriad dense non-folliculocentric pustules, primarily in skin folds and on the trunk (**Figure 132**). A total of 80% of cases are caused by antibiotics. Most cases are self-limited and resolve within 2 weeks. Treatment consists of ces-sation of the causative agent and supportive care, but topical and systemic glucocorticoids may be helpful for symptomatic relief. The condition carries a mortality rate of less than 5%.

Erythroderma

Erythroderma is defined as diffuse erythema covering 80% to 90% body surface area and is commonly associated with pruri-tus, peripheral edema, erosions, scaling, and lymphadenopathy

(**Figure 133**). The most common causes are idiopathic (up to 40%), exacerbation of a preexisting rash, or medication reaction (**Table 31**). Atopic dermatitis or psoriasis can flare to erythro-derma following injudicious usage and abrupt cessation of sys-temic glucocorticoids. Alopecia, nail dystrophy, and thickening of the palms and soles are indicative of a long-standing cause such as cutaneous T-cell lymphoma, graft-versus-host disease,

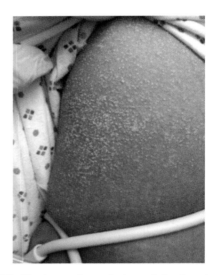

FIGURE 132. Pinpoint pustules on a background of erythema in a patient with acute generalized exanthematous pustulosis.

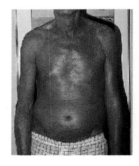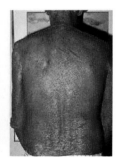

FIGURE 133. Erythroderma with redness and scaling secondary to pityriasis rubra pilaris.

TABLE 31. Causes of Acute and Chronic Erythroderma	
Causes of Acute Erythroderma	**Causes of Chronic Erythroderma**
Atopic dermatitis (flare)	Atopic dermatitis
Psoriasis (flare)	Psoriasis
Medication reaction	Cutaneous T-cell lymphoma
Autoimmune disease	Graft-versus-host disease
Staphylococcal scalded skin syndrome	Pityriasis rubra pilaris
Toxic shock syndrome	
Sézary syndrome (will transition to chronic)	

CONT.

psoriasis, or pityriasis rubra pilaris. Drug reactions, staphylococcal scalded skin syndrome, and autoimmune bullous diseases often have a more acute onset without a long-standing history of preceding dermatosis. When erythroderma is acute, thick scaling of the palms and soles or nail changes do not occur. Complications may result from heat and fluid loss across the inflamed skin.

Management of erythroderma involves treatment of infection and managing fluid and electrolyte imbalance. Emollients will help to restore the skin barrier, and topical glucocorticoids and systemic antihistamines will improve pruritus.

KEY POINTS

- Erythroderma is defined as diffuse erythema covering 80% to 90% body surface area and is commonly associated with pruritus, peripheral edema, erosions, scaling, and lymphadenopathy.

(Continued)

KEY POINTS *(continued)*

- Most cases of erythroderma are idiopathic; however, it may also be caused by exacerbation of a preexisting rash or a medication reaction.

- Management of erythroderma involves treatment of the infection and managing fluid and electrolyte imbalance; emollients will help to restore the skin barrier, and topical glucocorticoids and systemic antihistamines will improve pruritus.

Hair Disorders

Hypertrichosis/Hirsutism

Hypertrichosis is the abnormal growth of hair on an area of the body. Although it's typically a cosmetic concern, hypertrichosis can also be a cutaneous sign of an underlying systemic condition (**Table 32**). Hirsutism is a subclass of hypertrichosis

TABLE 32. Diagnosing Excessive Hair Growth in Women		
Differential Diagnosis of Excess Hair Growth	**Associated Causes and Findings**	**Initial Testing/Assessment**
Hirsutism (androgen-dependent sites)	Polycystic ovary syndrome: chronic anovulation, hyperandrogenemia, menstrual irregularities, infertility, obesity	Medical history (oligo- or anovulation); clinical or biochemical signs of hyperandrogenism; and echogenic evidence of polycystic ovaries and exclusion of other causes
	Ovarian tumors (many types): persistent bloating, early satiety, abdominal pain	Testosterone, DHEAS, pelvic ultrasound
	Cushing syndrome: acne, striae, moon facies, abdominal obesity, muscle wasting	Overnight low-dose dexamethasone suppression test, 24-hour urine free cortisol, or late-night salivary cortisol
	Congenital adrenal hyperplasia: salt-losing crisis, ambiguous genitals, precocious puberty, oligo- or amenorrhea	17-hydroxyprogesterone
	Prolactinoma: galactorrhea, visual changes, amenorrhea	Serum prolactin level
	Drug-induced: testosterone, DHEAS, danazol, corticotropin, high-dose glucocorticoids, androgenic progestins, acetazolamide, anabolic steroids	Medication history
Idiopathic/familial	Present since puberty	Serum testosterone, 17-hydroxyprogesterone, DHEAS
	Slow development/progression	
	Normal menses	
	Family history	
Hypertrichosis (non-androgen-responsive hair)	Porphyria: blistering, skin fragility, scarring	24-hour urine porphyrins
	Hyperthyroidism: weight loss, anxiety, tachycardia, increased sweating	TSH, T_3, and free T_4
	Drug-induced: cyclosporine, phenytoin, diazoxide, minoxidil, hexachlorobenzene, penicillamine, methyldopa, metoclopramide, reserpine	Medication history
Acquired hypertrichosis lanuginosa (rare)	Excessive growth of fine lanugo hair (white or blonde, 1-2 cm long) on all hair-bearing surfaces, including the face. Associated with malignancy, especially colorectal cancer	Age-appropriate and symptom-directed cancer screening

DHEAS = dehydroepiandrosterone; TSH = thyroid stimulating hormone; T_3 = triiodothyronine; T_4 = thyroxine.

that specifically affects androgen-sensitive hair. It is characterized by excessive hair growth in a male pattern distribution in women or children, often associated with hyperandrogenism (**Figure 134**). Androgen-sensitive hair is located in the groin, lower abdomen, breasts, chin, lateral cheeks, and upper cutaneous lip. It is seen in about 8% to 10% of women. Other signs of hyperandrogenism such as acne, androgenic alopecia, and virilism should be sought. In suspicious cases, selected laboratory testing and imaging should be done (see MKSAP 18 Endocrinology and Metabolism).

Treatment involves addressing the underlying condition. For women with hirsutism, estrogen-progestin contraceptives are a common and effective initial therapy. Additional antiandrogens such as spironolactone or finasteride may be added in 6 months if there is suboptimal response to the oral contraceptive. Antiandrogen therapy should not be used as monotherapy because of potential teratogenic effects on the male fetus. Therapeutic options for the hair itself include hair removal (shaving, depilatories, waxing, or tweezing), camouflaging with bleach, and eflornithine cream. Eflornithine cream inhibits hair growth and must be used indefinitely to be effective. Other methods of destroying the hair bulb include electrolysis and laser hair removal, and although these results may last longer, both of these methods can be painful, costly, and require multiple treatments.

Alopecia

Alopecia is the loss of hair that is either localized or generalized. When evaluating alopecia, first determine if it is localized (patchy) or generalized (diffuse). Then determine if hair loss is scarring or nonscarring (**Table 33**). Scarring alopecia results in permanent hair loss, whereas nonscarring alopecia is usually reversible. Scarring alopecia can be distinguished by the absence of follicular openings (ostia). The diagnosis of most cases can be determined by history and physical examination and confirmed with a 4-mm punch

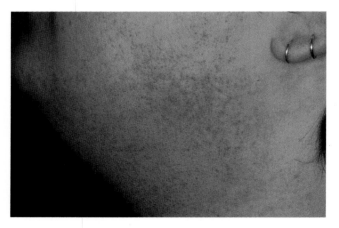

FIGURE 134. Terminal hair growth on the lateral cheeks in a patient with hirsutism secondary to polycystic ovary syndrome.

biopsy. The area of the scalp with active hair loss (not an area of scar) should be chosen for biopsy. Scalp and hair biopsies may require special processing techniques and referral to a dermatopathologist.

KEY POINTS

- When evaluating alopecia, first determine if it is localized (patchy) or generalized (diffuse); then determine if the hair loss is scarring or nonscarring.
- Scarring alopecia results in permanent hair loss, whereas nonscarring alopecia is usually reversible.

Nonscarring Localized and Generalized Alopecia

Alopecia areata is characterized by round or oval patches of nonscarring acute hair loss. It affects both women and men, and onset occurs before the age of 30. It presents as well-circumscribed round patches with no hair. The scalp is smooth and scaleless. The rim of the patches has characteristic "exclamation point" hairs that narrow close to the skin surface (**Figure 135**). The exact cause is unknown; however, an autoimmune mechanism is postulated due to the high association with other autoimmune conditions such as type 1 diabetes mellitus and autoimmune thyroiditis. In about 10% to 15% of patients, there is complete loss of scalp hair (alopecia totalis) and all of the body hair (alopecia universalis).

Traumatic alopecia includes traction alopecia, trichotillomania, and iatrogenic damage from chemicals and heat. Traumatic alopecia can begin as nonscarring; however, with continuing trauma, the alopecia can become permanent and scarring.

Androgenic alopecia, or patterned baldness, is due to the postpubertal terminal hair replacement, first with miniaturized follicles and eventually with atrophic follicles. It is seen in both men and women. Prevalence varies by populations studied. In comparison to white persons, pattern baldness is less common in Chinese, Japanese, and American Indians. The onset begins after puberty and can be gradual. In men, it presents as bitemporal hairline recession followed by vertex baldness (**Figure 136**). In women, it more often presents as generalized thinning rather than baldness and is often first recognized as widening of the part on the crown (**Figure 137**).

Telogen effluvium is caused by a traumatic event (emotionally or physiologically) that disrupts the natural hair cycle resulting in diffuse hair shedding. The hairs on the scalp are all in different stages of the hair cycle, mostly anagen (growing) and telogen (resting). After a traumatic event, the hairs in the anagen phase are prematurely converted into the telogen phase. Hair shedding occurs about 3 months after the inciting event. This is most commonly seen in women in the postpartum period. In most cases, telogen effluvium is self-limiting with resumption of normal hair growth with resolution of the inciting factor.

TABLE 33. Management of Selected Types of Alopecia		
Type of Alopecia	**Treatment Options**	**Possible Systemic Associations**
Androgenetic alopecia	Men: Topical minoxidil 5%,[a] 5-α reductase inhibitors (finasteride,[a] dutasteride)	Men: Increased rate of prostate cancer (if onset in the 20s)
	Women: Topical minoxidil 5% foam,[a] spironolactone (spironolactone should not be administered during pregnancy and should be used with a highly effective contraceptive in premenopausal women)	Women: Polycystic ovary syndrome
	Both: Hair transplant, cosmetic camouflage	
Alopecia areata	<50% scalp involvement: watchful waiting, topical glucocorticoids ± topical minoxidil, anthralin, intralesional glucocorticoid	Autoimmune disease (hyperthyroidism, hypothyroidism, vitiligo, pernicious anemia, diabetes mellitus)
	>50% scalp involvement: topical immunotherapy (squaric acid or DPCP), topical glucocorticoids, ± topical minoxidil, phototherapy, wigs or other cosmetic camouflage, intralesional triamcinolone for brows, bimatoprost for eyelashes	Atopic eczema
Telogen effluvium	Remove or correct potential trigger	Anemia, thyroid disease, significant weight loss, eating disorders, parturition, high fever, major surgery, blood loss, mental stress
	Watchful waiting	Medications:
		Anabolic steroids or supplemental androgens
		Antithyroid medications
		Antiepileptics
		β-blockers
		Oral retinoids
		Warfarin
Tinea capitis	Oral therapy with terbinafine, fluconazole, or itraconazole for about 6 weeks	Screen close contacts
	Oral therapy with griseofulvin for ~12 weeks	
Discoid lupus erythematosus	Sunscreen or other sun-protection	Systemic lupus erythematosus (5%-10%)
	Glucocorticoids:	ROS for symptoms
	Topical are first line	Examination for signs
	Intralesional for recalcitrant or thick lesions	Urinalysis, ANA
	Oral reserved for patients with rapid progression	
	Antimalarial agents	
	Retinoids: topical or oral if severe	
Traumatic alopecia	Traction/styling alopecia: decrease tension from styling practices	Concomitant psychiatric disorder is more common in adults than children
	Trichotillomania: Cognitive behavioral therapy	Consider referral to psychiatrist or psychologist
	If severe or recalcitrant, antidepressants or anxiolytics may be helpful	
Lichen planopilaris	Topical, intralesional, or oral glucocorticoids, antimalarial agents, immunosuppressants	Check for concomitant lichen planus on the skin, nails, and oral and genital mucosa
Frontal fibrosing alopecia	Antimalarial agents, 5-α reductase inhibitors	
Central centrifugal cicatricial alopecia	Topical and intralesional glucocorticoids, oral tetracyclines, antimalarial agents, immunosuppressants, minimal hair grooming	

ANA = antinuclear antibody; DPCP = diphenylcyclopropenone; ROS = review of systems.

[a]FDA-approved treatment for that condition/indication.

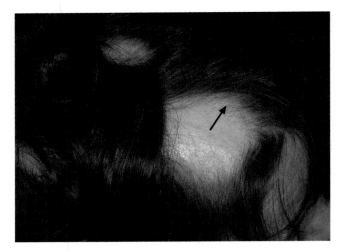

FIGURE 135. Well-demarcated, smooth, oval patches of hair loss. Note the smooth scalp and short hairs near the rim of the balding patch (arrow). Closer examination of these hairs will reveal "exclamation point" hairs (hairs that narrow close to the skin surface).

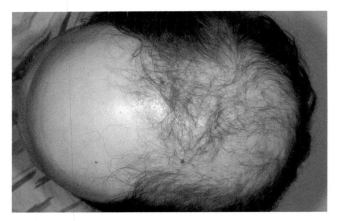

FIGURE 136. Typical distribution of androgenic alopecia in a male. Note the bitemporal hairline recession and vertex hair loss.

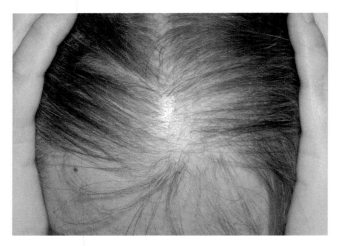

FIGURE 137. Androgenic alopecia in a female. Note the widening of the part width at the crown.

KEY POINT

- Alopecia areata, a nonscarring alopecia, presents as well-circumscribed round patches with no hair; the rim of the patches has characteristic "exclamation point" hairs that narrow close to the skin surface.

Scarring Localized and Generalized Alopecia

Discoid lupus erythematous on the scalp can result in scarring localized alopecia. It presents as multiple pink, scaling hypo- and hyperpigmented scarring plaques (**Figure 138**) (see Common Rashes).

Acne keloidalis nuchae is a chronic inflammatory disorder of the follicles causing an alopecic scar on the nape of the neck (**Figure 139**). It can be pruritic. Pseudofolliculitis barbae occurs on the face and anterior neck. It is likely due to the curvature of the hair shaft and repeated trauma such as from shaving. When the curved hairs grow out after shaving, they curve downward into the skin, inciting an inflammatory response. This causes small pustules that can become keloidal. These conditions most commonly affect black men.

Lichen planopilaris is a diffuse scarring alopecia that more commonly affects postmenopausal women. It presents as mild scaling and limited erythema and scale surrounding the follicle (**Figure 140**). Associated symptoms are pain, burning, and pruritus.

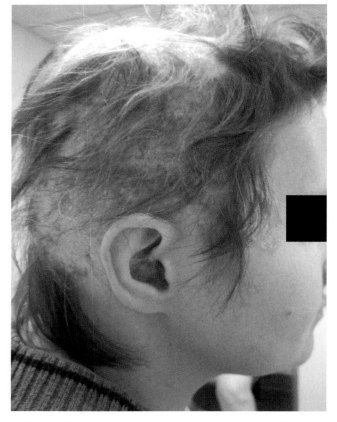

FIGURE 138. Multiple pink scarring plaques of hair loss in discoid lupus.

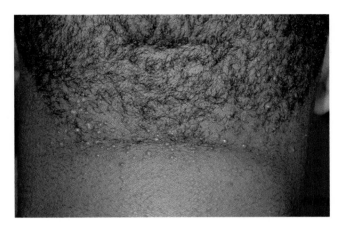

FIGURE 139. Multiple papules and pustules at the nape of the neck characteristic of early acne keloidalis nuchae.

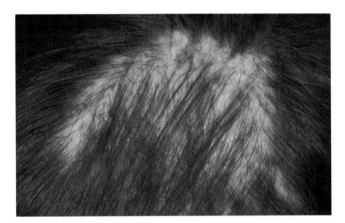

FIGURE 140. Lichen planopilaris is a cause of scarring alopecia and often demonstrates redness around the follicles.

Nail Disorders

The nail complex is composed of the nail plate, hyponychium, proximal and lateral nail folds, cuticle, nail bed, and matrix. The hyponychium is the skin underneath the distal free edge of the nail plate. It seals the junction between the distal nail plate and the nail bed. The nail fold protects the nail matrix and produces the cuticle. The nail bed is adherent to the bottom of the nail plate. Nail disorders can be caused by various diseases, infections, trauma, and drugs (**Table 34**).

Infection

Onychomycosis is a fungal (dermatophyte) infection of the nail commonly seen in elderly persons, especially those with comorbidities such as diabetes mellitus, peripheral vascular disease, or immunosuppression. The most common sites of infection are the toenails. It can appear as distal subungual and proximal subungual onychomycosis. Distal subungual

onychomycosis is the most common pattern. The distal nail plate becomes discolored (yellow, white, or brown) and thickened. Under the nail plate, there is an accumulation of subungual debris, resulting in separation of the plate from the bed (onycholysis) (**Figure 141**). Proximal subungual onychomycosis appears similar except that it starts at the proximal nail fold. This pattern is rare and can be associated with HIV and immunosuppression.

Onychomycosis is treated mostly for cosmetic reasons. Confirmation of infection with potassium hydroxide preparation, staining with periodic acid-Schiff, or fungal culture should be done before treatment. Topical antifungal agents are of limited efficacy. Oral therapy with terbinafine or itraconazole is more effective.

KEY POINTS

- Onychomycosis is a fungal (dermatophyte) infection of the nail commonly seen in elderly persons, especially those with comorbidities such as diabetes mellitus, peripheral vascular disease, or immunosuppression.

- Oral therapy with terbinafine or itraconazole is the preferred treatment for onychomycosis; confirmation of infection should be done before treatment. **HVC**

Paronychia

Paronychia is an infection of the nail fold. Infection is caused by trauma or chronic maceration leading to an incompetent cuticle. Acute paronychia is painful swelling of the nail fold, most commonly caused by *Staphylococcus aureus*. It typically affects only one nail. Chronic paronychia tends to be more insidious and involve multiple fingers. In adults, it is most often seen in those with frequent hand immersion in water. There is tender swelling in the nail folds with missing or dystrophic cuticles (**Figure 142**). Chronic paronychia can cause ridging of the nail plate. It is a multifactorial condition with several inciting factors including water, irritants, and possibly *Candida* species. Treatment of acute paronychia includes the use of warm compresses, incision and drainage, and in severe cases, oral antibiotics. For chronic paronychia, minimizing inciting factors is key. Treatment includes topical glucocorticoids and antifungal agents to reduce inflammation and minimizing inciting factors.

KEY POINT

- Acute paronychia is a painful swelling of the nail fold, most commonly caused by *Staphylococcus aureus*, typically affecting one nail; chronic paronychia tends to be more insidious and involve multiple fingers.

Inflammatory Dermatosis

Psoriasis affects fingernails more commonly than toenails. If the nail matrix is affected, tiny multiple pits will be seen on

TABLE 34. Nail Findings Associated with Possible Systemic Conditions

Nail Finding	Description	Associated Diseases
Nail Plate		
Koilonychia (spoon nails)	Thin curving up nail with everted edges (spoon)	Iron disorders (Plummer-Vinson syndrome, hemochromatosis, iron deficiency anemia); chronic injury
Trachyonychia	Rough sandpaper nails on all 20 nails	Lichen planus; psoriasis; eczema; idiopathic
Onychogryphosis	Curved, hypertrophic nails resembling claw	Trauma; peripheral vascular disease; neglect
Onychomadesis	Periodic shedding of the nail beginning at its proximal end due to temporary arrest of the matrix	Severe systemic illness (high fever, toxic epidermal necrosis, erythroderma, scarlet fever, surgery, medications)
Transverse indentations (Beau lines)	Transverse furrows beginning in the matrix	Systemic illness or major trauma (childbirth, measles, acute febrile illnesses, drug reaction)
Pitted nails	Tiny indentations on the nail plate due to abnormal keratinization of the proximal nail matrix	Psoriasis; alopecia areata; lichen planus
Nail Color		
Half and half (Lindsey) nails	Proximal nail is white and the distal nail is red, pink, brown with a sharp line of demarcation	Chronic kidney disease
Terry nails	Distal 1-2 mm of nails have normal pink color but proximal end has abnormal white appearance	Liver disease; chronic heart failure; diabetes mellitus; normal aging
Melanonychia	Diffuse/partial brown-black	Chemotherapy agents, antimalarial agents, minocycline, gold; common in dark skin types; trauma
	Longitudinal melanonychia – vertical brown band	Nevus; lentigo; drugs; melanoma; trauma
Green nail syndrome	Onycholytic toenails with green discoloration	Prolonged immersion in fresh water and infection with *Pseudomonas aeruginosa*
Blue nails	Blue lunulae	Argyria, antimalarials, hepatolenticular degeneration
		5-Fluorouracil and azidothymidine
Yellow	Yellow nail syndrome	Aging, dermatophyte infection
		Lymphedema; chronic pulmonary disease
Red lunulae		Carbon monoxide poisoning; subungual digital myxoid cyst; heart failure
Periungual/Cuticle		
Ragged cuticles (Samitz sign)	Dystrophic, ragged-appearing cuticles	Dermatomyositis
Periungual erythema	Alternating areas of capillary dilated, torturous vessels and capillary dropout; red cuticles	Dermatomyositis; scleroderma; lupus erythematosus (less common)

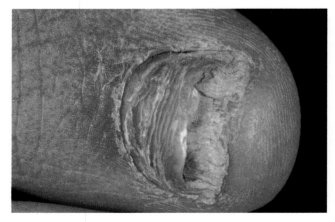

FIGURE 141. Yellow hypertrophic nail plate and subungual debris from onychomycosis.

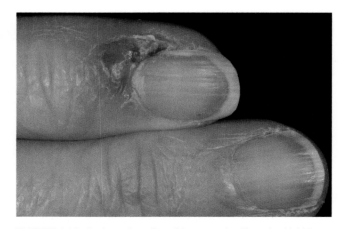

FIGURE 142. Tender, pink swelling of the proximal and lateral nail fold due to chronic paronychia. Note the dystrophic cuticle.

the nail plate (**Figure 143**). In cases of nail bed involvement, yellow-brown discoloration (oil stains) can occur. Other findings include nail plate thickening, separation of the nail plate from the nail bed, distal nail plate crumbling, and splinter hemorrhages (**Figure 144**). Patients with psoriatic nail involvement are often affected by psoriatic arthritis.

Lichen planus, in about 10% of cases, can affect the nails. It causes nail plate dystrophy including thinning, red-streaking, and pterygium unguis formation, which is the scarring of the proximal nail fold and matrix (**Figure 145**).

Ingrown Toenail

An ingrown toenail is the result of the nail plate growing into the lateral nail fold causing an inflammatory response.

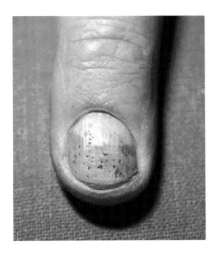

FIGURE 143. Nail pitting in a patient with psoriasis.

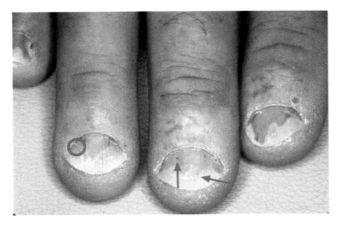

FIGURE 144. Other characteristic features of nail psoriasis include distal onycholysis (separation of the nail plate from the underlying nail bed) [arrow] and splinter hemorrhages, which represent the "Auspitz sign" (punctuate bleeding) in the nail bed. In addition, some patients may display the "oil-drop sign" (circle), which is characterized by a localized tan to brown discoloration of the nail. In more severe forms of psoriatic involvement, there can be thickening and crumbling of the nails.

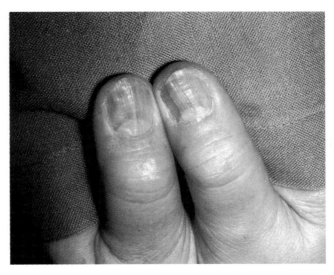

FIGURE 145. Lichen planus can cause pitting, onycholysis, and nail dystrophy. Lichen planus is a common cause of 20-nail dystrophy (trachyonychia) characterized by roughness and longitudinal ridging of the nail plate on all 20 nails.

Ingrown toenails of the great toe are most common, presenting as painful swelling of the lateral nail fold (**Figure 146**). There may be some weeping granulation tissue.

Conservative treatment for mild to moderate ingrown nails involve wider shoes, trimming the nail plate straight across, antiseptic application, and inserting a cotton pledget under the nail edge. For severe cases, partial or complete nail avulsion with matricectomy may be necessary.

Melanonychia

Melanonychia is a brown banded pigmentation of the nail plate that can be caused by increased melanin production of the melanocytes in the nail matrix, benign hyperplasia, and melanoma (see Common Neoplasms). Longitudinal melanonychia is

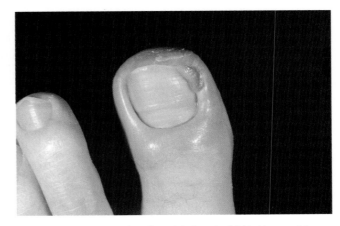

FIGURE 146. Tender pink swelling of the lateral nail fold with some pink granulation tissue growing on the lateral distal end suggesting an ingrown toenail.

the transverse brown-black band on the nail plate (**Figure 147**), most commonly found on dark-skinned patients. Multiple nails are usually involved. Longitudinal, irregular melanonychia on a single nail can be a sign of melanoma.

Squamous Cell Carcinoma

Squamous cell carcinoma of the nail unit often presents with pain, swelling, and erythema. It commonly arises in the nail fold and appears as a hyperkeratotic papule and plaque similar to warts (**Figure 148**). If treatment of a wart does not progress as expected, a biopsy is warranted to rule out squamous cell carcinoma, which is strongly associated with human papillomavirus infection.

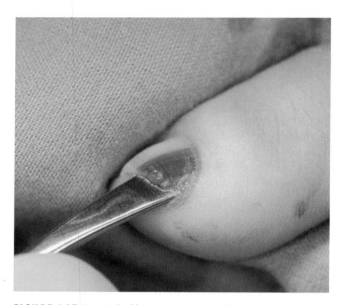

FIGURE 147. Longitudinal brown pigmentation with transverse streaks on the nail plate characteristic of melanonychia.

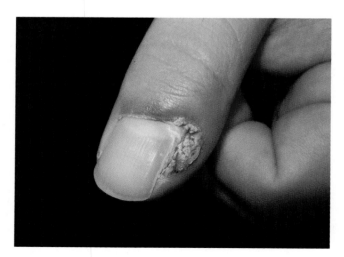

FIGURE 148. Verruca plaque on the lateral nail fold that looks like a wart but biopsy demonstrated squamous cell carcinoma.

Disorders of the Mucous Membranes

Melanotic Macule

A melanotic macule is a small, well-circumscribed, brown-to-black mucosal lesion. The most common location is the lower lip (**Figure 149**), but they may also be found on the gingival, buccal mucosa, or tongue, or within the genital mucosa. If large, papular, or not well-circumscribed, biopsy should be performed to rule out melanoma. Solitary lesions are the rule, and multiple lesions suggest the possibility of rare inherited disorders such as Peutz-Jeghers syndrome.

Amalgam Tattoo

Amalgam dental fillings contain metals that can be inadvertently implanted into the adjacent mucosa at the time of dental filling. They present as blue-gray macules and do not change over time. In cases of uncertainty, a mucosal biopsy should be performed.

Leukoplakia and Erythroplakia

Leukoplakia is a premalignant lesion that presents as white patches on the oral mucosa (**Figure 150**). It should be differentiated from oral candidiasis and oral hairy leukoplakia. Oral hairy leukoplakia (Epstein-Barr virus induced) occurs in patients with HIV infection and presents as adherent linear white plaques on the lateral surface of the tongue. Erythroplakia, appearing as red mucosal patches, has a high risk of malignant transformation. Both leukoplakia and erythroplakia require biopsy to rule out dysplasia. These conditions are seen most frequently in tobacco users.

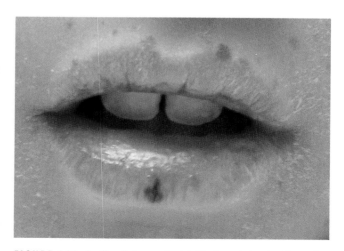

FIGURE 149. Small, well-circumscribed darkly pigmented melanotic macule occurring on the vermilion border of the lower lip.

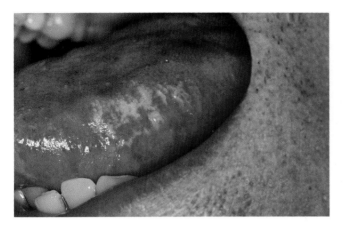

FIGURE 150. Oral hairy leukoplakia is a precancerous lesion that presents as linear white patches or plaques on the lateral surface of the tongue with changes in the surface texture.

Oral Candidiasis

Oropharyngeal candidiasis presents as white-to-red plaques that are painful (**Figure 151**). The white surface of the plaques can be scraped off. *Candida* is also responsible for angular cheilitis (perleche) presenting as fissuring and maceration of the angle of the mouth due to drooling and poorly fitting dentures. Risk factors for oral candidiasis include immunosuppression, diabetes mellitus, use of antibiotics, oral and inhaled glucocorticoids, and smoking. First-line treatment includes azole troches or nystatin swish and swallow mouthwash. Oral fluconazole may be required for severe, recalcitrant, or recurrent cases.

Aphthous Ulcers

Aphthous ulcers ("canker sores") are recurrent ulcers with a gray pseudomembrane base and an erythematous halo that affect lips, buccal mucosa, and tongue (**Figure 152**). Diagnosis

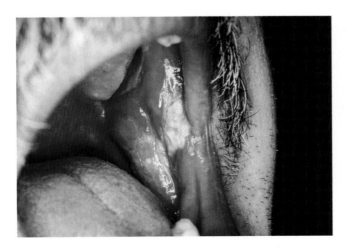

FIGURE 151. Oral candidiasis most commonly presents as painful white, fluffy, nonadherent film on the tongue, buccal mucosa, or palate.

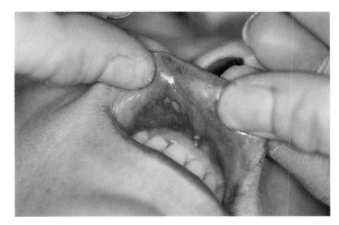

FIGURE 152. Aphthous ulcer is characterized by painful, discrete shallow, round to oval ulcer with a gray base and red surrounding halo typically less than 1 cm in diameter.

is by clinical findings and history of self-healing. Severe, recurrent oral ulcers suggest the possibility of infection or a systemic disease such as Behçet syndrome, Crohn disease, HIV infection, or erythema multiforme.

> **KEY POINT**
> - Severe, recurrent oral aphthous ulcers may suggest a systemic disease such as Behçet syndrome, Crohn disease, HIV infection, or erythema multiforme.

Lichen Planus

Oral lichen planus can be isolated or associated with skin lesions or be part of a vulvovaginal syndrome. Oral lesions appear as erythematous patches with an overlying white lacelike pattern (Wickham striae), typically on the buccal mucosa (**Figure 153**). Treatment often requires systemic

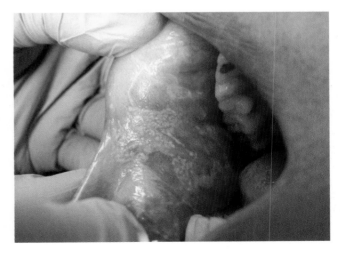

FIGURE 153. Lichen planus is an autoimmune disease of unknown cause that can affect the skin, mucous membranes, scalp, or nails. Common clinical findings of mucosal lichen planus are a white reticulated network on the buccal mucosa (Wickham striae); desquamative gingivitis; and chronic, painful erosions on the oral or vulvar mucosa.

steroid-sparing agents in addition to medium- to high-potency topical glucocorticoids.

Actinic Cheilitis and Squamous Cell Carcinoma

Actinic cheilitis is a premalignant condition that presents as scaly patches with erosions on the lower lip and is the result of chronic sun damage. Management is with topical chemotherapy agents (5-fluorouracil), imiquimod, laser therapy, photodynamic therapy, or cryotherapy.

The development of a nodule or ulcer suggests squamous cell carcinoma, most often found on the lower lip of older men (see Common Neoplasms). Risk factors include tobacco, alcohol use, and ultraviolet radiation. Other predisposing conditions include lichen planus and lichen sclerosus. In all cases of suspected squamous cell carcinoma, biopsy is required to establish the diagnosis.

> **KEY POINT**
> - Actinic cheilitis is a premalignant condition that presents as scaly patches with erosions on the lower lip; the development of a nodule or ulcer suggests squamous cell carcinoma.

Lichen Sclerosus

Lichen sclerosus is a chronic inflammatory disease that most often affects women in the fifth or sixth decade of life. It presents as a white, atrophic patch that circumferentially involves the vaginal introitus and perianal area with a "figure 8" morphology (**Figure 154**). Extragenital lesions can occur. Biopsy is required for the diagnosis. Treatment is with potent topical glucocorticoids. If left untreated, permanent scarring can occur, and chronic lesions are at risk for squamous cell carcinoma.

Black Hairy Tongue

Black hairy tongue is characterized by elongation and defective desquamation of filiform papillae (**Figure 155**). It is more common in men and with advancing age. Management includes good oral hygiene and tongue brushing.

Geographic Tongue

Geographic tongue is fairly common and may be sporadic, familial, or associated with psoriasis. These migratory patterned patches of smooth red surfaces and white patches on the dorsal tongue (**Figure 156**) are usually asymptomatic, but discomfort and burning may be reported, which are exacerbated by hot or spicy foods. About 40% of patients will develop tongue fissures.

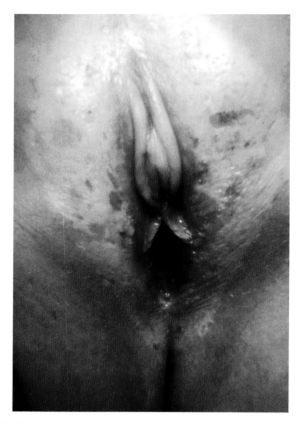

FIGURE 154. Lichen sclerosus is a chronic inflammatory mucocutaneous disease characterized by "parchment-like" or "cigarette paper" skin that circumferentially involves the vaginal introitus and perianal area with a "figure 8" morphology; some patients may have thickened or lichenified areas. It may predispose the patient to subsequent development of squamous cell carcinoma. Image reproduced from the CDC Public Health Image Library.

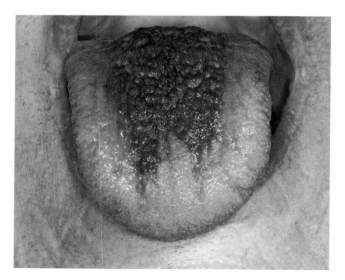

FIGURE 155. Black hairy tongue is a benign self-limited disorder. The clinical appearance of black discoloration and thickened papillae without other symptoms is characteristic.

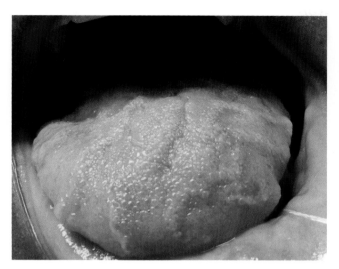

FIGURE 156. Geographic tongue (benign migratory glossitis) showing irregularly shaped, map-like migratory patches on the dorsal tongue.

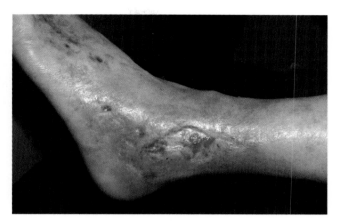

FIGURE 157. Venous stasis ulcers of the medial lower extremity with associated changes of edema, hyperpigmentation, and evidence of previous healed ulcers.

Foot and Lower Leg Ulcers

Venous stasis ulcers, arterial insufficiency ulcers, and neuropathic ulcers are the most common ulcerations of the feet and lower extremities. The proper diagnosis is important since treatments are directed at the underlying cause.

Venous Stasis Ulcers

Venous stasis ulcers account for up to 70% of all leg ulcers. They occur on the lower extremities in the area from the mid-calf to the ankle, most commonly near the medial malleolus, and are associated with signs of chronic venous insufficiency. Venous stasis ulcers can be single or multiple and are typically irregularly shaped, shallow, and often weep serous fluid **(Figure 157)**. The presence of fibrinous tissue is common, and ulcers are rarely necrotic. Pain may or may not be present.

Physical findings suggestive of venous stasis ulcers include edema, varicosities, eczematous changes, brown pigmentation from hemosiderin deposition, lipodermatosclerosis (fibrosis of subcutaneous tissue), atrophie blanche (pale plaques of scar tissue), and evidence of healed ulcers. Diagnosis is usually made clinically, although duplex ultrasonography can be helpful in evaluating venous reflux and obstruction, or if the diagnosis is unclear. Ankle-brachial indexes should be measvured to rule out concurrent arterial disease.

Treatment consists of compression therapy, which improves venous flow, reduces edema, and promotes fibrinolysis. Compression therapy is best administered through the use of high-compression, multicomponent bandaging; other options include elastic or inelastic compression bandages (Unna boots, compression stockings) or intermittent pneumonic compression devices. Compression is avoided if the

ankle-brachial index is less than 0.8, and referral to a vascular specialist should be considered.

Local wound care includes debridement of devitalized tissue. Simple nonadherent dressings appear to be as effective as other more expensive dressings, and the addition of topical cadexomer iodine may improve healing. When added to standard care, oral pentoxifylline, simvastatin, and aspirin have been shown to increase ulcer healing. Lower quality evidence suggests that flavonoids and hydroxyethyl rutoside may also improve healing. Routine use of systemic antibiotics is not recommended except for patients with suspected infection (increased pain, drainage, surrounding cellulitis). Superficial venous surgery reduces 1-year ulcer recurrence rate in patients with superficial venous reflux. Bilayer artificial skin replacement may improve healing of venous ulcers compared to compression and simple dressings. 🅗

KEY POINTS

- Venous stasis ulcers occur on the lower extremities in the area from the midcalf to the ankle and are associated with signs of chronic venous insufficiency.

- The mainstay of venous ulcer treatment consists of compression therapy, which improves venous flow, reduces edema, and promotes fibrinolysis.

- Routine use of systemic antibiotics is not recommended **HVC** for the treatment of venous stasis ulcers except for patients with suspected infection (increased pain, drainage, surrounding cellulitis).

Arterial Insufficiency Ulcers 🅗

Arterial leg ulcers account for up to 25% of leg ulcers. Arterial insufficiency is typically due to atherosclerosis, which leads to inadequate oxygenation of the tissue and ulcer formation. Common risk factors are smoking, obesity, diabetes, hyperlipidemia, hypertension, and increased age. Common locations are the distal toes, on the anterior portion of the lower leg where minimal collateral arterial circulation is present, and at sites of trauma. Arterial ulcers are usually painful and have sharply demarcated borders with a dry, pale gray or yellow wound base without evidence of granulation tissue (**Figure 158**). Claudication and rest pain are commonly present. If tissue necrosis is present, the wound may be covered by an eschar. Other findings include cool extremities with digital hair loss; shiny, taunt skin around the ulcer; and delayed capillary refill time. The key diagnostic test is an ankle-brachial index less than or equal to 0.9.

Treatment must involve aggressive risk factor management and measures to increase blood supply to the affected area. Surgical revascularization, percutaneous balloon angioplasty, or stent placement is usually necessary. Arterial ulcers are treated with local wound care similar to venous stasis ulcers.

KEY POINTS

- Arterial insufficiency ulcers are usually located at the distal extremities, such as the distal toes and anterior portion of the lower leg, where minimal collateral arterial circulation is present.
- Arterial ulcers are painful and usually have sharply demarcated borders with a dry, pale gray or yellow wound bed.
- Treatment of arterial ulcers must involve risk factor management and measures to increase blood supply to the affected area.

Neuropathic Ulcers

Neuropathic ulcers arise secondary to repetitive trauma to the skin, typically in patients with diabetic peripheral neuropathy and a reduced awareness of pressure or trauma to the

skin. Diabetic ulcers are painless, are most common on the plantar surface of the feet, and have associated callus and foot deformity (Charcot foot) (**Figure 159**). The skin is warm and dry with signs of fissuring and breakdown. Polymicrobial infections are common, and patients are at increased risk of osteomyelitis (see MKSAP 18 Infectious Disease). Surgical debridement of necrotic tissue along with redistributing pressure is important to achieve healing. Offloading measures include foot inserts, therapeutic shoes, and removable cast walkers.

KEY POINTS

- Neuropathic ulcers arise secondary to repetitive trauma to the skin, typically in patients with diabetes mellitus.
- Treatment of neuropathic ulcers includes surgical debridement and redistributing or offloading pressure.

Other Causes of Lower Extremity Ulcers

Pressure ulcers of the heels and lateral ankles are common in bedridden patients due to necrosis from persistent pressure. Rarer causes of ulcers (**Table 35**) should be suspected based on a suggestive history, physical findings, and lack of response to traditional therapies. In these cases, a punch or incisional biopsy should be considered. The sampled tissue should include both ulcer edge and bed, and the tissue should also be sent for bacterial, fungal, and mycobacterial cultures. Further workup and treatment are directed at the underlying cause.

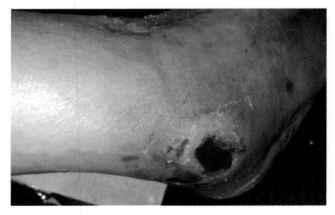

FIGURE 158. Arterial insufficiency ulcers appear sharply demarcated or "punched out" with a dry pale, gray or yellow base and the surrounding skin is red, taunt, and tender.

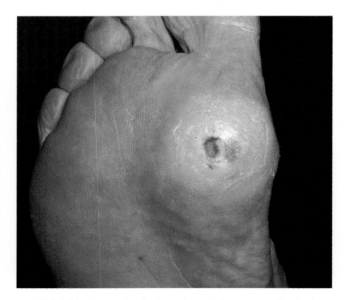

FIGURE 159. Neuropathic ulcer located over the first metatarsal head with associated callus in a patient with diabetes mellitus.

TABLE 35. Other Causes of Leg Ulcers	
Diagnosis	**Characteristics/Associations**
Pyoderma gangrenosum	Often follows trauma
	Undermined or violaceous borders
	Associated with inflammatory bowel disease, rheumatoid arthritis, and monoclonal gammopathy
Vasculitis	Findings may include palpable purpura, livedo reticularis
	Associated with autoimmune disorders, infections, and other causes of vasculitis
Calciphylaxis	Advanced disease is characterized by painful angulated necrotic ulcers with eschars most commonly found on buttocks, abdomen, and thighs in patients with end-stage kidney disease
Vasculopathy (microthrombi)	Painful, necrotic, and usually multiple ulcers associated with hypercoagulable states
Malignant ulcer	Chronic, nonhealing ulcer at site of chronic inflammation or prior trauma
	Most commonly squamous cell carcinoma, basal cell carcinoma, or melanoma
Necrobiosis lipoidica diabeticorum	Typically starts as a yellow-brown plaque that ulcerates
	Higher incidence in patients with diabetes mellitus
Sickle cell disease	Painful ulcers on the medial and lateral malleoli
	May occur spontaneously or after trauma
	Can be associated with hydroxyurea therapy

Dermatologic Conditions of Pregnancy and Aging

Pregnancy and Lactation

Women who are pregnant or lactating can present with unique skin findings, some of which are physiologic (**Table 36**) and others that may require treatment (**Table 37**). Preexisting skin conditions may be exacerbated during pregnancy or uniquely arise during pregnancy. Pruritic urticarial papules and plaques of pregnancy (PUPPP) is the most common specific dermatosis of pregnancy (**Figure 160**). Clinically, PUPPP appears late in the third trimester as erythematous plaques in the distribution of striae typically with sparing of the periumbilical skin. While the lesions may be restricted to abdominal striae, they may also appear on the arms and legs. Persistent and bothersome pruritus is a symptomatic hallmark of the condition. The condition usually resolves shortly after delivery. For symptom control, low- to medium-potency topical glucocorticoids are often first-line therapy; nonsedating antihistamines are sometimes required to control pruritus.

Pemphigoid gestationis (herpes gestationis) is a pruritic blistering disease typically appearing during the second or third trimester. Urticarial plaques, papules, and vesicles first appear surrounding the umbilicus, but can involve the palms and soles. It usually spares the mucous membranes (**Figure 161**). A skin biopsy demonstrating a subepidermal bulla with neutrophils can confirm the diagnosis. Treatment with topical glucocorticoids is usually initiated for pruritus, and the lesions spontaneously remit following delivery. Pemphigoid gestationis is associated with an increased risk of fetal growth restriction and prematurity. ⊞

Treatment of dermatologic conditions during pregnancy can be challenging, as special consideration needs to be made for potential medication-induced teratogenicity. The FDA has published changes in pregnancy and lactation labeling for prescription drugs, effective June 30, 2015. The pregnancy letter categories will be removed with the new labeling requirements; however, for prescription drugs that were previously approved, these changes will be phased in gradually. This section will refer to previously approved drugs and their letter categories of risk (**Table 38**). It is important to consider these drugs when prescribing for women of childbearing age. For some drugs, there are regulatory programs to monitor medications such as iPledge for isotretinoin, STEPs for thalidomide, and mycophenolate REMS for mycophenolate mofetil.

Dermatologic surgery under local anesthesia (lidocaine) can be safely done during pregnancy if necessary; however, opiates and sedatives should be avoided in pregnant and lactating women.

Aging

Similar to other organs, the skin's functional capacity diminishes with age, thus increasing its susceptibility to cutaneous disorders such as dermatoses and skin cancer. Clinically and histologically, the skin structure changes (**Table 39**) from both intrinsic and extrinsic mechanisms (ultraviolet light, smoking). Nails can change as well. The nail growth rate begins to decline after the age of 25. Decreased lipophilic sterols and free fatty acids cause nails to develop some ridging and become

TABLE 36. Physiologic Changes Associated with Pregnancy

Category	Finding	Treatment After Pregnancy
Pigmentary	Melasma (mask of pregnancy) characterized by ill-defined brown macules on face	Sun protection
	Linea nigra appears as a vertical linear hyperpigmentation on abdomen	Spontaneous resolution over time
	Areolae, axillae, and genitals darken	Spontaneous resolution over time
	Moles may darken	Melanoma can occur during pregnancy; biopsy if there is significant change
Vascular	Angiomas develop commonly on the face, neck, and extremities	Spontaneous resolution over time for most lesions
	Palmar erythema may be diffuse or limited to thenar and hypothenar eminences	Spontaneous resolution over time
	Saphenous, vulvar, and hemorrhoidal varicosities	Medical or surgical therapy for unresolved extremity varicosities after pregnancy
	Pyogenic granulomas can develop on the gingiva and fingers. Gingival hyperemia is universally present.	Spontaneous resolution
Hair	Hypertrichosis can develop on the face, but arms, back, and suprapubic regions may also be affected. Terminal hair growth is likely to be permanent without treatment.	See Hair Disorders; lanugo hairs resolve spontaneously
	Postpartum telogen effluvium is common and recognized as hair shedding. Hair may become sparse.	Spontaneous resolution over time
Nail	Onycholysis appears as white discoloration at end with separation of the nail plate from the nail bed	Spontaneous resolution in most cases
Connective Tissue	Striae gravidarum (stretch marks) appears as linear atrophic scars that may start as pink/red then become paler on abdomen, breasts, and thighs	No effective treatment

TABLE 37. Pregnancy Dermatoses

	Description/Area	Timing/Course	Treatment	Fetal Involvement
Prurigo of pregnancy	Prurigo nodules (firm, pruritic nodules); extremities more often than abdomen	After first trimester; resolves after pregnancy	None indicated; can consider topical glucocorticoids	None
Pemphigoid gestationis (herpes gestationis)	Pruritic, vesiculobullous eruption Abdomen, umbilicus; can generalize	Late pregnancy, but can occur in any trimester, or immediately postpartum Spontaneously remits weeks to months after delivery	Self-limited; topical and systemic glucocorticoids, antihistamines Commonly recurs in subsequent pregnancies	Increase risk of prematurity; small for gestational age infants; neonatal pemphigoid gestationis
Pruritic urticarial papules and plaques of pregnancy	Pruritic erythematous and edematous papules and plaques that may become vesicular Within abdominal striae; can generalize Spares umbilicus, face, palms, soles	End of third trimester, immediately postpartum	Self-limited, resolving shortly after delivery; topical glucocorticoids; antihistamines	None
Intrahepatic cholestasis of pregnancy	Pruritus with excoriations; jaundice	Late second trimester, third trimester	Resolves within days of delivery; ursodeoxycholic acid for pruritus Recurs in subsequent pregnancies	Increased risk of premature labor; fetal distress; stillbirth
Generalized pustular psoriasis of pregnancy (impetigo herpetiformis)	Peripheral pustules on pink polycyclic patches	Third trimester	Systemic glucocorticoids; resolves postpartum Recurs in subsequent pregnancies	Low birth weight; intrauterine growth restriction; premature rupture of membranes; stillbirth

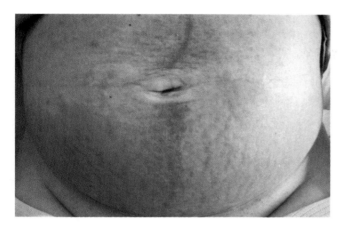

FIGURE 160. Characteristic appearance of pruritic urticarial papules and plaques of pregnancy (PUPPP) in a gravid woman with edematous, erythematous plaques on the abdomen involving the striae. Note the relative sparing of the umbilicus.

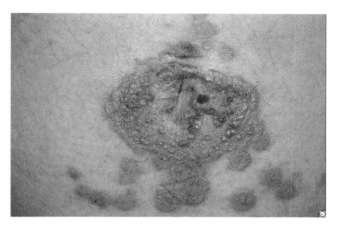

FIGURE 161. Classic appearance of pemphigoid gestationis with pruritic vesicles and pink plaques surrounding the umbilicus in a gravid woman.

more brittle. Generally, chest, axillary, and pubic hair all decrease with age. In men, there is increased hair in eyebrows, the nostrils, and external auditory meati. In women, the vellus hairs on the chin and upper lip convert into course terminal hairs possibly due to reduced estrogen levels. Hair graying can occur due to depletion of hair bulb melanocytes.

Dryness (xerosis cutis) is one of the most prevalent skin conditions in an aging population. While pilo-sebaceous glands become larger with age, there is a 50% reduction in sebum production. Excessive xerosis can cause xerotic dermatitis (eczema). It occurs more often in the winter (low humidity) and on the lower legs. It presents as dry fissured patches

TABLE 38. Selected Systemic Medications to Avoid During Pregnancy and Lactation Commonly Used in Dermatology

Medication	FDA Category	Risks
Tetracyclines	D	Dental staining and enamel hypoplasia in the second and third trimester
		Acute fatty liver of pregnancy
Trimethoprim-Sulfamethoxazole	C	Interference with folic acid metabolism
Isotretinoin	X	Increased fetal loss during first trimester
		Microtia; external ear canal stenosis; cleft palate; hydrocephalus; cardiac outflow trace defects
Acitretin	X	Craniofacial, cardiac, thymic, and central nervous system malformation
Tazarotene (topical)	X	Similar retinoid anomalies in animal studies
Spironolactone	C	Delayed sexual maturation in female rats and feminization of male rat fetuses
		No reported risk in humans in case reports
Methotrexate	X	Increased risk of miscarriage
		Micrognathia; developmental delays; craniosynostosis, small low-set ears; limb abnormalities; growth retardation
		Potential fathers should not be on medication
Glucocorticoids	C	In high doses, possible growth retardation and inhibition of endogenous corticosteroid production
Mycophenolate mofetil	D	Increased risk of miscarriage
		Anomalies of distal limbs, hearts, esophagus, kidney, external ear, and face

FDA categories: (A) Studies on pregnant women show no risk (safe); (B) No clinical data of human risk but uncertain; (C) Risk cannot be ruled out; (D) Evidence of risk; (X) Contraindicated during pregnancy.

The FDA has published changes in pregnancy and lactation labeling for prescription drugs, effective June 30, 2015 (see www.fda.gov/Drugs/DevelopmentApprovalProcess/DevelopmentResources/Labeling/ucm093307.htm). The pregnancy letter categories will be removed with the new labeling requirements; however, for prescription drugs that were previously approved, these changes will be phased in gradually. Labeling will include information relevant to the use of the drug in pregnant women (such as dosing and potential risks to the developing fetus), information about using the drug while breastfeeding (such as the amount of drug in breast milk and potential effects on the breastfed infant), and information regarding potential risks to females and males of reproductive potential who take the drug. Prescribing information for individual preparations should be consulted for more specific information.

TABLE 39.	Skin Changes Due to Intrinsic and Extrinsic Aging	
	Intrinsic	**Extrinsic (Photoaging, Smoking)**
Pigmentation	Skin pallor	Diffuse pigmentation
		Lentigines
Epidermis	Thinned	
	Xerosis	
Dermis	Fine wrinkles	Coarse furrows
	Decreased elasticity	Pebbly texture (elastosis)
	Decreased skin temperature	Solar purpura
		Telangiectasia
Other	Subcutaneous fat loss	
	Decreased skin temperature	
Nails	Brittle and ridging	
Hair	Graying	

with a scalelike appearance (**Figure 162**). Severe xerosis can cause pruritus. Subsequent itching can result in actinic purpura. Good skin care measures are recommended, including the frequent application of emollients, especially immediately after bathing, to reduce dryness. Topical glucocorticoids can be applied to areas of inflamed skin.

Actinic purpura appears as purpuric macules or patches, most commonly on the forearms, due to minor trauma such as scratching (**Figure 163**). There may be associated stellate pseudoscars that are atrophic scars occurring after the skin tears. Actinic purpura is due to blood vessel fragility and dermal atrophy from aging. No additional testing needs to be done. There is no therapy for the purpura but sun protection is recommended to prevent further damage.

KEY POINT

- Actinic purpura is due to blood vessel fragility and dermal atrophy from aging; no additional testing needs to be done.

HVC

Infection

Group living arrangements such as skilled nursing facilities can predispose elderly persons to infestations with scabies, lice, or bedbugs (see Infestations). Herpes zoster and postherpetic neuralgia can occur more frequently in the elderly (see Common Skin Infections). Onychomycosis is more common in elderly populations (see Nail Disorders).

Chronic Wounds/Poor Wound Healing

Elderly persons with mobility impairments and comorbidities (cardiovascular disease, diabetes mellitus) are predisposed to chronic wounds such as venous, pressure, and diabetic foot ulcers (see Foot and Leg Ulcers).

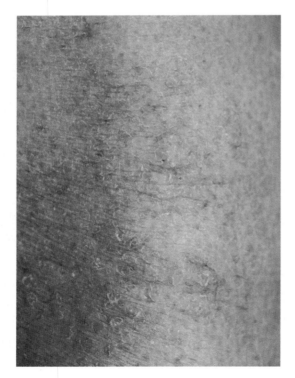

FIGURE 162. Characteristic findings of xerotic eczema located on the anterior leg showing fine, porcelain-like cracks on eczematous skin.

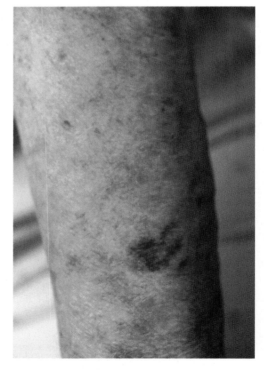

FIGURE 163. Purpuric ill-defined patches (actinic purpura) and ill-defined tan macules (solar lentigines) on atrophic skin demonstrating signs of aging.

Bibliography

Approach to the Patient with Dermatologic Disease

Bibbins-Domingo K, Grossman DC, Curry SJ, Davidson KW, Ebell M, Epling JW Jr, et al; US Preventive Services Task Force. Screening for Skin Cancer: US Preventive Services Task Force Recommendation Statement. JAMA. 2016;316:429-35. [PMID: 27458948] doi:10.1001/jama.2016.8465

Fenske NA, Cohen LE. The dermatologic exam. Emerg Med Clin North Am. 1985;3:643-58. [PMID: 2414092]

Jackson R. The importance of being visually literate. Observations on the art and science of making a morphological diagnosis in dermatology. Arch Dermatol. 1975;111:632-6. [PMID: 1130808]

Therapeutic Principles in Dermatology

du Vivier A. Tachyphylaxis to topically applied steroids. Arch Dermatol. 1976;112:1245-8. [PMID: 999300]

Miller JA, Munro DD. Topical corticosteroids: clinical pharmacology and therapeutic use. Drugs. 1980;19:119-34. [PMID: 7363838]

Smith ES, Fleischer AB Jr, Feldman SR. Nondermatologists are more likely than dermatologists to prescribe antifungal/corticosteroid products: an analysis of office visits for cutaneous fungal infections, 1990-1994. J Am Acad Dermatol. 1998;39:43-7. [PMID: 9674396]

Walsh P, Aeling JL, Huff L, Weston WL. Hypothalamus-pituitary-adrenal axis suppression by superpotent topical steroids. J Am Acad Dermatol. 1993;29:501-3. [PMID: 8349876]

Wilson R, Camacho F, Clark AR, Young T, Inabinet R, Yentzer BA, et al. Adherence to topical hydrocortisone 17-butyrate 0.1% in different vehicles in adults with atopic dermatitis [Letter]. J Am Acad Dermatol. 2009;60:166-8. [PMID: 19103374] doi:10.1016/j.jaad.2008.09.031

Common Rashes

Antonov D, Schliemann S, Elsner P. Hand dermatitis: a review of clinical features, prevention and treatment. Am J Clin Dermatol. 2015;16:257-70. [PMID: 25920436] doi:10.1007/s40257-015-0130-z

Atzmony L, Reiter O, Hodak E, Gdalevich M, Mimouni D. Treatments for cutaneous lichen planus: a systematic review and meta-analysis. Am J Clin Dermatol. 2016;17:11-22. [PMID: 26507510] doi:10.1007/s40257-015-0160-6

Borda LJ, Wikramanayake TC. Seborrheic dermatitis and dandruff: a comprehensive review. J Clin Investig Dermatol. 2015;3. [PMID: 27148560] doi:10.13188/2373-1044.1000019

Cassler NM, Burris AM, Nguyen JC. Asteatotic eczema in hypoesthetic skin: a case series. JAMA Dermatol. 2014;150:1088-90. [PMID: 25029204] doi:10.1001/jamadermatol.2014.394

Eichenfield LF, Tom WL, Berger TG, Krol A, Paller AS, Schwarzenberger K, et al. Guidelines of care for the management of atopic dermatitis: section 2. Management and treatment of atopic dermatitis with topical therapies. J Am Acad Dermatol. 2014;71:116-32. [PMID: 24813302] doi:10.1016/j.jaad.2014.03.023

Grover RW. Transient acantholytic dermatosis. Arch Dermatol. 1970;101:426-34. [PMID: 5440816]

Kouris A, Christodoulou C, Efstathiou V, Platsidaki E, Tsatovidou R, Torlidi-Kordera E, et al. Comparative study of quality of life and obsessive-compulsive tendencies in patients with chronic hand eczema and lichen simplex chronicus. Dermatitis. 2016;27:127-30. [PMID: 27172307] doi:10.1097/DER.0000000000000180

Metin A, Dilek N, Demirseven DD. Fungal infections of the folds (intertriginous areas). Clin Dermatol. 2015;33:437-47. [PMID: 26051058] doi:10.1016/j.clindermatol.2015.04.005

Nast A, Jacobs A, Rosumeck S, Werner RN. Efficacy and safety of systemic long-term treatments for moderate-to-severe psoriasis: a systematic review and meta-analysis. J Invest Dermatol. 2015;135:2641-8. [PMID: 26046458] doi:10.1038/jid.2015.206

Warshaw EM, Maibach HI, Taylor JS, Sasseville D, DeKoven JG, Zirwas MJ, et al. North American contact dermatitis group patch test results: 2011-2012. Dermatitis. 2015;26:49-59. [PMID: 25581671] doi:10.1097/DER.0000000000000097

Yim KM, Armstrong AW. Updates on cardiovascular comorbidities associated with psoriatic diseases: epidemiology and mechanisms. Rheumatol Int. 2017;37:97-105. [PMID: 27221457] doi:10.1007/s00296-016-3487-2

Disorders of Pigmentation

Alikhan A, Felsten LM, Daly M, Petronic-Rosic V. Vitiligo: a comprehensive overview Part I. Introduction, epidemiology, quality of life, diagnosis, differential diagnosis, associations, histopathology, etiology, and work-up. J Am Acad Dermatol. 2011;65:473-91. [PMID: 21839315] doi:10.1016/j.jaad.2010.11.061

Felsten LM, Alikhan A, Petronic-Rosic V. Vitiligo: a comprehensive overview Part II: treatment options and approach to treatment. J Am Acad Dermatol. 2011;65:493-514. [PMID: 21839316] doi:10.1016/j.jaad.2010.10.043

Sheth VM, Pandya AG. Melasma: a comprehensive update: part I. J Am Acad Dermatol. 2011;65:689-97; quiz 698. [PMID: 21920241] doi:10.1016/j.jaad.2010.12.046

Sheth VM, Pandya AG. Melasma: a comprehensive update: part II. J Am Acad Dermatol. 2011;65:699-714; quiz 715. [PMID: 21920242] doi:10.1016/j.jaad.2011.06.001

Silverberg JI, Silverberg NB. Clinical features of vitiligo associated with comorbid autoimmune disease: a prospective survey [Letter]. J Am Acad Dermatol. 2013;69:824-6. [PMID: 24124820] doi:10.1016/j.jaad.2013.04.050

Stollery N. Pigmentation disorders. Practitioner. 2015;259:30-1. [PMID: 26738250]

Drug Reactions

Calabrese LH, Michel BA, Bloch DA, Arend WP, Edworthy SM, Fauci AS, et al. The American College of Rheumatology 1990 criteria for the classification of hypersensitivity vasculitis. Arthritis Rheum. 1990;33:1108-13. [PMID: 2202309]

Monteiro AF, Rato M, Martins C. Drug-induced photosensitivity: Photoallergic and phototoxic reactions. Clin Dermatol. 2016;34:571-81. [PMID: 27638435] doi:10.1016/j.clindermatol.2016.05.006

Svensson CK, Cowen EW, Gaspari AA. Cutaneous drug reactions. Pharmacol Rev. 2001;53:357-79. [PMID: 11546834]

Acneiform Eruptions

Das S, Reynolds RV. Recent advances in acne pathogenesis: implications for therapy. Am J Clin Dermatol. 2014;15:479-88. [PMID: 25388823] doi:10.1007/s40257-014-0099-z

Mehdizadeh A, Hazen PG, Bechara FG, Zwingerman N, Moazenzadeh M, Bashash M, et al. Recurrence of hidradenitis suppurativa after surgical management: A systematic review and meta-analysis. J Am Acad Dermatol. 2015;73:S70-7. [PMID: 26470621] doi:10.1016/j.jaad.2015.07.044

Micheletti RG. An update on the diagnosis and treatment of hidradenitis suppurativa. Cutis. 2015;96:7-12. [PMID: 27051885]

Oge LK, Muncie HL, Phillips-Savoy AR. Rosacea: diagnosis and treatment. Am Fam Physician. 2015;92:187-96. [PMID: 26280139]

van Zuuren EJ, Fedorowicz Z. Interventions for rosacea: abridged updated Cochrane systematic review including GRADE assessments. Br J Dermatol. 2015;173:651-62. [PMID: 26099423] doi:10.1111/bjd.13956

Woodruff CM, Charlie AM, Leslie KS. Hidradenitis Suppurativa: a guide for the practicing physician. Mayo Clin Proc. 2015;90:1679-93. [PMID: 26653298] doi:10.1016/j.mayocp.2015.08.020

Zaenglein AL, Pathy AL, Schlosser BJ, Alikhan A, Baldwin HE, Berson DS, et al. Guidelines of care for the management of acne vulgaris. J Am Acad Dermatol. 2016;74:945-73.e33. [PMID: 26897386] doi:10.1016/j.jaad.2015.12.037

Common Skin Infections

Amin AN, Cerceo EA, Deitelzweig SB, Pile JC, Rosenberg DJ, Sherman BM. Hospitalist perspective on the treatment of skin and soft tissue infections. Mayo Clin Proc. 2014;89:1436-51. [PMID: 24974260] doi:10.1016/j.mayocp.2014.04.018

Blaise G, Nikkels AF, Hermanns-Lê T, Nikkels-Tassoudji N, Piérard GE. Corynebacterium-associated skin infections. Int J Dermatol. 2008;47:884-90. [PMID: 18937649] doi:10.1111/j.1365-4632.2008.03773.x

Chen X, Anstey AV, Bugert JJ. Molluscum contagiosum virus infection. Lancet Infect Dis. 2013;13:877-88. [PMID: 23972567] doi:10.1016/S1473-3099(13)70109-9

Chipolombwe J, Török ME, Mbelle N, Nyasulu P. Methicillin-resistant Staphylococcus aureus multiple sites surveillance: a systemic review of the literature. Infect Drug Resist. 2016;9:35-42. [PMID: 26929653] doi:10.2147/IDR.S95372

Huang SS, Rifas-Shiman SL, Warren DK, Fraser VJ, Climo MW, Wong ES, et al; Centers for Disease Control and Prevention Epicenters Program. Improving methicillin-resistant Staphylococcus aureus surveillance and reporting in intensive care units. J Infect Dis. 2007;195:330-8. [PMID: 17205470]

Laureano AC, Schwartz RA, Cohen PJ. Facial bacterial infections: folliculitis. Clin Dermatol. 2014;32:711-4. [PMID: 25441463] doi:10.1016/j.clindermatol.2014.02.009

Kaushik N, Pujalte GG, Reese ST. Superficial fungal infections. Prim Care. 2015;42:501-16. [PMID: 26612371] doi:10.1016/j.pop.2015.08.004

Kullar R, Vassallo A, Turkel S, Chopra T, Kaye KS, Dhar S. Degowning the controversies of contact precautions for methicillin-resistant Staphylococcus aureus: a review. Am J Infect Control. 2016;44:97-103. [PMID: 26375351] doi:10.1016/j.ajic.2015.08.003

Oh CC, Ko HC, Lee HY, Safdar N, Maki DG, Chlebicki MP. Antibiotic prophy-laxis for preventing recurrent cellulitis: a systematic review and meta-analysis. J Infect. 2014;69:26-34. [PMID: 24576824] doi:10.1016/j.jinf.2014.02.011

Stevens DL, Bisno AL, Chambers HF, Dellinger EP, Goldstein EJ, Gorbach SL, et al; Infectious Diseases Society of America. Practice guidelines for the diag-nosis and management of skin and soft tissue infections: 2014 update by the Infectious Diseases Society of America. Clin Infect Dis. 2014;59:e10-52. [PMID: 24973422] doi:10.1093/cid/ciu444

Pedrosa AF, Lisboa C, Gonçalves Rodrigues A. Malassezia infections: a medical conundrum. J Am Acad Dermatol. 2014;71:170-6. [PMID: 24569116] doi:10.1016/j.jaad.2013.12.022

Pereira LB. Impetigo - review. An Bras Dermatol. 2014;89:293-9. [PMID: 24770507]

Talan DA, Mower WR, Krishnadasan A, Abrahamian FM, Lovecchio F, Karras DJ, et al. Trimethoprim-Sulfamethoxazole versus placebo for uncompli-cated skin abscess. N Engl J Med. 2016;374:823-32. [PMID: 26962903] doi:10.1056/NEJMoa1507476

He L, Zhang D, Zhou M, Zhu C. Corticosteroids for preventing postherpetic neuralgia. Cochrane Database Syst Rev. 2008:CD005582. [PMID: 18254083] doi:10.1002/14651858.CD005582.pub2

Infestations

Dadabhoy I, Butts JF. Parasitic skin infections for primary care physicians. Prim Care. 2015;42:661-75. [PMID: 26612378] doi:10.1016/j.pop.2015.07.004

Drugs for sexually transmitted infections. Treat Guidel Med Lett. 2013;11:87-94; quiz 96. [PMID: 23979529]

Johnstone P, Strong M. Scabies. BMJ Clin Evid. 2014;2014. [PMID: 25544114]

Vasievich MP, Villarreal JD, Tomecki KJ. Got the travel bug? A review of com-mon infections, infestations, bites, and stings among returning travelers. Am J Clin Dermatol. 2016;17:451-462. [PMID: 27344566]

Bites and Stings

Foulke GT, Anderson BE. Bed bugs. Semin Cutan Med Surg. 2014;33:119-22. [PMID: 25577850]

Kang JK, Bhate C, Schwartz RA. Spiders in dermatology. Semin Cutan Med Surg. 2014;33:123-7. [PMID: 25577851]

Prickett KA, Ferringer TC. Helminths: a clinical review and update. Semin Cutan Med Surg. 2014;33:128-32. [PMID: 25577852]

Rosamilia LL. Scabies. Semin Cutan Med Surg. 2014;33:106-9. [PMID: 25577847]

Steen CJ, Carbonaro PA, Schwartz RA. Arthropods in dermatology. J Am Acad Dermatol. 2004;50:819-42, quiz 842-4. [PMID: 15153881]

Cuts, Scrapes, and Burns

Lloyd EC, Rodgers BC, Michener M, Williams MS. Outpatient burns: preven-tion and care. Am Fam Physician. 2012 Jan 1;85(1):25-32. Review. Erratum in: Am Fam Physician. 2012 Jun 15;85(12):1127. PubMed PMID: 22230304

Monseau AJ, Reed ZM, Langley KJ, Onks C. Sunburn, thermal, and chemical injuries to the skin. Prim Care. 2015;42:591-605. [PMID: 26612374] doi:10.1016/j.pop.2015.07.003

Singer AJ, Dagum AB. Current management of acute cutaneous wounds. N Engl J Med. 2008;359:1037-46. [PMID: 18768947] doi:10.1056/NEJMra0707253

Common Neoplasms

Davis J, Bordeaux J. Squamous cell carcinoma. JAMA Dermatol. 2013;149:1448. [PMID: 24352728] doi:10.1001/jamadermatol.2013.6947

Duffy K, Grossman D. The dysplastic nevus: from historical perspective to management in the modern era: part I. Historical, histologic, and clinical aspects. J Am Acad Dermatol. 2012;67:1.e1-16; quiz 17-8. [PMID: 22703915] doi:10.1016/j.jaad.2012.02.047

Higgins JC, Maher MH, Douglas MS. Diagnosing common benign skin tumors. Am Fam Physician. 2015;92:601-7. [PMID: 26447443]Wick MR. Cutaneous melanoma: A current overview. Semin Diagn Pathol. 2016;33:225-41. [PMID: 27229301] doi:10.1053/j.semdp.2016.04.007

Sobanko JF, Lynm C, Rosenbach M. Basal cell carcinoma. JAMA Dermatol. 2013;149:766. [PMID: 23783161] doi:10.1001/jamadermatol.2013.368

Wick MR, Gru AA. Metastatic melanoma: pathologic characterization, current treatment, and complications of therapy. Semin Diagn Pathol. 2016;33:204-18. [PMID: 27234321] doi:10.1053/j.semdp.2016.04.005

Wiznia LE, Federman DG. Treatment of Basal Cell Carcinoma in the Elderly: What nondermatologists need to know. Am J Med. 2016;129:655-60. [PMID: 27046242] doi:10.1016/j.amjmed.2016.03.003

Pruritus

Pereira MP, Kremer AE, Mettang T, Ständer S. Chronic pruritus in the absence of skin disease: pathophysiology, diagnosis and treatment. Am J Clin Dermatol. 2016;17:337-48. [PMID: 27216284] doi:10.1007/s40257-016-0198-0

Silverberg JI. Practice gaps in pruritus. Dermatol Clin. 2016;34:257-61. [PMID: 27363881] doi:10.1016/j.det.2016.02.008

Urticaria

Bernstein JA, Lang DM, Khan DA, Craig T, Dreyfus D, Hsieh F, et al. The diag-nosis and management of acute and chronic urticaria: 2014 update. J Allergy Clin Immunol. 2014;133:1270-7. [PMID: 24766875] doi:10.1016/j.jaci.2014.02.036

Fine LM, Bernstein JA. Guideline of chronic urticaria beyond. Allergy Asthma Immunol Res. 2016;8:396-403. [PMID: 27334777] doi:10.4168/aair.2016.8.5.396

Maurer M, Church MK, Marsland AM, Sussman G, Siebenhaar F, Vestergaard C, et al. Questions and answers in chronic urticaria: where do we stand and where do we go? J Eur Acad Dermatol Venereol. 2016;30 Suppl 5:7-15. [PMID: 27286498] doi:10.1111/jdv.13695

Staubach P, Zuberbier T, Vestergaard C, Siebenhaar F, Toubi E, Sussman G. Controversies and challenges in the management of chronic urticaria. J Eur Acad Dermatol Venereol. 2016;30 Suppl 5:16-24. [PMID: 27286499] doi:10.1111/jdv.13696

Autoimmune Bullous Diseases

Huang A, Madan RK, Levitt J. Future therapies for pemphigus vulgaris: rituxi-mab and beyond. J Am Acad Dermatol. 2016;74:746-53. [PMID: 26792592] doi:10.1016/j.jaad.2015.11.008

Jaleel T, Kwak Y, Sami N. Clinical approach to diffuse blisters. Med Clin North Am. 2015;99:1243-67, xii. [PMID: 26476251] doi:10.1016/j.mcna.2015.07.009

Krishnareddy S, Lewis SK, Green PH. Dermatitis herpetiformis: clinical pres-entations are independent of manifestations of celiac disease. Am J Clin Dermatol. 2014;15:51-6. [PMID: 24293087] doi:10.1007/s40257-013-0051-7

Stavropoulos PG, Soura E, Antoniou C. Drug-induced pemphigoid: a review of the literature. J Eur Acad Dermatol Venereol. 2014;28:1133-40. [PMID: 24404939] doi:10.1111/jdv.12366

Cutaneous Manifestations of Internal Disease

Balwani M, Desnick RJ. The porphyrias: advances in diagnosis and treatment. Blood. 2012;120:4496-504. [PMID: 22791288] doi:10.1182/blood-2012-05-423186

Braswell SF, Kostopoulos TC, Ortega-Loayza AG. Pathophysiology of pyoderma gangrenosum (PG): an updated review. J Am Acad Dermatol. 2015;73:691-8. [PMID: 26253362] doi:10.1016/j.jaad.2015.06.021

Cacoub P, Comarmond C, Domont F, Savey L, Saadoun D. Cryoglobulinemia vasculitis. Am J Med. 2015;128:950-5. [PMID: 25837517] doi:10.1016/j.amjmed.2015.02.017

Goeser MR, Laniosz V, Wetter DA. A practical approach to the diagnosis, evalua-tion, and management of cutaneous small-vessel vasculitis. Am J Clin Dermatol. 2014;15:299-306. [PMID: 24756249] doi:10.1007/s40257-014-0076-6

Grönhagen CM, Fored CM, Linder M, Granath F, Nyberg F. Subacute cutaneous lupus erythematosus and its association with drugs: a population-based matched case-control study of 234 patients in Sweden. Br J Dermatol. 2012;167:296-305. [PMID: 22458772] doi:10.1111/j.1365-2133.2012.10969.x

Iaccarino L, Ghirardello A, Bettio S, Zen M, Gatto M, Punzi L, et al. The clinical features, diagnosis and classification of dermatomyositis. J Autoimmun. 2014;48-49:122-7. [PMID: 24467910] doi:10.1016/j.jaut.2013.11.005

Kim SW, Kim MS, Lee JH, Son SJ, Park KY, Li K, et al. A clinicopathologic study of thirty cases of acquired perforating dermatosis in Korea. Ann Dermatol. 2014;26:162-71. [PMID: 24882969] doi:10.5021/ad.2014.26.2.162

Larson KN, Gagnon AL, Darling MD, Patterson JW, Cropley TG. Nephrogenic systemic fibrosis manifesting a decade after exposure to gadolinium. JAMA Dermatol. 2015;151:1117-20. [PMID: 26017458] doi:10.1001/jamaderma-tol.2015.0976

Molina-Ruiz AM, Cerroni L, Kutzner H, Requena L. Cutaneous deposits. Am J Dermatopathol. 2014;36:1-48. [PMID: 23249837] doi:10.1097/DAD.0b013e3182740122

Murphy-Chutorian B, Han G, Cohen SR. Dermatologic manifestations of dia-betes mellitus: a review. Endocrinol Metab Clin North Am. 2013;42:869-98. [PMID: 24286954] doi:10.1016/j.ecl.2013.07.004

Nigwekar SU, Kroshinsky D, Nazarian RM, Goverman J, Malhotra R, Jackson VA, et al. Calciphylaxis: risk factors, diagnosis, and treatment. Am J Kidney Dis. 2015;66:133-46. [PMID: 25960299] doi:10.1053/j.ajkd.2015.01.034

Petri M, Orbai AM, Alarcón GS, Gordon C, Merrill JT, Fortin PR, et al. Derivation and validation of the Systemic Lupus International Collaborating Clinics classification criteria for systemic lupus erythematosus. Arthritis Rheum. 2012;64:2677-86. [PMID: 22553077] doi:10.1002/art.34473

Reunala T, Salmi TT, Hervonen K, Laurila K, Kautiainen H, Collin P, et al. IgA antiepidermal transglutaminase antibodies in dermatitis herpetiformis: a significant but not complete response to a gluten-free diet treatment [Letter]. Br J Dermatol. 2015;172:1139-41. [PMID: 25196300] doi:10.1111/bjd.13387

Rochet NM, Chavan RN, Cappel MA, Wada DA, Gibson LE. Sweet syndrome: clinical presentation, associations, and response to treatment in 77 patients. J Am Acad Dermatol. 2013;69:557-64. [PMID: 23891394] doi:10.1016/j.jaad.2013.06.023

Rose TA Jr, Choi JW. Intravenous imaging contrast media complications: the basics that every clinician needs to know. Am J Med. 2015;128:943-9. [PMID: 25820169] doi:10.1016/j.amjmed.2015.02.018

Sharma A, Dhooria A, Aggarwal A, Rathi M, Chandran V. Connective tissue disorder-associated vasculitis. Curr Rheumatol Rep. 2016;18:31. [PMID: 27097818] doi:10.1007/s11926-016-0584-x

Thrash B, Patel M, Shah KR, Boland CR, Menter A. Cutaneous manifestations of gastrointestinal disease: part II. J Am Acad Dermatol. 2013;68:211.e1-33; quiz 244-6. [PMID: 23317981] doi:10.1016/j.jaad.2012.10.036

Tilstra JS, Lienesch DW. Rheumatoid nodules. Dermatol Clin. 2015;33:361-71. [PMID: 26143419] doi:10.1016/j.det.2015.03.004

Volkmann ER, Furst DE. Management of systemic sclerosis-related skin disease: a review of existing and experimental therapeutic approaches. Rheum Dis Clin North Am. 2015;41:399-417. [PMID: 26210126] doi:10.1016/j.rdc.2015.04.004

Werth VP. Clinical manifestations of cutaneous lupus erythematosus. Autoimmun Rev. 2005;4:296-302. [PMID: 15990077]

Dermatologic Emergencies

Darlenski R, Kazandjieva J, Tsankov N. Systemic drug reactions with skin involvement: Stevens-Johnson syndrome, toxic epidermal necrolysis, and DRESS. Clin Dermatol. 2015;33:538-41. [PMID: 26321400] doi:10.1016/j.clindermatol.2015.05.005

Law EH, Leung M. Corticosteroids in Stevens-Johnson syndrome/toxic epidermal necrolysis: current evidence and implications for future research. Ann Pharmacother. 2015;49:335-42. [PMID: 25406459] doi:10.1177/1060028014560012

Marzano AV, Borghi A, Cugno M. Adverse drug reactions and organ damage: the skin. Eur J Intern Med. 2016;28:17-24. [PMID: 26674736] doi:10.1016/j.ejim.2015.11.017

Mistry N, Gupta A, Alavi A, Sibbald RG. A review of the diagnosis and management of erythroderma (generalized red skin). Adv Skin Wound Care. 2015;28:228-36; quiz 237-8. [PMID: 25882661] doi:10.1097/01.ASW.0000463573.40637.73

Roujeau JC. Re-evaluation of 'drug-induced' erythema multiforme in the medical literature [Letter]. Br J Dermatol. 2016;175:650-1. [PMID: 27373787] doi:10.1111/bjd.14841

Wysong A, Venkatesan P. An approach to the patient with retiform purpura. Dermatol Ther. 2011;24:151-72. [PMID: 21410606] doi:10.1111/j.1529-8019.2011.01392.x

Hair Disorders

Housman E, Reynolds RV. Polycystic ovary syndrome: a review for dermatologists: part I. Diagnosis and manifestations. J Am Acad Dermatol. 2014;71:847.e1-847.e10; quiz 857-8. [PMID: 25437977] doi:10.1016/j.jaad.2014.05.007

Mubki T, Rudnicka L, Olszewska M, Shapiro J. Evaluation and diagnosis of the hair loss patient: part I. History and clinical examination. J Am Acad Dermatol. 2014;71:415.e1-415.e15. [PMID: 25128118] doi:10.1016/j.jaad.2014.04.070

Mubki T, Rudnicka L, Olszewska M, Shapiro J. Evaluation and diagnosis of the hair loss patient: part II. Trichoscopic and laboratory evaluations. J Am Acad Dermatol. 2014;71:431.e1-431.e11. [PMID: 25128119] doi:10.1016/j.jaad.2014.05.008

Schmidt TH, Shinkai K. Evidence-based approach to cutaneous hyperandrogenism in women. J Am Acad Dermatol. 2015;73:672-90. [PMID: 26138647] doi:10.1016/j.jaad.2015.05.026

Wendelin DS, Pope DN, Mallory SB. Hypertrichosis. J Am Acad Dermatol. 2003;48:161-79; quiz 180-1. [PMID: 12582385]

Nail Disorders

Cohen PR, Scher RK. Geriatric nail disorders: diagnosis and treatment. J Am Acad Dermatol. 1992;26:521-31. [PMID: 1597537]

Goydos JS, Shoen SL. Acral lentiginous melanoma. Cancer Treat Res. 2016;167:321-9. [PMID: 26601870] doi:10.1007/978-3-319-22539-5_14

Hay RJ, Baran R. Onychomycosis: a proposed revision of the clinical classification [Editorial]. J Am Acad Dermatol. 2011;65:1219-27. [PMID: 21501889] doi:10.1016/j.jaad.2010.09.730

Hinshaw MA, Rubin A. Inflammatory diseases of the nail unit. Semin Cutan Med Surg. 2015;34:109-16. [PMID: 26176289] doi:10.12788/j.sder.2015.0132

Holzberg M. Common nail disorders. Dermatol Clin. 2006;24:349-54. [PMID: 16798432]

Disorders of the Mucous Membranes

Dubach P, Caversaccio M. Images in clinical medicine. Amalgam tattoo. N Engl J Med. 2011;364:e29. [PMID: 21488760] doi:10.1056/NEJMicm1011669

Fernandes D, Ferrisse TM, Navarro CM, Massucato EM, Onofre MA, Bufalino A. Pigmented lesions on the mucosa: a wide range of diagnoses. Oral Surg Oral Med Oral Pathol Oral Radiol. 2015;119:374-8. [PMID: 25687194] doi:10.1016/j.oooo.2014.11.015

Stoopler ET, Sollecito TP. Oral mucosal diseases: evaluation and management. Med Clin North Am. 2014;98:1323-52. [PMID: 25443679] doi:10.1016/j.mcna.2014.08.006

Foot and Lower Leg Ulcers

Alavi A, Sibbald RG, Phillips TJ, Miller OF, Margolis DJ, Marston W, et al. What's new: Management of venous leg ulcers: approach to venous leg ulcers. J Am Acad Dermatol. 2016;74:627-40; quiz 641-2. [PMID: 26979354] doi:10.1016/j.jaad.2014.10.048

Alavi A, Sibbald RG, Phillips TJ, Miller OF, Margolis DJ, Marston W, et al. What's new: management of venous leg ulcers: treating venous leg ulcers. J Am Acad Dermatol. 2016;74:643-64; quiz 665-6. [PMID: 26979355] doi:10.1016/j.jaad.2015.03.059

Kirsner RS, Vivas AC. Lower-extremity ulcers: diagnosis and management. Br J Dermatol. 2015;173:379-90. [PMID: 26257052] doi:10.1111/bjd.13953

Morton LM, Phillips TJ. Wound healing and treating wounds: differential diagnosis and evaluation of chronic wounds. J Am Acad Dermatol. 2016;74:589-605; quiz 605-6. [PMID: 26979352] doi:10.1016/j.jaad.2015.08.068

O'Donnell TF Jr, Passman MA, Marston WA, Ennis WJ, Dalsing M, Kistner RL, et al; Society for Vascular Surgery. Management of venous leg ulcers: clinical practice guidelines of the Society for Vascular Surgery ® and the American Venous Forum. J Vasc Surg. 2014;60:3S-59S. [PMID: 24974070] doi:10.1016/j.jvs.2014.04.049

Powers JG, Higham C, Broussard K, Phillips TJ. Wound healing and treating wounds: chronic wound care and management. J Am Acad Dermatol. 2016;74:607-25; quiz 625-6. [PMID: 26979353] doi:10.1016/j.jaad.2015.08.070

Dermatologic Conditions of Pregnancy and Aging

Blume-Peytavi U, Kottner J, Sterry W, Hodin MW, Griffiths TW, Watson RE, et al. Age-associated skin conditions and diseases: current perspectives and future options. Gerontologist. 2016;56 Suppl 2:S230-42. [PMID: 26994263] doi:10.1093/geront/gnw003

Kroumpouzos G, Cohen LM. Dermatoses of pregnancy. J Am Acad Dermatol. 2001;45:1-19; quiz 19-22. [PMID: 11423829]

Murase JE, Heller MM, Butler DC. Safety of dermatologic medications in pregnancy and lactation: Part I. Pregnancy. J Am Acad Dermatol. 2014;70:401.e1-14; quiz 415. [PMID: 24528911] doi:10.1016/j.jaad.2013.09.010

Sheth VM, Pandya AG. Melasma: a comprehensive update: part I. J Am Acad Dermatol. 2011;65:689-97; quiz 698. [PMID: 21920241] doi:10.1016/j.jaad.2010.12.046

Tyler KH, Zirwas MJ. Pregnancy and dermatologic therapy. J Am Acad Dermatol. 2013;68:663-71. [PMID: 23182064] doi:10.1016/j.jaad.2012.09.034

Tobin DJ. Introduction to skin aging. J Tissue Viability. 2017;26:37-46. [PMID: 27020864] doi:10.1016/j.jtv.2016.03.002

Dermatology Self-Assessment Test

This self-assessment test contains one-best-answer multiple-choice questions. Please read these directions carefully before answering the questions. Answers, critiques, and bibliographies immediately follow these multiple-choice questions. The American College of Physicians (ACP) is accredited by the Accreditation Council for Continuing Medical Education (ACCME) to provide continuing medical education for physicians.

The American College of Physicians designates MKSAP 18 Dermatology for a maximum of 16 *AMA PRA Category 1 Credits*™. Physicians should claim only the credit commensurate with the extent of their participation in the activity.

Successful completion of the CME activity, which includes participation in the evaluation component, enables the participant to earn up to 16 medical knowledge MOC points in the American Board of Internal Medicine's Maintenance of Certification (MOC) program. It is the CME activity provider's responsibility to submit participant completion information to ACCME for the purpose of granting MOC credit.

Earn Instantaneous CME Credits or MOC Points Online

Print subscribers can enter their answers online to earn instantaneous CME credits or MOC points. You can submit your answers using online answer sheets that are provided at mksap.acponline.org, where a record of your MKSAP 18 credits will be available. To earn CME credits or to apply for MOC points, you need to answer all of the questions in a test and earn a score of at least 50% correct (number of correct answers divided by the total number of questions). Please note that if you are applying for MOC points, you must also enter your birth date and ABIM candidate number.

Take either of the following approaches:

- Use the printed answer sheet at the back of this book to record your answers. Go to mksap.acponline.org, access the appropriate online answer sheet, transcribe your answers, and submit your test for instantaneous CME credits or MOC points. There is no additional fee for this service.

- Go to mksap.acponline.org, access the appropriate online answer sheet, directly enter your answers, and submit your test for instantaneous CME credits or MOC points. There is no additional fee for this service.

Earn CME Credits or MOC Points by Mail or Fax

Pay a $20 processing fee per answer sheet and submit the printed answer sheet at the back of this book by mail or fax, as instructed on the answer sheet. Make sure you calculate your score and enter your birth date and ABIM candidate number, and fax the answer sheet to 215-351-2799 or mail the answer sheet to Member and Customer Service, American College of Physicians, 190 N. Independence Mall West, Philadelphia, PA 19106-1572, using the courtesy envelope provided in your MKSAP 18 slipcase. You will need your 10-digit order number and 8-digit ACP ID number, which are printed on your packing slip. Please allow 4 to 6 weeks for your score report to be emailed back to you. Be sure to include your email address for a response.

If you do not have a 10-digit order number and 8-digit ACP ID number, or if you need help creating a username and password to access the MKSAP 18 online answer sheets, go to mksap.acponline.org or email custserv@acponline.org.

CME credits and MOC points are available from the publication date of July 31, 2018, until July 31, 2021. You may submit your answer sheet or enter your answers online at any time during this period.

Directions

*Each of the numbered items is followed by lettered answers. Select the **ONE** lettered answer that is **BEST** in each case.*

Item 1

A 63-year-old man is evaluated for a skin eruption that is itchy and worsening for the past several weeks. Medical history is unremarkable, and he takes no medications.

On physical examination, vital signs are normal. There are tense bullae on an erythematous base and scattered erosions on the trunk and extremities.

Which of the following is the most appropriate diagnostic test to perform next?

(A) Biopsy of lesional skin for direct immunofluorescence

(B) Biopsy of lesional skin for histology

(C) Biopsy of lesional skin for histology and perilesional skin for direct immunofluorescence

(D) Biopsy of perilesional skin for histology and direct immunofluorescence

Item 2

A 25-year-old man is evaluated for recurrent skin eruption with oval lesions on the chest and upper back, which are occasionally itchy. The lesions began in late spring and worsened over the summer. Medical history is unremarkable, and he takes no medications.

On physical examination, vital signs are normal. Skin findings on the chest are shown.

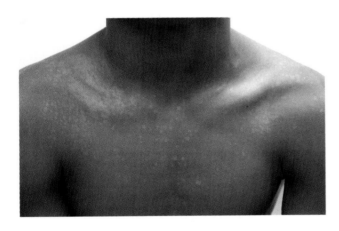

Extremities and feet are unaffected.

Which of the following is the most likely diagnosis?

(A) *Candida albicans* infection

(B) Erythrasma

(C) Pityriasis versicolor

(D) Tinea corporis

Item 3

A 32-year-old man is evaluated for an intermittent pruritic rash of 8 years' duration. Medical history is significant for mild persistent asthma. His only medications are an albuterol inhaler and an inhaled glucocorticoid.

On physical examination, vital signs are normal. There is mild xerosis with erythematous plaques on the bilateral antecubital fossae, volar wrists, and anterior lower legs. Lichenification is present on the dorsal hands. Linear excoriations are found within many of the erythematous plaques on the arms.

Which of the following is the most appropriate treatment?

(A) Oral cephalexin

(B) Oral prednisone

(C) Topical glucocorticoids

(D) Topical ketoconazole

(E) Topical mupirocin

Item 4

A 43-year-old woman is evaluated for painful wheals on the upper legs and back that have been present for 2 weeks. Individual lesions resolve with bruising in 3 to 4 days. The patient also reports some associated joint pain, particularly of the small joints in her hands. Medical history is unremarkable, and she takes no medications.

On physical examination, vital signs are normal. There are polycyclic edematous plaques on the back and upper legs. The remainder of the examination, including joint examination, is normal.

Which of the following is the most appropriate management?

(A) Epicutaneous patch testing

(B) Ice cube provocation test

(C) Oral prednisone

(D) Skin biopsies

(E) Topical triamcinolone

Item 5

A 25-year-old man is evaluated for asymptomatic skin changes on his thighs. He has a 1-year history of plaque psoriasis on his elbows and knees for which he uses triamcinolone cream and calcipotriene cream. The patient has been applying these medications to the entire leg and arm. Prior to treatment, the patient's thighs were normal. He is otherwise in good health.

On physical examination, vital signs are normal. A thigh lesion is shown (see top of next page).

Which of the following is the most appropriate treatment for the patient's thighs?

(A) Add clobetasol cream

(B) Add terbinafine cream

(C) Discontinue calcipotriene cream

(D) Discontinue triamcinolone cream

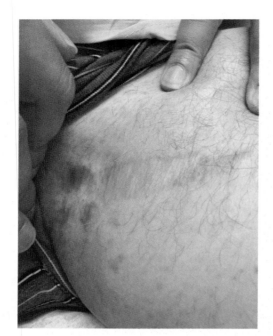

ITEM 5

Item 6

A 35-year-old woman is evaluated for severe pain on the left side of the chest for 1 week followed by increased redness and the development of small blisters. Medical history is significant for rheumatoid arthritis. Medications are naproxen as needed, methotrexate folic acid, and an oral contraceptive.

On physical examination, skin findings are shown.

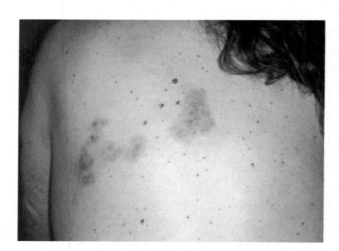

The remainder of the examination is unremarkable.

Which of the following is the most likely diagnosis?

(A) Chicken pox (varicella)
(B) Eczema herpeticum
(C) Herpes simplex virus
(D) Herpes zoster

Item 7

A 58-year-old woman was evaluated for dark brown pigmentation on her thumb nail. She noticed it was getting darker and wider. She is otherwise healthy and takes no medications.

On physical examination, vital signs are normal. The other nails are uninvolved. Nail findings are shown.

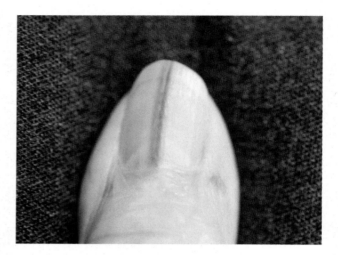

The remainder of the examination is normal.

Which of the following is the most likely diagnosis?

(A) Lichen planus
(B) Melanonychia
(C) Normal aging
(D) Onychomycosis

Item 8

A 25-year-old woman is evaluated for finger pain that began approximately 6 weeks ago. She works as a hairdresser. She is otherwise healthy and takes no medications.

On physical examination, vital signs are normal. Skin findings reveal ragged cuticles on most of her digits. On the third digit of the left hand, the nail fold is tender. Skin and nail findings are shown (see top of next page).

Which of the following is the most likely cause of this patient's tender finger lesion?

(A) Acute paronychia
(B) Chronic paronychia
(C) Onychomycosis
(D) Psoriasis

Item 9

A 60-year-old woman is evaluated for follow-up treatment of long-standing psoriasis. Medical history is significant for hypertension and hypercholesterolemia. Family history includes multiple family members with psoriasis. She has no joint symptoms, and her medications are atenolol and simvastatin.

On physical examination, vital signs are normal. There is no joint swelling.

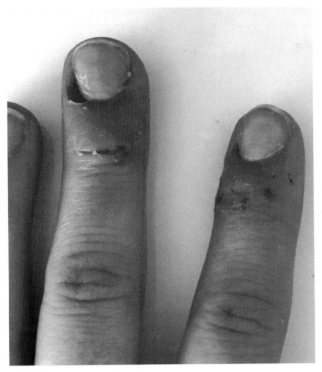

ITEM 8

She has a total of 30% body surface area involvement with psoriasis without nail involvement.

Which of the following is the most appropriate treatment?

(A) Methotrexate
(B) Oral prednisone
(C) Tacrolimus ointment
(D) Topical calcitriol

Item 10

A 27-year-old woman is evaluated for itchy bumps on her abdomen. The patient is pregnant and in her third trimester. She was diagnosed with pruritic urticarial papules and plaques of pregnancy (PUPPP).

On physical examination, vital signs are normal. Skin findings are shown.

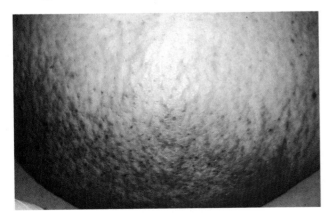

Which of the following is the most appropriate treatment?

(A) Early delivery
(B) Topical glucocorticoids
(C) Topical imiquimod
(D) Ursodeoxycholic acid

Item 11

A 65-year-old man is evaluated in the ICU for a rash limited to his back that was first noticed this morning. He was admitted to the ICU for hospital-acquired pneumonia following hip replacement surgery 3 days ago. Because of deteriorating respiratory function, he was intubated and placed on mechanical ventilation. His current medications are fentanyl and piperacillin-tazobactam.

On physical examination, temperature is 38.3 °C (100.9 °F), blood pressure is 110/60 mm Hg, pulse rate is 115/min, and respiration rate is 18/min (ventilator set rate is 14/min). Pulmonary examination reveals diffuse crackles. Skin findings are shown.

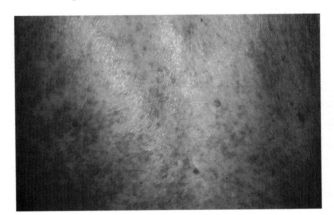

Which of the following is the most likely diagnosis?

(A) Acute generalized exanthematous pustulosis
(B) *Candida albicans* infection
(C) Miliaria
(D) Povidone iodine contact dermatitis

Item 12

An 18-year-old man is evaluated for a 6-month history of acne on his face, chest, and upper back. He is otherwise in good health. He has been treated with doxycycline, tretinoin cream, and topical clindamycin lotion for 6 months with minimal improvement.

On physical examination, vital signs are normal. Skin findings are shown (see top of next page).

The remainder of the examination is unremarkable.

Which of the following is the most appropriate treatment?

(A) Add topical benzoyl peroxide gel
(B) Add topical dapsone
(C) Change doxycycline to trimethoprim-sulfamethoxazole
(D) Discontinue current treatment and start oral isotretinoin
(E) Start oral prednisone

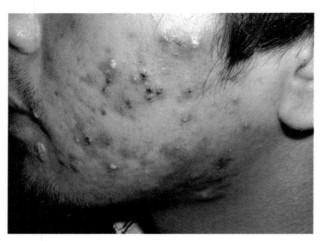

ITEM 12

Item 13

A 62-year-old woman is evaluated for a "sun allergy," manifesting as a rash on her scalp, eyelids, upper back, and knuckles. This started 2 years ago, but is less pronounced over the winter months. Medical history is unremarkable. Her only medication is hydrocortisone cream.

On physical examination, vital signs are normal. Pink-violet edematous macules are present on the eyelids. The scalp has pink-violet diffuse scaly macules with some thinning of the hair. There is a poikilodermatous pink scaly plaque on the upper back and posterior neck. The metacarpophalangeal and proximal interphalangeal joints have pink-violet flat-topped papules on their dorsal surface. There are dilated periungual capillary loops on each finger, and all 10 cuticles are dystrophic. There are no swollen joints, no abnormalities on strength testing, and no oral ulcerations.

Laboratory studies show antinuclear antibody titer of 1:640. All other laboratory values, including creatine kinase, aldolase, aspartate aminotransferase, and gamma-glutamyl transferase, are normal.

Which of the following is the most likely diagnosis?

(A) Amyopathic dermatomyositis
(B) Mixed connective tissue disease
(C) Polymorphus light eruption
(D) Systemic lupus erythematosus

Item 14

A 42-year-old man reported to the emergency department yesterday with a painful blistering rash, mouth sores, and eye pain. He started taking allopurinol 10 days ago for gout. He developed flu-like symptoms and skin pain 2 days ago. He was admitted last night with a diagnosis of toxic epidermal necrolysis. His allopurinol was discontinued, fluid and electrolyte resuscitation was initiated, and he was started on intravenous glucocorticoids.

On physical examination, heart rate is 95/min; the remaining vital signs are normal. Oxygen saturation is 98%

breathing ambient air. The patient appears to be in pain. Extensive oral ulcerations are present but do not extend across the vermillion border. Large sheets of his skin are denuding, affecting more than 35% of his body surface area. His conjunctivae are injected and red. He has generalized lymphadenopathy.

Laboratory studies:

Aspartate aminotransferase	92 IU/L
Alanine aminotransferase	87 IU/L
Bicarbonate	22 mEq/L (22 mmol/L)
Blood urea nitrogen	27 mg/dL (9.6 mmol/L)
Plasma glucose	210 mg/dL (11.6 mmol/L)

Which of the following factors has the greatest impact on this patient's prognosis?

(A) Age
(B) Heart rate
(C) Affected body surface area
(D) Plasma glucose level
(E) Serum bicarbonate level

Item 15

A 25-year-old woman is evaluated for pruritic lesions on the legs and in the groin area that first appeared several months ago. The patient is otherwise in good health and takes no medications.

On physical examination, vital signs are normal. Skin findings are shown.

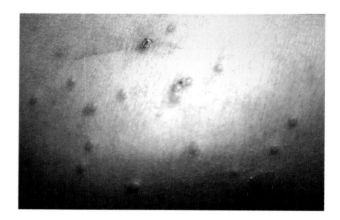

Which of the following is the most likely diagnosis?

(A) Condylomata acuminata
(B) Herpes simplex virus infection
(C) Molluscum contagiosum infection
(D) Seborrheic keratoses

Item 16

A 65-year-old man is evaluated for pruritic hive-like lesions on the trunk and upper legs that are worsening and starting to blister. He has no oral or mucous membrane involvement. He has no significant medical history and takes no medications.

CONT.

On physical examination, vital signs are normal. Skin findings are shown.

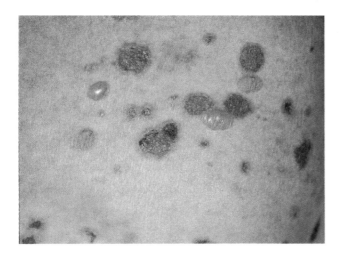

Which of the following is the most likely diagnosis?

(A) Bullous pemphigoid
(B) Dermatitis herpetiformis
(C) Pemphigus foliaceus
(D) Pemphigus vulgaris

Item 17

A 24-year-old woman is evaluated for a 4-day history of a worsening pruritic rash on the chin. She is a kindergarten teacher. Medical history is unremarkable, and she takes no medications.

On physical examination, vital signs are normal. Skin findings are shown.

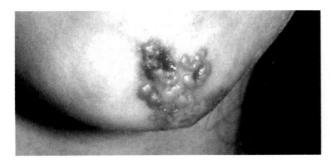

Which of the following is the most appropriate treatment?

(A) Oral doxycycline
(B) Topical hydrocortisone
(C) Topical mupirocin
(D) Topical neomycin/polymyxin B/bacitracin

Item 18

A 68-year-old man is evaluated for 3 weeks of painful "blood blisters" on his legs and feet. He has noticed burning and tingling of his right foot and three toes over the last 2 weeks. Medical history is significant for rheumatoid arthritis for 22 years. He is a 60-pack-year cigarette smoker. He occasionally uses cocaine. He denies fever, chills, and night sweats, anorexia, or weight loss. Medications are hydroxychloroquine and methotrexate.

On physical examination, temperature is 36.6 °C (97.8 °F), blood pressure is 134/79 mm Hg, and pulse rate is 82/min. Changes typical of destructive rheumatoid arthritis are apparent in the hands, wrists, elbows, and feet. Palpable purpura is present over the legs and ankles. Periungual purpura is present on three fingers. There is reduced sensitivity to pinprick and fine touch over the lateral right foot and dorsal lateral three toes. There is no murmur on his cardiac examination.

Laboratory studies show substantially elevated rheumatoid factor titer. Antinuclear antibody titer is less than 1:40. ANCA screen is negative. Complement levels are normal. Results of kidney and liver chemistry tests are normal.

Which of the following is the most likely cause of the patient's skin findings?

(A) Actinic purpura
(B) Illicit drug use
(C) Infective endocarditis
(D) Rheumatoid vasculitis

Item 19

A 38-year-old woman is evaluated for a new rash on the chest, arms, and back. It appeared 3 weeks ago. It burns and itches and has not responded to over-the-counter hydrocortisone cream. The rash substantially worsened following a vacation at the beach. Medical history is significant for psoriasis vulgaris with involvement of the elbows and knees with psoriatic arthritis for 3 years' duration. Her only medication is adalimumab, which she started 2 months ago. It cleared her elbows and knees in about 3 weeks.

On physical examination, vital signs are normal. Representative skin findings are shown.

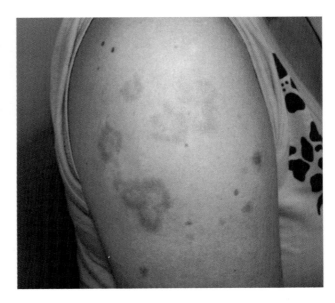

There is no facial rash, hair loss, rash in the ears, oral ulcerations, or swollen joints.

Laboratory studies show antinuclear antibody titer less than 1:40.

Which of the following is the most appropriate treatment for this patient?

(A) Add hydroxychloroquine

(B) Add methotrexate

(C) Add oral prednisone taper

(D) Discontinue adalimumab

Item 20

A 71-year-old man is evaluated for erythema and tenderness of the left lower leg for 1 week's duration. This is the second similar episode of the left lower leg. The last episode was 2 months ago. He was previously treated successfully with antibiotics.

On physical examination, temperature is 38.1 °C (100.6 °F), blood pressure is 125/75 mm Hg, respiration rate is 16/min, and pulse rate is 85/min. There is a well-demarcated, warm and tender erythematous patch on the anterior lower left leg extending from dorsal foot to mid shin. There is tissue maceration and fissuring between second and third toe spaces bilaterally. The remainder of the physical examination is normal.

In addition to initiating antibiotic therapy, which of the following is the most appropriate management?

(A) Following acute therapy, start prophylactic antibiotics

(B) Obtain blood cultures

(C) Obtain skin punch biopsy

(D) Staphylococcal decolonization with intranasal mupirocin

(E) Treat the interdigital intertrigo

Item 21

An 82-year-old woman is evaluated for a spot on her left cheek. Six months ago, she was diagnosed with an actinic keratosis. This lesion was treated with cryotherapy two times; however, the lesion is still persistent. On palpation, it is indurated. The lesion is shown.

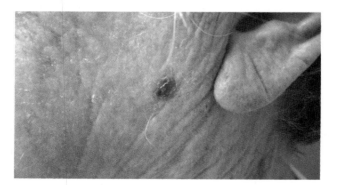

Which of the following is the most appropriate next step in management?

(A) Cryotherapy

(B) Biopsy

(C) Topical imiquimod

(D) Wide local excision

Item 22

A 44-year-old man is evaluated for a new lesion on the side of his face. It has been present for several months and is asymptomatic. When he shaves he cuts it, and it starts bleeding. He is otherwise healthy and takes no medications.

On physical examination, vital signs are normal. Skin findings are shown.

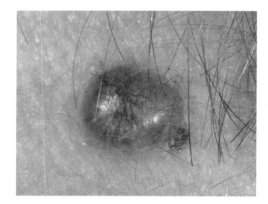

The remainder of the examination is normal.

Which of the following is the mostly likely diagnosis?

(A) Basal cell carcinoma

(B) Dermal nevus

(C) Keratoacanthoma

(D) Nodular melanoma

(E) Squamous cell carcinoma

Item 23

A 54-year-old woman is evaluated for lumps that have appeared around the outside of her nostrils over the last 5 months. She has had arthralgias for the past 6 months. She takes no medications.

On physical examination, vital signs are normal. Skin findings are shown (see top of next page).

The remainder of the skin examination is normal.

Skin biopsy shows granulomas without necrosis or lymphocytic infiltration in the dermis.

Which of the following is the most likely diagnosis?

(A) Lepromatous leprosy

(B) Lupus pernio (cutaneous sarcoidosis)

(C) Lupus vulgaris (cutaneous tuberculosis)

(D) Systemic lupus erythematosus

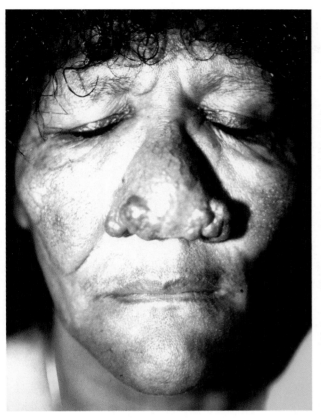

ITEM 23

Item 24

A 63-year-old woman is evaluated for a lesion on her nose that is slowly enlarging and nonhealing. She is otherwise in good health and takes no medications.

On physical examination, vital signs are normal. The skin examination demonstrates a 0.8 × 0.6-cm pearly ulcerated papule with arborizing telangiectasias. The remainder of the examination is normal.

Biopsy of the lesion demonstrates basal cell carcinoma with high-risk micronodular and infiltrative histologic features.

Which of the following is the most appropriate treatment of this lesion?

(A) Cryotherapy
(B) Electrodesiccation and curettage
(C) Mohs micrographic surgery
(D) Topical 5-fluorouracil
(E) Vismodegib

Item 25

A 23-year-old woman is evaluated in the emergency department. Four days ago she developed a cold sore on her lower lip. This was followed by the development of painful sores throughout her mouth. The next day she developed a rash on her hands, arms, legs, and face, and eventually on her palms and soles. She takes no medications.

On physical examination, vital signs are normal. The patient has pain in her mouth, but is in no acute distress. Erosions are present in the oropharynx. There are five distinct monomorphic clustered 2- to 3-mm erosions on the left lower lip. Skin findings on the palm are shown.

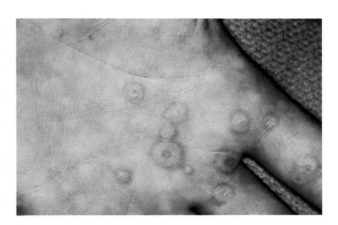

The arms and face have lesions similar to those on the palm. There is no sloughing of the skin when shearing force is applied. The lesions affect about 7% body surface area. There is no corneal injection or tearing and no genital erosion or ulceration.

Which of the following is the most likely diagnosis?

(A) Disseminated gonococcemia
(B) Erythema multiforme major
(C) Stevens-Johnson syndrome
(D) Toxic epidermal necrolysis

Item 26

An 89-year-old woman is evaluated in the office for an annual examination. She has dementia. She was brought to the appointment by her caregiver who noted "bruises" on her arms. The patient says she does not remember what happened.

On physical examination, vital signs are normal. Skin findings are shown.

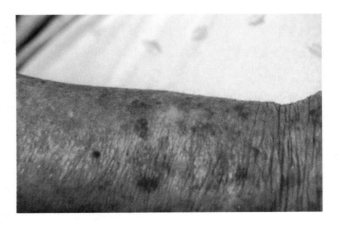

Which is the following is the most appropriate management?

(A) Biopsy the lesion
(B) Call adult protective services
(C) Obtain coagulation studies
(D) Prescribe triamcinolone ointment
(E) No intervention needed

Item 27

A 68-year-old woman is evaluated for a 12-month history of swelling of both of her lower legs. Over the past 4 months, there was worsening edema, erythema, scaling, and itching of the lower legs. She has not used any prescription or over-the-counter topical medications or emollients. Medical history is significant for hypertension and type 2 diabetes mellitus. Medications are lisinopril, amlodipine, hydrochlorothiazide, and metformin.

On physical examination, vital signs are normal. BMI is 32. Skin findings are shown.

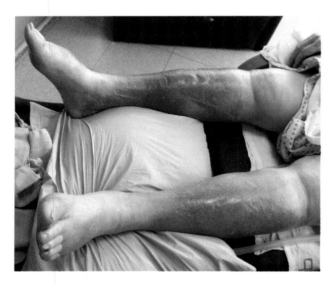

There is no tenderness. Pedal pulses are strong bilaterally.

Laboratory studies, including leukocyte count, are within normal range.

Which of the following is the most likely diagnosis?

(A) Allergic contact dermatitis
(B) Cellulitis
(C) Leukocytoclastic vasculitis
(D) Psoriasis
(E) Stasis dermatitis

Item 28

A 40-year-old man is evaluated for a firm, flesh-colored lesion that has been growing on the back for several months. Foul-smelling material can be expressed from the lesion. The patient is bothered by the periodic drainage. He is otherwise healthy and takes no medications.

On physical examination, vital signs are normal. There is a 3-cm subepidermal nodule with a central punctum on the upper back. There is no erythema or warmth of surrounding skin.

Which of the following is the most appropriate treatment for this patient?

(A) Excision
(B) Incision
(C) Incision and drainage
(D) Oral antibiotics

Item 29

A 27-year-old woman is evaluated in the office for generalized hair loss. She has not had any similar episodes previously. The patient is 3 months postpartum and does not take any medications.

On physical examination, vital signs are normal. The scalp skin itself appears normal with no erythema, scale, or scarring. The hair shafts are normal as well. As the hair was combed through, several hairs fell out at the root. The remainder of the examination is unremarkable.

Which of the following is the most appropriate management?

(A) Intralesional glucocorticoids
(B) Oral finasteride
(C) Topical minoxidil
(D) Reassurance

Item 30

A 24-year-old woman is evaluated for a rash on her face for several months' duration. It is asymptomatic but has gotten worse over the summer. She washes her face with soap and water twice daily and has recently changed soaps. Previously her skin was normal. She is otherwise healthy. Her only medication is an oral contraceptive pill, which she started 3 months ago.

On physical examination, vital signs are normal. Skin findings are shown.

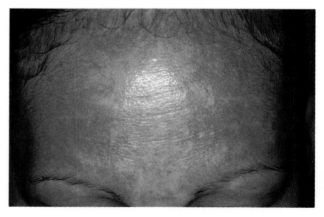

Which of the following is the most likely diagnosis?

(A) Irritant contact dermatitis
(B) Melasma

(C)   Morbilliform drug eruption

(D)   Postinflammatory hyperpigmentation

Item 31

A 45-year-old man is evaluated for an explosive onset of a rash with greasy scale on the chin, nasolabial folds, scalp, and chest that is getting worse. He has never had this condition before. He has tried over-the-counter selenium sulfide shampoo and hydrocortisone cream without success. Medical history is otherwise unremarkable, and he takes no additional medications.

On physical examination, vital signs are normal. Skin findings are shown.

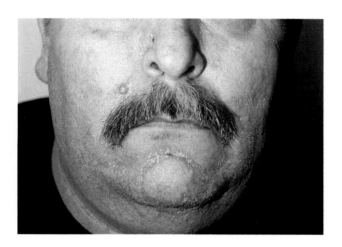

Which of the following is the most appropriate diagnostic test to perform next?

(A)   Fasting blood glucose

(B)   Fasting lipid panel

(C)   Hepatitis C testing

(D)   HIV testing

Item 32

A 60-year-old man is evaluated for dry skin and a pruritic rash of 6 months' duration. He is a farmer and has extensive exposure to the sun. The rash is transient, occurring most frequently during the winter and spring when his skin is dry, and is worsened by heat and sweating during the summer. The patient is otherwise well, has no other medical problems, and takes no medications.

On physical examination, vital signs are normal. Skin findings on the upper torso are shown (see top of next column).

The arms, legs, face, and mucous membranes are unaffected. The remainder of the examination is unremarkable.

Which of the following is the most likely diagnosis?

(A)   Allergic contact dermatitis

(B)   Atopic dermatitis

(C)   Lichen planus

(D)   Transient acantholytic dermatosis

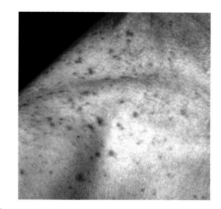

ITEM 32

Item 33

A 30-year-old woman is evaluated for a dark spot on the lower lip for several months' duration. Medical history is unremarkable, and she takes no medications.

On physical examination, vital signs are normal. There is 2 × 3-mm perfectly round, well-circumscribed brown-to-black macule on the lower mucosal lip. Oral mucosa is otherwise normal.

Which of the following is the most likely diagnosis?

(A)   Actinic cheilitis

(B)   Amalgam tattoo

(C)   Melanoma in-situ

(D)   Melanotic macule

Item 34

A 47-year-old woman is evaluated for her skin "turning to leather." She notes that she had originally developed an itchy pink rash on the skin over her forearms, elbows, and upper arms. Eventually the rash turned to thick hard skin. She has similar skin findings in the area of her waistband. She denies symptoms of Raynaud phenomenon.

On physical examination, vital signs are normal. Skin findings are shown.

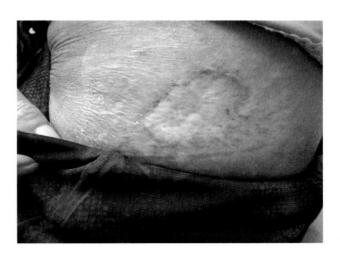

There are no changes over the face or lips.

Which of the following is the most likely diagnosis?

(A) Diffuse cutaneous systemic sclerosis
(B) Limited cutaneous systemic sclerosis (CREST)
(C) Localized scleroderma (morphea)
(D) Scleredema
(E) Scleromyxedema

Item 35

A 69-year-old man is evaluated for a new lesion behind his ear. It is asymptomatic. His wife noted that it first appeared last year and is growing. The patient is a farmer and has had many sunburns over his lifetime. He has no other medical problems and takes no medications.

On physical examination, vital signs are normal. Skin findings are shown.

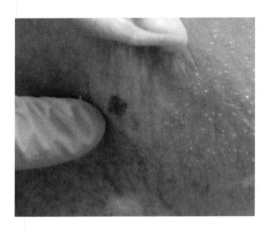

Which of the following is the most likely diagnosis?

(A) Junctional melanocytic nevus
(B) Melanoma in situ, lentigo maligna
(C) Nodular melanoma
(D) Solar lentigo

Item 36

A 30-year-old woman is evaluated for an acne flare on her face. She is 12 weeks pregnant. When she was younger, she was on a course of isotretinoin, and it cleared her acne. She is otherwise in good health and has not been on any medications other than a prenatal vitamin since she became pregnant.

On physical examination, her vital signs are normal. Skin findings are shown (see top of next column).

The remainder of the examination is normal.

Which of the following is the most appropriate treatment for the patient?

(A) Oral doxycycline
(B) Oral isotretinoin
(C) Oral spironolactone
(D) Topical erythromycin
(E) Topical tazarotene

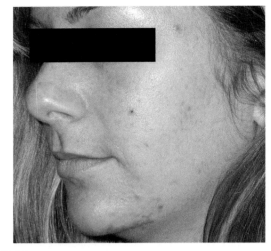

ITEM 36

Item 37

A 35-year-old man is evaluated after 3 weeks of worsening sinus pain and congestion. He was prescribed amoxicillin-clavulanate. Four days into his treatment, he developed a rash.

On physical examination, vital signs are normal. Skin findings are shown.

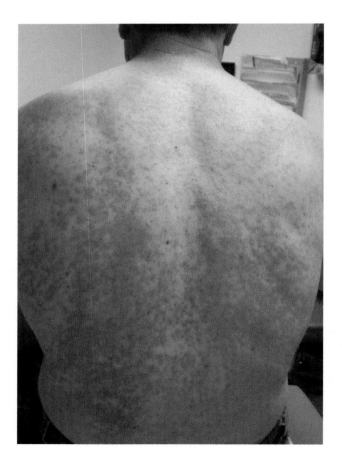

There is purulent postnasal drainage noted in the oropharynx. There are no oral, genital, or corneal erosions. There are no findings on the palms, soles, wrists, or ankles. The patient has no skin pain, mouth ulcers, or dysuria. His conjunctivae are injected, but there is no ocular pain.

Laboratory studies show peripheral eosinophilia. Other laboratory values, including creatinine, blood urea nitrogen, and liver chemistry tests, are unremarkable.

Which of the following is the most likely diagnosis?

(A) Drug reaction with eosinophilia and systemic symptoms (DRESS)
(B) Morbilliform drug reaction
(C) Stevens-Johnson syndrome
(D) Viral exanthem

Item 38

A 20-year-old woman is evaluated for white spots on her eyelids, hands, elbows, and knees for several months' duration. There was no previous rash. She is otherwise healthy and takes no medications.

On physical examination, vital signs are normal. Representative skin findings on the eyelids are shown.

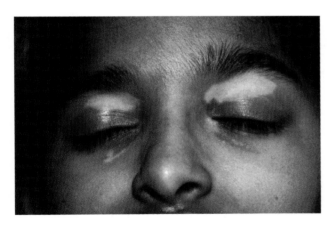

The remainder of the examination is normal.

Which of the following is the most likely diagnosis?

(A) Pityriasis alba
(B) Tinea versicolor
(C) Tuberous sclerosis
(D) Vitiligo

Item 39

A 36-year-old woman is evaluated for a 6-year history of tender, foul-smelling, draining nodules in the inguinal folds. She has had occasional nodules in the axillae. She has taken multiple courses of oral clindamycin with only temporary improvement. She has a 14-pack-year smoking history. Medical history is otherwise unremarkable.

On physical examination, vital signs are normal. BMI is 34. There are tender nodules, draining sinus tracts, and comedones in the inguinal folds. Scarring is present in

right and left axillae. Additional inguinal skin findings are shown.

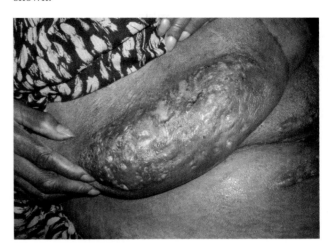

Which of the following is the most likely diagnosis?

(A) Carbuncles
(B) Chancroid
(C) Epidermal inclusion cysts
(D) Hidradenitis suppurativa

Item 40

A 34-year-old woman is evaluated for a painful leg ulceration on her left anterior shin. The patient notes that the lesion began 2 weeks ago as a red papule after hitting her leg on her stairs at home. The initial papule expanded and ulcerated over the past 2 weeks. Medical history is significant for ulcerative colitis. Her only medication is mesalamine.

On physical examination, vital signs are normal. Skin findings are shown.

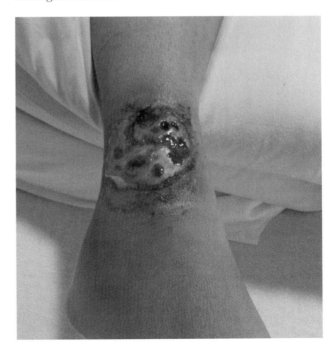

Which of the following is the most likely diagnosis?

(A) Acrodermatitis enteropathica

(B) Calciphylaxis

(C) Pyoderma gangrenosum

(D) Venous stasis ulcer

Item 41

A 64-year-old man is evaluated for treatment of extensive psoriasis on 20% body surface area, covering the knees, elbows, scalp, and trunk. Medical history is otherwise unremarkable, and he takes no medications.

On physical examination, vital signs are normal. He has no fingernail changes and no arthritis. Skin findings are shown.

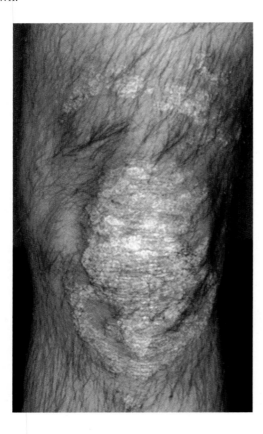

Which of the following forms of phototherapy is the most appropriate initial treatment?

(A) Narrowband ultraviolet B (UVB) phototherapy

(B) Photodynamic therapy

(C) Psoralen plus ultraviolet A (PUVA) photochemotherapy

(D) Retinoid plus PUVA (RePUVA) photochemotherapy

(E) Ultraviolet A (UVA) phototherapy

 ## Item 42

A 44-year-old woman is evaluated for painful nodules, ulcers, and skin changes on the lower legs of 2 years' duration. She takes no medications.

On physical examination, vital signs are normal. Tender subcutaneous nodules, stellate ulcerations, and livido reticularis are evenly distributed bilaterally over her lower legs. The dorsalis pedis and posterior tibial pulses are normal. There are no varicosities present on the legs. The remainder of the examination is normal.

Laboratory studies show an erythrocyte sedimentation rate of 65 mm/h. Skin biopsy shows vasculitis of a mid-sized arteriole in the subcutis. ANCA screen is negative. Antinuclear antibodies titer is 1:40. C3 and C4 values are normal. Rheumatoid factor and hepatitis B and C tests are negative. Stool is negative for occult blood, and urinalysis is unremarkable.

Which of the following is the most likely diagnosis?

(A) Granulomatosis with polyangiitis

(B) Leukocytoclastic vasculitis

(C) Microscopic polyangiitis

(D) Polyarteritis nodosa

(E) Takayasu arteritis

Item 43

A 23-year-old woman is evaluated for 2 weeks of painful lumps on her legs. The lumps persist for several days and make it difficult for her to go to work as a waitress. She is a college student in Ohio where she has lived her whole life. She has not traveled outside of the state for the last 2 years. She has no swollen or painful joints. She denies abdominal pain, diarrhea, weight loss, night sweats, and fever. She is sexually active with one partner for the past 2 years. She is taking oral contraceptive pills.

On physical examination, vital signs are normal. There are tender faint pink-brown nodules on the shins bilaterally. The throat and tonsils appear normal. There is no joint swelling.

Pregnancy test is negative. Complete blood count, erythrocyte sedimentation rate, and antistreptolysin O titers are pending.

Barrier contraceptive methods are recommended in lieu of oral contraceptives.

Which of the following tests should be done next?

(A) Biopsy of a nodule

(B) Chest radiography

(C) Colonoscopy

(D) Nucleic acid amplification testing for gonorrhea

Item 44

A 19-year-old man is evaluated for 4 to 5 months of persistent itching, thickening of the skin, and odor of the feet. He also has hyperhidrosis of the palms and soles. Medical history is otherwise unremarkable, and he takes no medications.

On physical examination, vital signs are normal. Skin findings are shown (see top of next page).

There is substantial odor of the feet. There are no changes to the toenails. The axillae and groin are unremarkable.

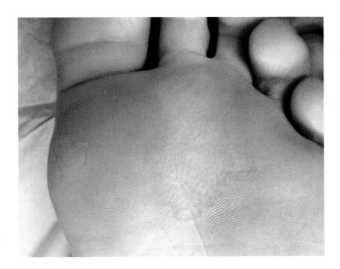

Potassium hydroxide preparation of skin scrapings does not reveal fungal elements.

Which of the following is the most likely diagnosis?

(A) Aquagenic keratoderma

(B) Erythrasma

(C) Keratoderma blenorrhagicum

(D) Pitted keratolysis

(E) Tinea pedis

Item 45

A 65-year-old man is evaluated for a 2-month history of an ulcer on the left lower leg that will not heal. While the ulcer has been painful, there has been no significant change in this symptom. The ulcer is minimally exudative and has not been associated with increased warmth, swelling, or expanding erythema. Medical history is significant for hypertension, hyperlipidemia, and type 2 diabetes mellitus. Medications are rosuvastatin, enalapril, hydrochlorothiazide, and metformin.

On physical examination vital signs are normal. Skin findings are shown.

Ankle-brachial index is 0.94 on both sides.

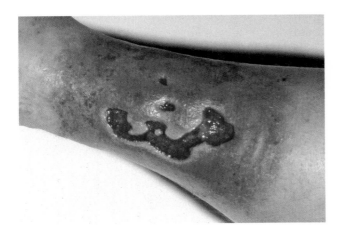

Which of the following is the most appropriate management for the ulcer?

(A) Compression therapy

(B) Oral cephalexin

(C) Oral cilostazol

(D) Topical povidone iodine

Item 46

A 52-year-old woman is evaluated in the emergency department for increasing redness, scaling, and itchiness of the skin. Over the last 2 days, it has expanded to cover most of her body. She complains of being cold and shivering. Her skin is flaking so badly she is embarrassed to go out in public. Medical history is significant for psoriasis since childhood and COPD for 5 years. She was treated for a COPD exacerbation last week with 5 days of 40-mg prednisone therapy. Medications are triamcinolone ointment, tiotropium, fluticasone/salmeterol, and albuterol as needed.

On physical examination, temperature is 37.8 °C (100 °F), blood pressure is 118/70 mm Hg, pulse rate is 100/min, and oxygen saturation is 97% breathing ambient air. BMI is 32. The patient is acutely uncomfortable, covered in many blankets and shivering. Her skin is leathery, indurated, and hot to the touch. Skin findings are shown.

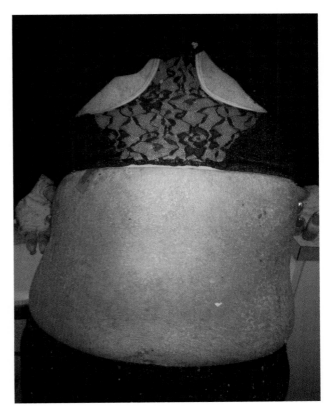

There is active bleeding at a few sites where some scale has detached. Nail pitting is present on most of her fingernails. There are no conjunctival, oral, or genital lesions.

CONT.

Which of the following is the most likely cause of the patient's new symptoms?

(A) Drug reaction with eosinophilia and systemic symptoms (DRESS)
(B) Prednisone
(C) Sézary syndrome
(D) Stevens-Johnson syndrome

Item 47

A 45-year-old man is evaluated for itching with dry scaling skin of 1 month's duration. His medical history is noncontributory, and he takes no medications.

On physical examination, vital signs are normal. Skin findings are shown.

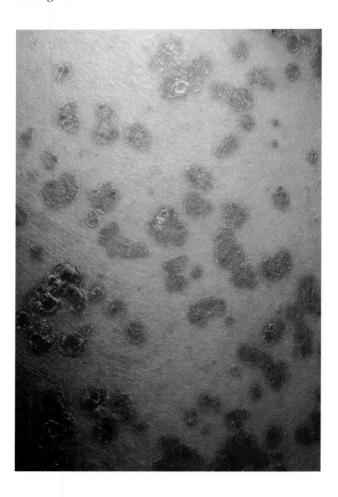

The remainder of the examination is unremarkable.

Which of the following is the most appropriate diagnostic test to perform next?

(A) Potassium hydroxide examination
(B) Scabies preparation
(C) Tzanck preparation
(D) Wood lamp examination

Item 48

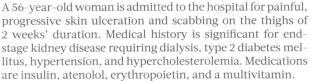

A 56-year-old woman is admitted to the hospital for painful, progressive skin ulceration and scabbing on the thighs of 2 weeks' duration. Medical history is significant for end-stage kidney disease requiring dialysis, type 2 diabetes mellitus, hypertension, and hypercholesterolemia. Medications are insulin, atenolol, erythropoietin, and a multivitamin.

On physical examination, she is afebrile. Blood pressure is 136/84 mm Hg, pulse rate is 108/min, respiration rate is 16/min, and oxygen saturation is 98% breathing ambient air. BMI is 32. Pedal pulses are normal. Skin findings are shown.

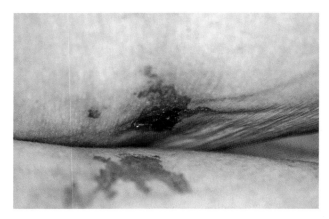

Laboratory studies show calcium level of 10.8 mg/dL (2.7 mmol/L), phosphorus level of 7.6 mg/dL (2.4 mmol/L), and parathyroid hormone level of 650 pg/mL (650 ng/L).

Blood cultures are negative.

Which of the following is the most likely diagnosis?

(A) Calciphylaxis
(B) Kyrle disease
(C) Nephrogenic systemic fibrosis
(D) Progressive systemic sclerosis

Item 49

A 28-year-old man is evaluated for a 4-day history of a tender nodule on the left dorsal hand. The patient thought the lesion started as a "spider bite," and it continued to increase in size and tenderness. He has no fever or chills. No other lesions are present.

Medical history is unremarkable, and he takes no medications.

On physical examination, vital signs are normal. Skin findings are shown (see top of next page).

The remainder of the examination is normal.

Laboratory values, including leukocyte count, are within normal range.

Which of the following is the most appropriate treatment?

(A) Antibiotic therapy based on culture result
(B) Incision and drainage
(C) Incision and drainage plus oral cephalexin
(D) Oral trimethoprim-sulfamethoxazole

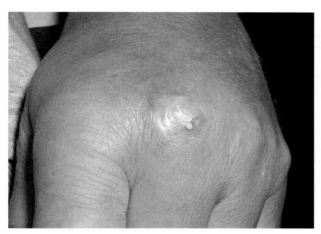

ITEM 49

Item 50

An 18-year-old woman is evaluated for a mole on her back that has been changing in color for several weeks. There are no other associated symptoms. She has no significant medical history and takes no medications.

On physical examination, vital signs are normal. Skin findings are shown.

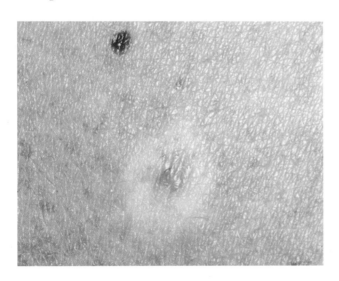

The remainder of the examination is unremarkable.

Which of the following is the most likely diagnosis?

(A) Compound melanocytic nevus
(B) Dysplastic nevus
(C) Halo nevus
(D) Malignant melanoma

Item 51

A 45-year-old man is evaluated for a 6-month history of pruritic rash in the inguinal and gluteal folds. He has used topical ketoconazole for 3 weeks with no improvement. Medical history is significant for type 2 diabetes mellitus. Medications are metformin and ketoconazole cream.

On physical examination, vital signs are normal. BMI is 32. Occipital scalp has erythematous plaque with scale. Skin findings are shown.

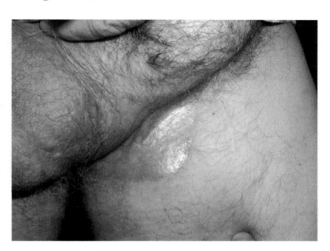

Similar findings are noted in the gluteal cleft. Elbows and knees are clear. Nail pitting is not present.

Which of the following is the most likely diagnosis?

(A) Allergic contact dermatitis
(B) Candidiasis
(C) Inverse psoriasis
(D) Seborrheic dermatitis
(E) Tinea cruris

Item 52

A 40-year-old man is evaluated during a follow-up visit for an extremely pruritic skin eruption for several months that was recently diagnosed as dermatitis herpetiformis. He denies gastrointestinal symptoms and is otherwise healthy and takes no medications.

On physical examination, vital signs are normal. There are numerous excoriations on elbows, knees, and buttocks with rare intact vesicles.

In addition to a gluten-free diet, which of the following is the most appropriate treatment for this patient?

(A) Betamethasone valerate
(B) Dapsone
(C) Diphenhydramine
(D) Prednisone
(E) Sulfasalazine

Item 53

A 68-year-old man is evaluated for a 3-year history of erythema of the bilateral lower extremities. The patient reports developing ulcerations 3 weeks ago and began applying neomycin/polymyxin B/bacitracin to the ulcerated area. Over the past week, he reports worsening erythema, weeping, and edema of the lower legs. His only medication is topical neomycin/polymyxin B/bacitracin ointment.

On physical examination, vital signs are normal. BMI is 34. There are strong pedal pulses. Skin findings are shown.

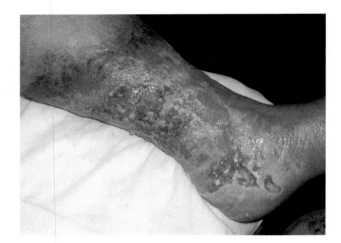

Laboratory studies show a leukocyte count of 8,200 µL (8.2 × 10⁹/L).

Which of the following is the most appropriate initial management?

(A) Discontinue neomycin/polymyxin B/bacitracin ointment
(B) Start intravenous vancomycin
(C) Start oral clindamycin
(D) Start oral terbinafine
(E) Start topical triamcinolone ointment

Item 54

A 32-year-old woman is evaluated for a 10-month history of pruritus and scaling of both her hands. She is a child care worker and washes her hands frequently. Medical history is unremarkable, and she takes no medications.

On physical examination, vital signs are normal. Skin findings are shown (see top of next column).

There is no scale or erythema of the feet. The remainder of the examination is normal.

Results of potassium hydroxide microscopy from the scale on her hands are negative.

Which of the following is the most appropriate management?

(A) Epicutaneous patch testing
(B) Oral fluconazole
(C) Oral prednisone
(D) Thick emollients

Item 55

A 16-year-old woman is evaluated for an acne breakout on her face for 6 months' duration. She has been using over-the-counter benzoyl peroxide products, but the acne is not

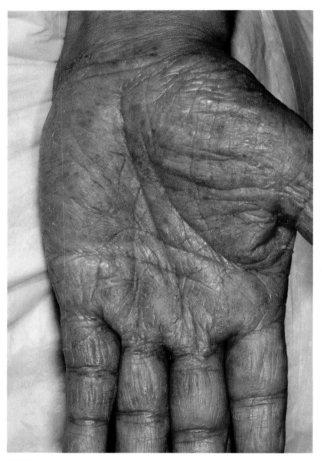

ITEM 54

improving. She is not sexually active. Medical history is unremarkable, and she takes no medications.

On physical examination, vital signs are normal. Skin findings show scattered open and closed comedones on the forehead, nose, and cheeks. There are no inflammatory pustules or nodules. The remainder of the examination is normal.

Which of the following is the most appropriate treatment?

(A) Isotretinoin
(B) Oral contraceptive pills
(C) Topical antibiotics
(D) Topical retinoids

Item 56

A 21-year-old man is evaluated 3 weeks following treatment of scabies. The patient lives alone, but his sexual partner had similar symptoms. Scabies was confirmed in both persons by microscopic examination of skin scrapings. Both were treated with two applications of 5% permethrin 2 weeks apart. Both patient and partner were adherent to the treatment protocol. The patient notes persistence of itching without the appearance of new lesions, whereas his partner is now asymptomatic.

Which of the following is the most appropriate next step?

(A) Begin an oral antihistamine and topical glucocorticoid
(B) Re-treat with 5% permethrin cream
(C) Treat with oral ivermectin
(D) Treat with combination oral ivermectin and 5% permethrin cream
(E) Treat with 1% lindane lotion

Item 57

A 45-year-old woman is evaluated for a 3-month history of ocular burning and a gritty sensation. Within the last day she has developed a red and swollen left upper eyelid. She has a 2-year history of facial flushing and intermittent pustules on the nose and cheeks. The flushing is worse during times of stress and with exercise. She is otherwise healthy and takes no medications.

On physical examination, vital signs are normal. There is erythema with telangiectasias on the bilateral cheeks, nasolabial folds, and nose. Several inflammatory pustules are on the nose and cheeks with no comedones. There is slight erythema of the left conjunctiva and prominent swelling of the left upper eyelid associated with a red to violet hue. The eyelash bases are coated with a fine crust.

The remainder of the examination is normal.

Which of the following is the most likely cause of her eye symptoms?

(A) Anterior scleritis
(B) Episcleritis
(C) Ocular rosacea
(D) Viral conjunctivitis

Item 58

A 28-year-old woman is evaluated for a rash on the bilateral shins for 1 month's duration. The lesions appeared suddenly and are slightly tender with palpation. She has no joint pain, fever, or cough. She has no diarrhea or abdominal problems. She is 4 months pregnant. Her only medication is prenatal vitamins.

On physical examination, vital signs are normal. Skin findings are shown.

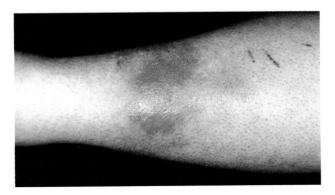

Which of the following is the most likely diagnosis?

(A) Erythema nodosum
(B) Granuloma annulare
(C) Lipodermatosclerosis
(D) Necrobiosis lipoidica
(E) Pyoderma gangrenosum

Item 59

A 62-year-old man is evaluated for painful ulcerations on the right lower leg at the site of previous minor trauma. Medical history is significant for hypertension, type 2 diabetes mellitus, and hyperlipidemia. He is a 50-pack–year smoker. Medications are hydrochlorothiazide, lisinopril, metformin, and atorvastatin.

On physical examination, vital signs are normal. BMI is 28. The leg ulcers are shown.

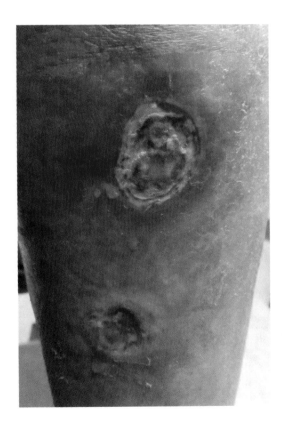

He has increased pain with elevation of the right leg. Pedal pulses are weak on left leg and absent on right leg. The right lower leg is cool to touch. Resting ankle-brachial index is 0.3 on the right leg and 0.7 on the left leg.

Which of the following is the most appropriate management of the ulcer?

(A) Compression stockings
(B) Oral cilostazol
(C) Skin grafting
(D) Surgical revascularization

Item 60

A 52-year-old man is evaluated for fragile skin and blisters on the dorsal hands of 2 years' duration. Medical history is significant for a 30-pack-year history of smoking and moderate alcohol consumption. He is a roofer and has had significant sun exposure. He is otherwise in good health and takes no medications.

On physical examination, vital signs are normal. He has hypertrichosis on the face. Skin findings are shown.

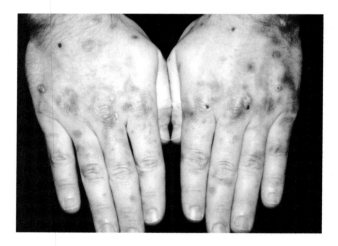

The remainder of the physical examination is normal.

Which of the following is the most likely diagnosis?

(A) Bullous pemphigoid
(B) Bullous tinea
(C) Dermatitis herpetiformis
(D) Pemphigus vulgaris
(E) Porphyria cutanea tarda

Item 61

A 26-year-old woman is evaluated for a changing mole on her left lower leg. She says it is getting bigger and darker. The patient is 5 weeks pregnant. Her only medication is a prenatal vitamin.

On physical examination, vital signs are normal. There is an 8-mm black and gray asymmetric papule with irregular borders on her left medial calf.

Which of the following is the most appropriate next step in management?

(A) Biopsy the lesion now
(B) Biopsy after delivery
(C) Cryotherapy
(D) Provide reassurance

Item 62

A 52-year-old man is evaluated for a rapidly enlarging, painful ulcer on the leg. It started as a small red "pimple" approximately 2 weeks ago and has been expanding over the past week. Medical history is significant for ulcerative colitis. His only medications are sulfasalazine and folic acid.

On physical examination, vital signs are normal. Skin findings are shown.

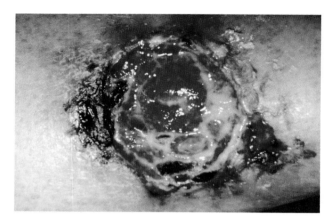

Tissue culture is negative.

Which of the following is the most appropriate initial treatment?

(A) Compression dressings
(B) Dapsone
(C) Prednisone
(D) Surgical debridement
(E) Topical hydrocortisone

Item 63

A 36-year-old woman is evaluated for a 3-day history of pruritic rash on the arms, legs, and face. She is very symptomatic and cannot concentrate on her tasks or sleep due to the intense itching. She is a summer camp counselor. Medical history is otherwise unremarkable, and she takes no medications.

On physical examination, vital signs are normal. Representative skin findings on the leg are shown.

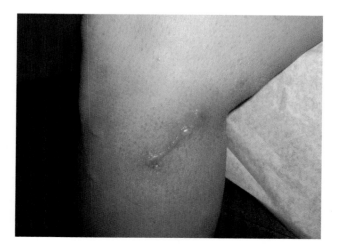

The remainder of the examination is normal.

Which of the following is the most appropriate treatment?

(A) 7-day course of oral acyclovir

(B) 10-day course of oral doxycycline

(C) 6-day taper of oral methylprednisolone

(D) 21-day taper of oral prednisone

(E) Topical hydrocortisone 1%

Item 64

A 50-year-old man is evaluated for a several month history of itchy, scaly feet. It has persisted despite the application of a moisturizing lotion. He has no significant medical history and takes no medications.

On physical examination, vital signs are normal. There are erythematous scaly patches on the sides of the feet and maceration between toes. Toenails are normal. Microscopic examination using potassium hydroxide preparation shows branching hyphae in the keratin (scale).

Which of the following is the most appropriate treatment?

(A) Imidazole cream

(B) Nystatin cream

(C) Oral ketoconazole

(D) Topical betamethasone and clotrimazole

Item 65

A 62-year-old man was admitted to the hospital following a motor vehicle accident. He underwent a craniotomy for treatment of intracranial hemorrhage following which he was started on carbamazepine. On postoperative day 19, the patient was noted to have a rash on his chest, arms, proximal legs, and buttocks, as well as redness on his face. The next day he had diffuse papules and macules on his trunk and proximal extremities, tachycardia, and hypotension. Hypotension and tachycardia responded to fluid resuscitation.

On physical examination, vital signs are normal. The patient is lethargic and confused. Skin findings are shown.

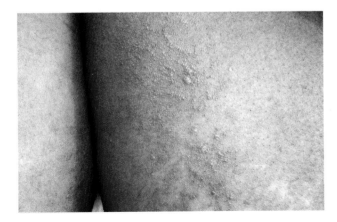

He has prominent swelling in his face. There is minimal skin erosion and no sloughing when shearing pressure is applied with the examiner's finger. There are a few erosions

in the oropharynx, but no eye or genital involvement. Generalized lymphadenopathy is present.

Which of the following is the most likely cause of this patient's clinical presentation?

(A) Drug reaction with eosinophilia and systemic symptoms (DRESS)

(B) Retiform purpura

(C) Stevens-Johnson syndrome

(D) Toxic epidermal necrolysis

Item 66

A 62-year-old man is evaluated for a 4-month history of itching all over his body. He has no fatigue, weight loss, or night sweats. His appetite is good. Medical history is significant for hypertension treated with hydrochlorothiazide. He has no risk factors for HIV infection.

On physical examination, vital signs are normal. There are a few scattered excoriations on the arms and lower legs. There are no other significant skin findings and no lymphadenopathy.

Laboratory studies, including complete blood count with differential, erythrocyte sedimentation rate, liver chemistry tests, serum creatinine, and thyroid-stimulating hormone level, are within normal range.

Which of the following is the most appropriate initial management?

(A) CT of the chest and abdomen

(B) Discontinue hydrochlorothiazide

(C) Start topical permethrin

(D) Start topical triamcinolone cream

Item 67

A 83-year-old man is seen in the office for routine follow-up. He has a history of hypertension and atrial fibrillation. Medications are hydrochlorothiazide and warfarin.

On physical examination, vital signs are normal. During lung auscultation, a 0.4×0.4-cm pink pearly papule with telangiectasias on his back is found.

Biopsy of the lesion reveals a basal cell carcinoma with low-risk histology.

Which of the follow is the most appropriate treatment?

(A) Electrodesiccation and curettage

(B) Mohs micrographic surgery

(C) Radiation

(D) Vismodegib

Item 68

An 18-year-old man is evaluated for an acute onset of hair loss on the scalp. The patient has a history of vitiligo. He is in good health and takes no medications.

On physical examination, vital signs are normal. His scalp findings are shown (see top of next page).

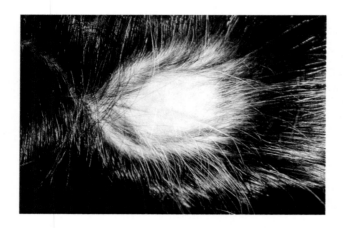

Which of the following is the most likely diagnosis?

(A) Alopecia areata
(B) Discoid lupus erythematosus
(C) Syphilis
(D) Tinea capitis
(E) Trichotillomania

Item 69

A 60-year-old woman is evaluated for easy bruising and bleeding after minor trauma, and a rash around her eyes. Medical history is unremarkable, and she takes no medications.

On physical examination, vital signs are normal. The patient has several ecchymoses located primarily on her arms and legs. Lesions around her eyes are shown.

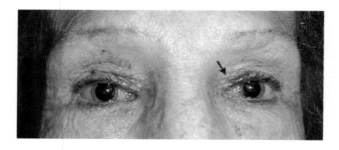

Hepatomegaly is present. The remainder of the physical examination is unremarkable. Urinalysis demonstrates 4+ proteinuria but is otherwise unremarkable.

Which of the following is the most likely diagnosis?

(A) Amyloidosis
(B) Dermatomyositis
(C) Hyperlipidemia
(D) Sarcoidosis

Item 70

A 40-year-old man is evaluated for a new skin rash of 10 days' duration. The rash appeared abruptly and is not tender or pruritic. The patient has poorly controlled type 2 diabetes mellitus. His current medications include metformin and glyburide. Family history is unremarkable.

On physical examination, vital signs are normal. BMI is 25. There are several grouped 1- to 5-mm yellow papules on extensor surfaces of extremities and buttocks. Some of the papules have surrounding erythema. The remainder of the examination is normal.

Laboratory studies show a hemoglobin A_{1c} value of 12%.

Which of the following disorders is associated with the patient's skin findings?

(A) Familial dysbetalipoproteinemia
(B) Familial hypercholesterolemia
(C) Hypertriglyceridemia
(D) No underlying disorder

Item 71

A 45-year-old woman is evaluated for a new growth on the leg. It has been present for several months. Medical history is unremarkable, and she takes no medications.

On physical examination, vital signs are normal. Skin finding is shown.

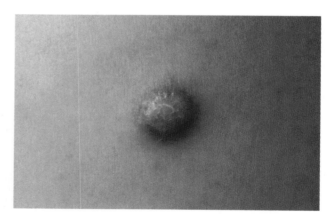

Which of the following is the most likely diagnosis?

(A) Acrochordon
(B) Dermatofibroma
(C) Neurofibroma
(D) Pyogenic granuloma

Item 72

A 40-year-old man is evaluated for skin changes around the neck that are asymptomatic, but have been worsening over the past year. Medical history is unremarkable. He takes no medications.

On physical examination, vital signs are normal. BMI is 30. Skin findings are shown (see top of next page).

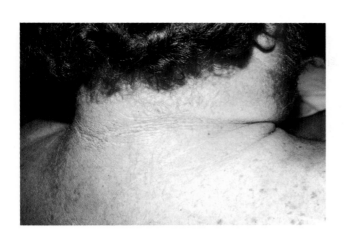

The remainder of the physical examination is unremarkable.

Which of the following is the most appropriate diagnostic test to perform next?

(A) Fasting blood glucose

(B) 24-Hour urine cortisol

(C) Thyroid-stimulating hormone and serum thyroxine

(D) Wood lamp evaluation

Answers and Critiques

H **Item 1** **Answer: C**

Educational Objective: Diagnose autoimmune bullous diseases.

This patient likely has an autoimmune bullous disease, and the most sensitive method for diagnosis is with two biopsies: one of lesional skin for histology, and one of perilesional skin for direct immunofluorescence, as shown.

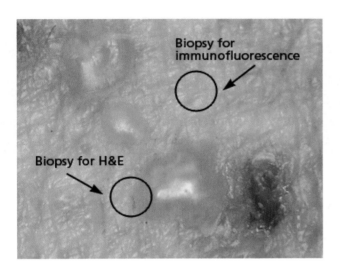

Autoimmune blistering diseases result from auto-antibodies to different antigens in the skin and have similar but distinct presentations. Clinically, they are characterized by persistent pruritic to painful blisters with erosions and variable mucosal and ocular involvement and scarring. These diseases often arise in older persons. Identification and diagnosis of these disorders are important because of the associated morbidity and mortality. Differentiation of the autoimmune blistering diseases can be made based on clinical features, but definitive diagnosis requires histopathologic examination and, in some patients, serologic testing for pathogenic antibodies.

Depending on the location of the targeted antigen, flaccid or tense bullae will be present clinically, and the corresponding separation can be appreciated using histopathology. In pemphigus, flaccid blisters correspond with suprabasilar separation, whereas tense bullae correspond with subepidermal blisters in bullous pemphigoid and epidermolysis bullosa acquisita.

A skin (shave or punch) biopsy of an intact, early vesicle or bullae with adjacent normal skin should be submitted in formalin and processed for hematoxylin and eosin to examine tissue histology. Each of the autoimmune bullous diseases has characteristic histologic findings that suggest a differential diagnosis. In addition, a perilesional skin biopsy

should be submitted for direct immunofluorescence, either in saline or Michel transport medium.

The histologic findings together with the pattern on direct immunofluorescence can usually render a diagnosis. Serum from affected patients also can assist in diagnosis. The blood can be reacted with different substrates and will determine if circulating antibodies are present (indirect immunofluorescence). Tests such as serum enzyme-linked immunosorbent assays have been developed that detect the presence of specific antibodies in pemphigus vulgaris, pemphigus foliaceus, and bullous pemphigoid, and may correlate with disease activity. Other studies such as salt-split skin immunofluorescence may be useful in selected instances, but overall serum studies have lower sensitivities than biopsy.

> **KEY POINT**
>
> - To diagnose an autoimmune bullous disease, two biopsies often are performed: one of lesional skin for histology and one of perilesional normal skin for direct immunofluorescence.

Bibliography

Elston DM, Stratman EJ, Miller SJ. Skin biopsy: Biopsy issues in specific diseases. J Am Acad Dermatol. 2016;74:1-16; quiz 17-8. [PMID: 26702794] doi:10.1016/j.jaad.2015.06.033

Item 2 **Answer: C**

Educational Objective: Diagnose pityriasis (tinea) versicolor.

Pityriasis versicolor, often referred to as tinea versicolor, is one of the most common, chronic, superficial fungal infections. It is most common in warm, humid environments. It typically presents in young adults as asymptomatic, oval-to-round, minimally scaly, hyperpigmented or hypopigmented macules that can coalesce into patches on the trunk and upper extremities. Hypopigmentation is more common in darker-skinned persons. These areas often become more noticeable after exposure to the sun because the organism prevents the skin from tanning.

The diagnosis of pityriasis versicolor can often be made by clinical presentation but may be confirmed by visualization of short rod-shaped hyphae and round yeast ("spaghetti and meatballs") on microscopic examination of skin scraping using a potassium hydroxide preparation. Treatment of pityriasis versicolor with topical antiseborrheic shampoos or lotions such as selenium sulfide or ketoconazole leads to resolution of erythema and scaling, but the pigmentation changes may persist for longer periods of time.

Candida albicans infections occur in hot, moist occluded areas, such as the armpits, groin, and beneath the breasts. *Candida* appears as erythematous patches with satellite pustules. Diagnosis is frequently made on clinical grounds alone, but a potassium hydroxide preparation can show spores and pseudohyphae.

Erythrasma is a superficial bacterial infection caused by *Corynebacterium minutissimum* that presents as mildly pruritic, thin erythematous-to-brown plaques with thin scale and an overlying wrinkled appearance and maceration in intertriginous areas such as the axillae, groin, and inframammary areas. The red-brown color and distribution in intertriginous areas distinguishes erythrasma from pityriasis versicolor. Diagnosis is typically made by clinical presentation but may be confirmed by coral-red fluorescence with a Wood lamp.

Tinea infections are superficial fungal infections caused by dermatophytes and classified by the site of infection. Tinea corporis appears in sites other than the feet, groin, face, or hand. It is characterized by annular patches with peripheral scale and central clearing that appear distinctly different from the hypo- or hyperpigmented patches of pityriasis versicolor. Diagnosis can often be made on clinical grounds, but a potassium hydroxide preparation of the scale shows fungal hyphae. A fungal culture can also be performed.

KEY POINT

- Pityriasis versicolor presents in young adults as asymptomatic, oval-to-round, minimally scaly, hyperpigmented or hypopigmented macules that can coalesce into patches on the trunk and upper extremities.

Bibliography

Kaushik N, Pujalte GG, Reese ST. Superficial fungal infections. Prim Care. 2015;42:501-16. [PMID: 26612371] doi:10.1016/j.pop.2015.08.004

Item 3   Answer: C

Educational Objective: Treat atopic dermatitis.

This patient has atopic dermatitis, and the most appropriate treatment is topical glucocorticoids. Eczematous dermatitis is a type of inflammation characterized by inflamed, dry, red, itchy skin. The terms *eczema* and *dermatitis* are often used interchangeably. There are multiple types of eczematous dermatoses. Atopic dermatitis is genetically driven and often affects areas such as the antecubital and popliteal fossae and typically presents in childhood. It is characterized by xerotic, pink, scaly skin and is most commonly seen on the periocular areas, posterior neck, antecubital and popliteal fossae, wrists, and ankles. The initial treatment for atopic dermatitis consists of good skin care with mild cleansers and thick emollients (petrolatum) along with topical glucocorticoids to decrease inflammation and pruritus.

Oral cephalexin is a first-generation cephalosporin antibiotic that can be used to treat selected skin infections. The use of oral antibiotics should be limited to conditions in which there is evidence of extensive bacterial infection. Clinical signs of bacterial infection typically include weeping of serous fluid, pustules, honey-colored crusting, unexplained worsening of dermatitis, or failure to respond to correct

therapy. There is no indication for treatment with systemic antibiotics in this patient.

Oral prednisone should be considered only in severe, acute exacerbations of atopic dermatitis and not for regular management. Chronic oral glucocorticoid treatment can lead to side effects such as diabetes, osteoporosis, and compromised immune function, so this treatment would not be appropriate before treatment with topical glucocorticoids.

Topical ketoconazole is a treatment for superficial fungal infections. This patient has atopic dermatitis, so antifungal creams would not be used.

Topical mupirocin is the treatment for localized bacterial infections of the skin, such as impetigo. Although patients with atopic dermatitis are often secondarily colonized or infected with *Staphylococcus aureus*, routine use of topical antibiotics is not recommended. There is no indication in this patient that the skin is infected.

KEY POINT

- The initial treatment for atopic dermatitis consists of good skin care with mild cleansers and thick emollients along with topical glucocorticoids to decrease inflammation and pruritus.

Bibliography

Eichenfield LF, Tom WL, Berger TG, Krol A, et al. Guidelines of care for the management of atopic dermatitis: section 2. Management and treatment of atopic dermatitis with topical therapies. J Am Acad Dermatol. 2014 Jul;71(1):116-32. [PMID: 24813302]

Item 4   Answer: D

Educational Objective: Diagnose urticarial vasculitis.

This patient has urticarial vasculitis, and the most appropriate management is to obtain skin biopsies to confirm the diagnosis. A routine skin biopsy (for histology) and a biopsy for direct immunofluorescence (for immunoglobulin and complement deposits) should both be obtained. Typical urticarial wheals last for less than 24 hours (with individual lesions lasting only a few hours), resolve without cutaneous sequelae, and are pruritic and not painful. Urticarial vasculitis differs from urticaria in that individual lesions persist longer than 24 hours. Urticarial vasculitis more commonly presents with painful or burning lesions instead of pruritus and leave bruise-like changes when they resolve, which is atypical for usual urticaria. Patients with urticarial vasculitis often have an underlying autoimmune disease, most often lupus erythematosus, but even in the absence of an associated autoimmune disease, patients with urticarial vasculitis (particularly hypocomplementemic urticarial vasculitis) are at risk of multisystem disease, including nephritis. The patient's joint pain suggests the possibility of an additional underlying disorder. Skin biopsies are important in making the diagnosis and guiding further work-up and treatment.

Epicutaneous patch testing is performed to diagnose allergic contact dermatitis. Allergic contact dermatitis can

CONT.

occasionally present as typical urticarial, but this patient's history suggests urticarial vasculitis.

Physical urticaria is induced by a physical stimulus such as the sun, sweating, physical pressure, or cold temperature. An ice cube provocation test is performed to help diagnose cold urticaria. This test would not be helpful in diagnosing urticarial vasculitis. Neither allergic contact dermatitis nor physical urticaria can explain the patient's joint symptoms.

Treatment of urticaria is most effective with long-acting antihistamines, since they help treat active disease and prevent new flares of urticaria. Systemic glucocorticoids and immunosuppressive agents have been used for urticaria, but in most patients, maximizing the dose of the long-acting antihistamines is equally effective and safer. Glucocorticoids are often the mainstay of treatment for urticarial vasculitis, but it would be inappropriate to commit a patient to this therapy without first confirming the diagnosis.

Topical glucocorticoids, such as triamcinolone, have limited efficacy in typical and urticarial vasculitis and are not the best management for either condition.

KEY POINT

- Skin biopsies should be performed to evaluate for urticarial vasculitis when individual urticarial lesions are present for longer than 24 hours.

Bibliography
Bernstein JA, Lang DM, Khan DA, et al. The diagnosis and management of acute and chronic urticaria: 2014 update. J Allergy Clin Immunol. 2014 May;133(5):1270-7. [PMID: 24766875]

Item 5   Answer: D

Educational Objective: Treat striae and atrophy from topical glucocorticoids.

This patient should discontinue the triamcinolone cream. He has striae distensae, or stretch marks, recognized as erythematous, violaceous, or hypopigmented linear striations secondary to topical glucocorticoid use. Topical glucocorticoids decrease the production of collagen resulting in atrophy, stretch marks, and telangiectasia. The application of any topical glucocorticoid to normal skin for prolonged periods of time, especially under occlusion, may lead to these changes. Some persons are more prone to these side effects, which may occur after a brief period, whereas others take months of usage before side effects appear. Areas of the skin especially prone to atrophy are the thighs, groin, axillae, and face. Potent topical glucocorticoids should be avoided in these areas to reduce the risk of atrophy, and the patient should be counseled to apply the topical glucocorticoids only to lesional skin, not normal-appearing skin. There is little data to support any therapy, including topical tretinoin, to reverse the side effects of topical glucocorticoids. Over time, patients will see an improvement in the atrophy as the effects of the glucocorticoids wear off and normal collagen production returns.

Triamcinolone is a medium-potency topical glucocorticoid. Adding a stronger topical glucocorticoid such as clobetasol would likely make the symptoms worse.

This patient's findings are most consistent with striae distensae. The scaly annular patch of a superficial fungal infection is not present, and therefore a topical antifungal agent such as terbinafine will not be of any benefit.

Calcipotriene is a vitamin D analogue used to treat psoriasis, and it has not been shown to cause atrophy, striae, or telangiectasia. Discontinuation of the calcipotriene would not result in improvement of the skin atrophy and striae in this patient.

KEY POINT

- Side effects from topical glucocorticoids include thinned skin, striae distensae (stretch marks), and easy bruising, and are likely to occur when they are used for extended periods of time, especially in skin folds or areas of occlusion.

Bibliography
Barnes L, Kaya G, Rollason V. Topical corticosteroid-induced skin atrophy: a comprehensive review. Drug Saf. 2015;38:493-509. [PMID: 25862024] doi:10.1007/s40264-015-0287-7

Item 6   Answer: D

Educational Objective: Diagnose herpes zoster.

Varicella zoster virus (VZV) is a DNA virus that causes two forms of cutaneous disease. This patient has symptoms of herpes zoster (shingles), recrudescent VZV, which typically presents as a painful, vesicular eruption confined to a single dermatome and is most commonly seen in immunocompromised or elderly patients. The clinical presentation of herpes zoster is characteristic. Prodromal symptoms, such as burning, stinging, or tingling, often occur in a localized region, followed by an eruption of grouped vesicles or pustules on an erythematous base. The outbreak is unilateral and does not cross the body's midline. The most common dermatomes affected are in the thoracic region. Diagnosis is based on clinical presentation but can be confirmed with a Tzanck preparation and/or viral direct fluorescent antibody or polymerase chain reaction testing. Oral antiviral agents (acyclovir, valacyclovir, or famciclovir) are typically used to treat herpes zoster infection and should be started within the first 72 hours of symptom onset for optimal response.

Primary infection with VZV causes chickenpox (varicella), a common disease in childhood. It is transmitted by aerosolized droplets; after a 2-week incubation period, it presents as pruritic papules and vesicles with an umbilicated center that appear in crops and heal with crusting. The virus becomes latent within dorsal root ganglia and can reactivate (10% to 20% risk), causing herpes zoster. A vaccine for primary VZV infection was approved for use in the United States in 1995.

Eczema herpeticum is a disseminated viral infection most often caused by primary infection of HSV and characteristically seen in patients with atopic dermatitis. It presents

CONT.

with disseminated punched-out erosions with crust, with a predilection for the face.

Cutaneous herpes simplex virus (HSV) infections have two common forms: herpes labialis (typically HSV1) or "cold sores/fever blisters" and genital herpes (typically HSV2). Herpes infection presents as vesicles on an erythematous base. Following primary infection, the virus lies dormant and can recur at the original site of infection. A prodrome of pain or burning often precedes recurrences.

> **KEY POINT**
>
> • Herpes zoster (shingles), recrudescent varicella zoster virus, typically presents as a painful, vesicular eruption confined to a single dermatome and is most commonly seen in immunocompromised or elderly patients.

Bibliography
Schmader K. Herpes Zoster. Clin Geriatr Med. 2016;32:539-53. [PMID: 27394022] doi:10.1016/j.cger.2016.02.011

Item 7   Answer: B
Educational Objective: Diagnose melanonychia.

This patient has melanonychia, a brown longitudinal pigmentation of the nail plate. It can be a normal variant in persons with darker skin types, but it may also occur as a result of systemic disease, medication, infection, or an underlying melanocytic lesion such as malignant melanoma. It is extremely difficult to clinically differentiate benign melanonychia from acral melanoma involving the nail. Certain findings may suggest a stronger likelihood of melanoma and the need for biopsy. These include: melanonychia that first appears in adulthood; involvement of a single digit (especially thumb or great toe); rapid growth; width greater than 3 to 4 mm; proximal width greater than distal width; variation in pigmentation; secondary nail changes such as splitting or dystrophy; pigmentation that extends beyond the nail fold; or personal history of melanoma. This patient has longitudinal melanonychia limited to the thumb that is changing in width. Furthermore, in this photo, there is a pigmented macule on the lateral nailfold that is called a Hutchinson sign. This is an important clinical clue for subungual melanoma. A biopsy should be performed.

Lichen planus can develop in the nails. The nail plate will become thinner or be completely destroyed, and the cuticle may attach to the nail plate (pterygium). Other findings may include longitudinal ridging, nail plate thinning, and longitudinal fissuring. Red streaking of the nail may also occur. Patients may have other cutaneous or mucosal findings of lichen planus. This patient lacks the dystrophic changes commonly associated with lichen planus.

With aging, the thickness, curvature, surface, and color of the nail plate can change. The underlying mechanisms are unknown. The nail plate may become thicker or thinner. The normal texture of the nail can become rougher and more friable, resulting in striations and splitting. The color of the nail may become paler or yellow. These changes may predispose nails to onychomycosis, pain, and subungual hemorrhage.

Normal aging is not associated with the occurrence of a growing, longitudinal stripe in one nail.

Onychomycosis is a fungal infection of the nail. The most common pattern is characterized by the distal corner of the nail becoming yellow and lifted, with the development of subungual debris. Eventually this process can spread proximally and laterally to involve the entire nail plate. Onychomycosis does not result in a well-defined dark brown longitudinal stripe as seen in this patient.

> **KEY POINT**
>
> • Melanonychia is a longitudinal brown pigmentation of the nail plate; it can be a normal variant in persons with darker skin types, but it may also occur as a result of systemic disease, medication, infection, or an underlying melanocytic lesion.

Bibliography
Goydos JS, Shoen SL. Acral lentiginous melanoma. Cancer Treat Res. 2016;167:321-9. [PMID: 26601870] doi:10.1007/978-3-319-22539-5_14

Item 8   Answer: B
Educational Objective: Diagnose chronic paronychia.

This patient has chronic paronychia. Chronic paronychia typically is present for 6 weeks or more and affects multiple fingers. Typical manifestations of chronic paronychia include red, swollen, and tender nail folds that lack a cuticle. It can also cause ridging and dystrophy of the nail plate. Chronic irritation from water or chemical contact is the primary cause. *Candida* species are often isolated. The cause of chronic paronychia is multifactorial, and an important component appears to be an eczematous process, which explains why patients with chronic paronychia respond better to topical glucocorticoid than topical antifungal therapy. The primary management includes minimizing wet work.

Acute paronychia is painful swelling of the nail fold, often following minor trauma, and most commonly is caused by *Staphylococcus aureus*. It typically only affects one nail. Management consists of warm compresses or soaks, incision and drainage, or topical or systemic antibiotics. This patient has chronic paronychia, which tends to be more insidious and involves multiple fingers.

Onychomycosis is a fungal infection of the nails. It affects 10% to 20% of adults and is the most common nail infection. Infection is more common in older men with comorbidities such as diabetes mellitus, peripheral vascular disease, and immunosuppression. Dermatophytes cause more than 90% of fungal nail infections. The most common pattern is distal subungual onychomycosis; the distal corner of the nail becomes yellow and lifted, and develops subungual debris. This can then spread proximally and laterally to involve the entire nail plate. Proximal subungual onychomycosis evolves similarly but begins at the proximal nail fold (the cuticle). This is a rare pattern and is associated with HIV infection or other severely immunocompromised patients. This patient's multiple nail involvement manifesting as red, tender, and swollen nail folds and absent cuticles is not compatible with onychomycosis.

Nail changes occur in about 75% of persons with psoriasis. The most common nail abnormality observed on both fingernails and toenails is subungual hyperkeratosis. Toenails more often demonstrate thickening and discoloration (whitening or yellowing), whereas pitting and ridging are more common on fingernails. Some of the nail damage can result from concomitant onychomycosis. This patient's findings are not compatible with psoriasis.

- Chronic paronychia appears as a loss of cuticle with tender, edematous nail folds involving multiple fingers; wet work can cause maceration and predispose to this condition.

Bibliography

Shafritz AB, Coppage JM. Acute and chronic paronychia of the hand. J Am Acad Orthop Surg. 2014;22:165-74. [PMID: 24603826] doi:10.5435/JAAOS-22-03-165

Item 9   Answer: A

Educational Objective: Treat moderate to severe psoriasis.

This patient has moderate to severe psoriasis (30% or more body surface area involvement) and should be treated with systemic agents. Patients with psoriasis covering more than 10% body surface area or those with psoriatic arthritis, recalcitrant palmoplantar psoriasis, pustular psoriasis, or psoriasis in challenging anatomic areas (groin, scalp) may be considered for systemic therapy. These include tumor necrosis factor inhibitors, acitretin, methotrexate, IL-23 and IL-17 inhibitors, and phototherapy. Tumor necrosis factor inhibitors, such as etanercept, adalimumab, and infliximab, are excellent options for treating patients with both severe psoriasis and psoriatic arthritis. The newer IL-12/IL-23 and IL-17 inhibitors have shown excellent efficacy in psoriasis treatment. Therapy with any of the systemic agents should be guided by a clinician experienced in their use, including appropriate evaluation for contraindications and careful monitoring.

Prednisone is not a good choice for the treatment of psoriasis, as the doses of prednisone required would lead to numerous side effects. Prednisone also has been shown to cause pustular and erythrodermic flares in a subset of patients with psoriasis. Oral glucocorticoids should also be avoided because they may worsen associated comorbidities such as hypertension and dyslipidemia.

Topical medications such as vitamin D analogues (for example, calcitriol), immunomodulators, and glucocorticoids can be used for the treatment of psoriasis; however, they are best used as solo agents in the treatment of mild disease with less than 10% body surface area involvement. These medications are often employed in conjunction with systemic therapy to treat small areas of psoriasis that remain after treatment with a systemic agent. Topical immunomod-

ulators, pimecrolimus cream, or tacrolimus ointment are best used on the face or in intertriginous regions to avoid the atrophy seen with topical glucocorticoids.

- Moderate to severe psoriasis is best treated with systemic agents; avoid prednisone as a therapy for psoriasis.

Bibliography

Mansouri Y, Goldenberg G. New systemic therapies for psoriasis. Cutis. 2015;95:155-60. [PMID: 25844781]

Item 10   Answer: B

Educational Objective: Treat pruritic urticarial papules and plaques of pregnancy (PUPPP).

The patient has pruritic urticarial papules and plaques of pregnancy (PUPPP), and the most appropriate treatment is topical glucocorticoids. PUPPP is a self-limiting condition that typically occurs in primiparous women at the end of the third trimester or immediately postpartum. Lesions are characterized as extremely pruritic, erythematous papules within striae, most often on the abdomen with sparing of the umbilicus. The lesions can be confined to the abdomen or spread to the extremities and torso. If the lesions coalesce, urticarial plaques within striae can be an additional finding. The symptoms typically last 4 to 6 weeks and usually abate by the second postpartum week.

Topical glucocorticoids can help relieve some of the symptoms. Glucocorticoids are pregnancy category C, but are generally thought to be safe, especially topical formulations.

Early delivery is rarely required to manage PUPPP. Most patients can be managed successfully with topical glucocorticoids and oral antihistamines. On rare occasions a burst of oral glucocorticoids with a quick taper can be used if the symptoms are particularly severe, and this approach is likely preferable to early delivery.

Topical imiquimod is an immunomodulator typically used for actinic keratoses, superficial basal cell carcinoma, and genital warts. It is not appropriate treatment for PUPPP.

Ursodeoxycholic acid is used in intrahepatic cholestasis of pregnancy (ICP). Symptoms include pruritus in most patients and jaundice in 10% to 25% of patients. Elevated serum bile acids are diagnostic of ICP. Ursodeoxycholic acid is effective for ICP. Fetal complications such as preterm labor, fetal distress, and intrauterine death are increased in ICP. Intrauterine deaths can occur late in gestation, and women with proven ICP typically are induced at 36 to 38 weeks of gestation. The patient's pruritic urticarial papules located on the abdomen are not compatible with the diagnosis of intrahepatic cholestasis of pregnancy, and ursodeoxycholic acid is not indicated.

- Low- to medium-potency topical glucocorticoids are first-line therapy for pruritic urticarial papules and plaques of pregnancy (PUPPP).

Bibliography

Kroumpouzos G, Cohen LM. Dermatoses of pregnancy. J Am Acad Dermatol. 2001;45:1-19; quiz 19-22. [PMID: 11423829]

Item 11   Answer: C

Educational Objective: Diagnose miliaria.

The patient has miliaria. Miliaria or "heat rash" can appear as superficial clear vesicles or as multiple discrete red papules due to occlusion of eccrine sweat ducts. When the gland is clogged superficially, there are minute pustules that rupture easily and can be wiped off (miliaria crystallina). Miliaria rubra causes deeper red papules and some pustules when the clog is deeper and more inflammation is present. Miliaria is often seen in the setting of fever and occlusion. A typical clinical situation is a patient who is immobilized, either from pain or following surgery, and the sweat glands are occluded as a result. Therapy is guided toward cooling the affected area, allowing air circulation.

Acute generalized exanthematous pustulosis (AGEP) is not an uncommon febrile drug reaction. It tends to occur 1 to 2 days after the offending agent is given. β-Lactam antibiotics are the most common cause of AGEP. It presents as punctate nonfollicular sterile pustules on a background of erythema. It starts on the face and intertriginous areas and spreads to the trunk and extremities. The pustular nature of this condition and its typical location argue against the diagnosis of AGEP.

Candidiasis occurs most often in intertriginous areas. An occluded, warm, moist area is an ideal setting for *Candida albicans*. The skin findings tend to be bright red plaques with surrounding red satellite papules and pustules. The location and appearance of this patient's rash are not consistent with a *Candida albicans* infection.

Postsurgical contact dermatitis to povidone iodine is not uncommon. It tends to occur at the surgical site about 1 to 2 days after surgery. It appears as pruritic, weeping vesicles with underlying erythema often in a well-delineated shape where the povidone was applied. Its appearance is quite unlike miliaria, and it is unlikely that the patient had povidone applied to his back, making this an untenable diagnosis.

KEY POINT

- Miliaria or "heat rash" can appear as superficial clear vesicles or as multiple discrete red papules due to the occlusion of eccrine sweat ducts.

Bibliography

Haas N, Martens F, Henz BM. Miliaria crystallina in an intensive care setting. Clin Exp Dermatol. 2004;29:32-4. [PMID: 14723716]

Item 12   Answer: D

Educational Objective: Treat severe nodulocystic acne.

This patient has severe nodulocystic acne with evidence of scarring. The most appropriate treatment is oral isotretinoin. Isotretinoin is approved for treatment of severe cystic acne or acne not responsive to traditional combination

therapy (topical antibiotics, oral antibiotics, and topical retinoids). This additional finding of scarring in this patient would also warrant treatment with isotretinoin. Isotretinoin is teratogenic and should be administered by a provider registered under the federal regulatory program iPLEDGE and who is familiar with the potential side effects of isotretinoin therapy.

Benzoyl peroxide is comedolytic and also has antibacterial properties. Benzoyl peroxide is available over the counter in a variety of formulations (lotion, gel, cream). Topical benzoyl peroxide is often used in combination therapy with topical antibiotics and topical retinoids to treat acne. Given the severity and duration of this patient's acne, topical benzoyl peroxide would not be the most effective treatment.

Topical dapsone is an approved treatment for mild to moderate acne but would likely provide minimal benefit to this patient with severe acne who is already on topical antibiotic therapy.

Changing doxycycline to trimethoprim-sulfamethoxazole is inappropriate treatment for this patient. Trimethoprim-sulfamethoxazole can be used for treatment of acne, but it is less effective than doxycycline or minocycline, and the potential risk of severe cutaneous drug reactions limits its long-term use. Guidelines recommend that the duration of oral antibiotic therapy be limited, specifically that oral antibiotics be used for 3 months and then discontinued for patients with good clinical improvement. The same antibiotic can be used again for patients with good clinical improvement who have a subsequent relapse. This patient has severe nodulocystic acne with scarring, so isotretinoin is the most appropriate treatment.

Oral prednisone should not be used for this patient. Systemic glucocorticoids are not an effective long-term treatment for acne. Steroid-induced acne is often a side effect of their use. Patients occasionally experience acute flares with the initiation of isotretinoin treatment, and a short course of oral prednisone can be added.

KEY POINT

- Isotretinoin is indicated for severe nodulocystic and recalcitrant acne; it is associated with severe birth defects and must be administered through the federal regulatory program iPLEDGE.

Bibliography

Zaenglein AL, Pathy AL, Schlosser BJ, Alikhan A, et al. Guidelines of care for the management of acne vulgaris. J Am Acad Dermatol. 2016 May;74(5):945-73. [PMID: 26897386]

Item 13   Answer: A

Educational Objective: Diagnose amyopathic dermatomyositis.

This patient has amyopathic dermatomyositis, an underrecognized presentation of dermatomyositis that does not include muscle disease. These patients experience characteristic cutaneous features of dermatomyositis, such as the heliotrope sign, shawl sign, and Gottron papules, but muscle enzymes and strength testing are normal. Skin findings in dermatomyositis are photosensitive and tend to flare after sun exposure. Amyopathic dermatomyositis carries similar risk for underlying malignancy and pulmonary fibrosis. There is no strong consensus on how to screen for malignancy.

Mixed connective tissue disease is an overlap syndrome that includes features of systemic lupus erythematosus (SLE), systemic sclerosis, and/or polymyositis in the presence of anti-U1-ribonucleoprotein antibodies. Skin manifestations include sclerodactyly, scleroderma, calcinosis, telangiectasias, photosensitivity, malar rash, and Gottron rash. The absence of findings consistent with SLE and systemic sclerosis make this diagnosis unlikely.

Polymorphous light eruption (PMLE) is the most common idiopathic photosensitivity disorder. PMLE typically manifests before the age of 30 and is most common in fair-skinned women, first appearing in the spring and early summer. The rash will persist for weeks and resolve without scarring, even with continued exposure to the sun. Lesions appear within hours of sun exposure and are found on sun-exposed body parts. Although many different types of eruptions may occur, the most common are pruritic skin-colored or pink papules. PMLE does not explain the positive antinuclear antibody titer or periungual findings.

The most specific skin manifestations of systemic lupus erythematosus are variations on interface dermatitis, with pink-to-violet macules or plaques and varying scale or atrophy. Cutaneous lupus as a rule spares the upper eyelids and the knuckles. Inflammatory joint involvement occurs in 90% of patients with SLE. The absence of joint findings, rash over the knuckles, and periungual findings are not consistent with SLE.

KEY POINT

- Amyopathic dermatomyositis presents with skin findings characteristic of dermatomyositis, but without clinical or laboratory evidence of muscle disease; it carries risks for underlying malignancy.

Bibliography

Iaccarino L, Ghirardello A, Bettio S, Zen M, Gatto M, Punzi L, et al. The clinical features, diagnosis and classification of dermatomyositis. J Autoimmun. 2014;48-49:122-7. [PMID: 24467910] doi:10.1016/j.jaut.2013.11.005

Item 14   Answer: C

Educational Objective: Evaluate the prognosis in toxic epidermal necrosis (TEN).

Body surface area is the strongest prognostic indicator in Stevens-Johnson syndrome/toxic epidermal necrosis (SJS/TEN). Stevens-Johnson syndrome (SJS) and TEN are related clinical syndromes that are characterized by acute epidermal necrosis. The classification of SJS and TEN is determined by the percentage of body surface area with epidermal detachment:

SJS involves less than 10%, SJS-TEN overlap involves 10% to 30%, and TEN involves greater than 30%. TEN is almost exclusively caused by medications, whereas SJS can also be triggered uncommonly by vaccines or infection. Patients may have flu-like symptoms for 1 to 3 days prior to the skin eruption. Initially, painful red-purple macules or patches develop on the trunk and extremities, which enlarge and coalesce. Two or more mucosal surfaces, such as the eyes, nasopharynx, mouth, and genitals, are involved in more than 80% of patients. Systemic inflammation can result in pneumonia, hepatitis, nephritis, arthralgia, and myocarditis. Loss of the skin barrier function can lead to infection, hypovolemia, electrolyte disturbances, and death. Prognosis for SJS/TEN can be estimated by application of the SCORTEN assessment tool at 24 hours after presentation. All of the listed answer choices are features of the SCORTEN, but the patient's body surface area has the greatest impact on the score.

SCORTEN is a severity-of-illness score validated for TEN. It incorporates blood Sugar (plasma glucose level >252 mg/dL [14.0 mmol/L]), presence of Cancer, Older age (>40 years), heart Rate (>120/min), Ten percent or more body surface area involvement on day 1, Electrolytes (serum bicarbonate <20 mEq/L [20 mmol/L]), and blood urea Nitrogen (>28 mg/dL [10 mmol/L]). Mortality is directly correlated with the number of SCORTEN variables that are fulfilled.

KEY POINT

- Body surface area involvement is the strongest prognostic indicator in Stevens-Johnson syndrome/toxic epidermal necrosis (SJS/TEN).

Bibliography

Bastuji-Garin S, Fouchard N, Bertocchi M, Roujeau JC, Revuz J, Wolkenstein P. SCORTEN: a severity-of-illness score for toxic epidermal necrolysis. J Invest Dermatol. 2000;115:149-53. [PMID: 10951229]

Item 15   Answer: C

Educational Objective: Diagnose molluscum contagiosum infection.

Molluscum contagiosum is a common cutaneous viral infection caused by the poxvirus molluscum contagiosum. It occurs in three settings: children, adults as a sexually transmitted disease, and AIDS patients. The lesions are flesh-colored to yellow smooth papules with a shiny surface and an umbilicated center. They can be located anywhere on the skin, but in adults they typically involve the genital area; in AIDS patients, they often involve the face. Diagnosis can be made by the clinical appearance. In immunocompromised patients, cryptococcosis, histoplasmosis, or *Penicillium marneffei* infections may resemble molluscum lesions and should be differentiated by skin biopsy. Although lesions can self-resolve, this may take months to years. Therapy includes destructive techniques including cryotherapy, salicylic acid, cantharidin, or physical removal with curettage.

Anogenital warts (condylomata acuminata) are the most common sexually transmitted infection and are most often caused by human papillomavirus types 6 and 11. They present as single or multiple papules on the penis, vulva, or perianal area and may be variably sized flat-topped or cauliflower-like papules. They do not have a shiny surface nor are they umbilicated. Lesions are diagnosed based on clinical appearance. Although warts may resolve spontaneously, treatment often is required. Treatment of anogenital warts may include chemical or physical destruction, immunologic therapy, or excision.

Herpes simplex virus (HSV) infection presents as localized, grouped pink macules and papules that progress to vesicles on an erythematous base and then evolve into pustules with subsequent ulcers and erosions. HSV1 traditionally causes orofacial lesions, and HSV2 most often causes genital lesions; however, both viruses can lead to either oral or genital lesions. Diagnosis of HSV can be made clinically, but several rapid tests are widely available, such as direct-fluorescent antibody and polymerase chain reaction. Oral antiviral agents including acyclovir, valacyclovir, and famciclovir are considered first-line therapies.

Seborrheic keratosis is a benign neoplasm of the skin that has a "stuck-on" appearance. They have a wide range of shades from tan to black, have different morphologies, and vary in size from a few millimeters to several centimeters. It is more common with advancing age and can be seen anywhere on the body, but they characteristically spare the palms and soles. This young patient's shiny papules are not compatible with the diagnosis of seborrheic keratoses.

KEY POINT

- Molluscum contagiosum is a common cutaneous viral infection that initially appears as firm, umbilicated flesh-colored to yellow papules; in adults it is considered a sexually transmitted infection that frequently involves the genital area.

Bibliography

Ramdass P, Mullick S, Farber HF. Viral Skin Diseases. Prim Care. 2015;42:517-67. [PMID: 26612372] doi:10.1016/j.pop.2015.08.006

Item 16   Answer: A
Educational Objective: Diagnose bullous pemphigoid.

This patient most likely has bullous pemphigoid, a chronic autoimmune blistering disease (ABD). ABDs should be suspected in any patient with persistent or recurrent blisters involving the skin, eyes, or oral and genital mucosa. The clinical presentation can vary depending on the underlying disorder, ranging from large urticarial plaques to flaccid blisters that may almost instantly rupture and appear as erosions to intact tense bullae. ABDs can be subdivided into intraepidermal and subepidermal disorders. Intraepidermal ABDs clinically present with flaccid vesicles that are seldom clinically visualized. They rupture easily leaving painful erosions, whereas subepidermal ABDs show intact, tense bullae. The intact, tense blisters seen in this patient suggest a subepidermal ABD, such as bullous pemphigoid, as the clinical diagnosis.

Bullous pemphigoid presents with urticarial and eczematous lesions on the trunk and upper legs that progress to tense bullae on an erythematous base. Onset is usually in elderly adults. Oral involvement is present in approximately 20% of patients. A thorough examination of the eyes, oral mucosa, and genital/perianal mucosa should be performed because mucosal and ocular involvement can lead to scarring, resulting in blindness and vaginal or oral contractures. There are varying degrees of pruritus with bullous pemphigoid.

Dermatitis herpetiformis is a subepidermal ABD that is extremely pruritic. There are small tense vesicles and papules, which are rarely intact due to the extreme pruritus and resultant scratching; therefore the usual presentation is excoriations on the elbows, knees, and buttocks.

Pemphigus foliaceus and pemphigus vulgaris are intraepidermal ABD. Pemphigus foliaceus is most common in middle-aged adults. There are crusted erosions ("corn flakes") on the scalp, head/neck, and trunk without mucous membrane involvement. It can be associated with other autoimmune diseases. Drug-induced pemphigus often has this pattern.

Pemphigus vulgaris is the most common intraepidermal ABD, and its incidence increases with age. It presents with oral and/or vaginal erosions and flaccid vesicles. Pemphigus vulgaris is associated with a positive Nikolsky sign whereby light friction on perilesional skin induces a blister.

KEY POINT

- Bullous pemphigoid is a chronic autoimmune blistering disease that predominantly affects elderly patients; it presents with urticarial plaques with tense bullae on the trunk and upper legs.

Bibliography

Schmidt E, della Torre R, Borradori L. Clinical features and practical diagnosis of bullous pemphigoid. Immunol Allergy Clin North Am. 2012;32:217-32, v. [PMID: 22560135] doi:10.1016/j.iac.2012.04.002

Item 17   Answer: C
Educational Objective: Treat impetigo.

This patient has nonbullous impetigo, and the most appropriate treatment is topical mupirocin. Impetigo is most commonly caused by *Staphylococcus aureus* or beta-hemolytic streptococci. It is very contagious and most commonly seen in children. Impetigo can be either nonbullous or bullous impetigo. Bullous impetigo is a toxin-mediated process usually caused by production of an exfoliative toxin by *S. aureus*, which induces erythema and loss of the superficial layer of the epidermis. Nonbullous impetigo is the more common type and often affects the face or extremities. It appears as erythematous papules or pustules that rupture and then progress to erosions with overlying honey-colored crust. The diagnosis of impetigo often can be made based on clinical presentation; however, culture of the honey-colored crust can confirm the pathologic organism and obtain sensitivity testing, which is

CONT.

important when treating extensive disease or staphylococcal scalded skin syndrome. This patient has only a few lesions, so the best treatment would be topical mupirocin. Mupirocin is a topical antibiotic that inhibits bacterial protein synthesis. It has good activity against both *S. aureus* and beta-hemolytic streptococci. There has been limited reported antibiotic resistance to mupirocin, and it is usually well tolerated. Washes with chlorhexidine and diluted bleach baths also can be used.

Oral doxycycline would be a treatment for patients with suspected or confirmed methicillin-resistant *Staphylococcus aureus* (MRSA) skin and soft tissue infection. Oral antibiotic therapy increases antibiotic resistance and has more potential side effects compared with topical therapy, so oral doxycycline would not be the most appropriate choice. Oral antibiotics should be reserved for patients with more extensive infection, involvement of deeper skin structures, or systemic symptoms such as fever. Cephalexin, dicloxacillin, erythromycin, amoxicillin-clavulanate, and clindamycin are the preferred initial systemic treatments for extensive impetigo.

Topical hydrocortisone is not appropriate to treat impetigo caused by *S. aureus* or beta-hemolytic streptococci. It may be used for eczematous dermatitis, but not for impetigo.

Topical neomycin/polymyxin B/bacitracin does have some activity again *S. aureus* and streptococci, but it is not as effective as mupirocin. Also, there is a higher risk of allergic contact dermatitis with topical antibiotics containing neomycin and bacitracin, so this would not be the most appropriate treatment in this patient.

> **KEY POINT**
>
> - A topical antibacterial agent, such as mupirocin, is the first-line therapy for localized impetigo.

Bibliography

Hartman-Adams H, Banvard C, Juckett G. Impetigo: diagnosis and treatment. Am Fam Physician. 2014 Aug 15;90(4):229-35. [PMID: 25250996]

 Item 18   Answer: D

Educational Objective: Diagnose rheumatoid vasculitis.

Elderly smokers with long-standing rheumatoid arthritis and high rheumatoid factor titers are at risk for rheumatoid vasculitis. Rheumatoid vasculitis commonly affects small to medium-sized vessels of the skin, digits, peripheral nerves, eyes, and heart. Small-vessel vasculitis (leukocytoclastic vasculitis) appears as palpable purpura. In medium-vessel disease, nodules, ulcerations, livedo reticularis, and digital infarcts can occur. Periungual purpura (Bywaters lesions) is the result of nailfold thrombosis and appears as purpuric papules on the digital pulp of a few digits and in the nail fold area.

Actinic purpura is caused by age- and sun damage-related capillary fragility and bleeding under atrophic skin. It is recognized as a flat, noninflamed ecchymosis typically in sun damaged skin on the forearms and dorsal hands.

Illicit drug use can result in leukocytoclastic vasculitis, most notably from cocaine adulterated with levami-

sole. These patients generally have palpable purpura, often with involvement of the ears. Laboratory studies typically show an elevated ANCA titer, with a mixed perinuclear and cytoplasmic pattern. These findings are absent in this patient.

Infective endocarditis can result in localized immune-mediated vasculitis secondary to vascular occlusion by infected microthrombi. Infective endocarditis is an unlikely diagnosis in this patient in the absence of heart murmur, fever (present in 90% of patients), or constitutional symptoms such as anorexia and weight loss.

> **KEY POINT**
>
> - Rheumatoid vasculitis typically occurs in elderly male smokers with long-standing rheumatoid arthritis and high titers of rheumatoid factor; it can appear as a small or medium-sized vasculitis and may affect nerves and other organs.

Bibliography

Sharma A, Dhooria A, Aggarwal A, Rathi M, Chandran V. Connective tissue disorder-associated vasculitis. Curr Rheumatol Rep. 2016 Jun;18(6):31. [PMID: 27097818]

Item 19   Answer: D

Educational Objective: Treat drug-induced subacute cutaneous lupus erythematosus.

This patient has subacute cutaneous lupus erythematosus (SCLE), and she should discontinue adalimumab. Approximately one third of SCLE cases are drug induced. Tumor necrosis factor inhibitors such as adalimumab are a leading cause of drug-induced SCLE. Unlike psoriasis, SCLE is photodistributed, tends to burn more than itch, and has a lighter pink-to-violet tone when compared with the red tones of psoriasis. Psoriasis improves with sun exposure, whereas SCLE worsens with sun exposure. This patient's rash at presentation is different from the distribution and appearance of her psoriasis, and it is worsened in the sun rather than improved. These features argue against psoriasis treatment failure and point toward drug-induced SCLE. Medications should be evaluated as a cause of all cases of SCLE, particularly those affecting young white men who have a very low risk of developing lupus spectrum disease. Other common causative medications are hydrochlorothiazide, ACE inhibitors, NSAIDs, proton pump inhibitors, and terbinafine. Drug withdrawal typically leads to improvement in drug-induced SCLE.

Hydroxychloroquine is a first-line therapy for native cutaneous lupus, but cessation of adalimumab is a better choice for drug-induced SCLE.

Methotrexate is an excellent agent to add to tumor necrosis factor inhibitors to prevent or manage the development of human antichimeric antibodies, which may lead to treatment failure or resistance in psoriasis or psoriatic arthritis. Such treatment failure may manifest as a sudden loss of efficacy of therapy with recurrence of skin or joint symptoms. This patient has no evidence of treatment failure, and the best management of the new rash is discontinuation of adalimumab.

A short prednisone taper might give the patient brief respite from her symptoms, but they would return shortly if adalimumab is not discontinued. Short prednisone tapers should be avoided in patients with psoriasis as significant rebound skin disease can occur, resulting in erythroderma in some patients.

KEY POINT

- Subacute cutaneous lupus erythematosus is frequently diagnosed as a drug-induced photosensitive rash characterized by erythematous annular scaly patches.

Bibliography

Grönhagen CM, Fored CM, Linder M, Granath F, Nyberg F. Subacute cutaneous lupus erythematosus and its association with drugs: a population-based matched case-control study of 234 patients in Sweden. Br J Dermatol. 2012;167:296-305. [PMID: 22458771] doi:10.1111/j.1365-2133.2012.10969.x

Item 20   Answer: E

Educational Objective: Manage recurrent cellulitis.

The most appropriate management of this patient is to treat the interdigital intertrigo. The diagnosis of cellulitis often is made based on the clinical presentation of a well-demarcated warm and tender erythematous plaque. Bacteria enter through superficial breaks in the skin or gain access by hematogenous spread. Treatment of the maceration and fissuring in the toe web spaces can decrease the risk of recurrent cellulitis. This fissuring, maceration, and scaling are often due to tinea pedis, which allows entry for *Streptococcus* and *Staphylococcus aureus* to infect the lower extremity. In addition, attempts should be made to identify and treat other predisposing conditions for cellulitis, such as edema, obesity, eczema, and venous insufficiency.

Because this is only the second episode of cellulitis for this patient, prophylactic antibiotics are inappropriate. There has been no attempt to address predisposing factors. Prophylactic antibiotics can be considered when a patient has three to four episodes of cellulitis per year. Treatment is usually with oral penicillin or erythromycin. Attempts to treat predisposing factors such as edema, obesity, venous insufficiency, and toe web abnormalities should be addressed first.

Blood culture is not recommended for cellulitis unless a patient has a malignancy and is on chemotherapy, or has neutropenia, severe immunodeficiency, an immersion injury, or an animal bite. This patient has none of these indications.

The patient has a classic presentation of cellulitis, and obtaining a skin biopsy is not necessary.

Staphylococcal decolonization with intranasal mupirocin can be considered for recurrent skin abscesses, but it is not effective for recurrent cellulitis.

KEY POINT

- Evaluation of the interdigital toe spaces and treatment of the maceration and fissuring in the web spaces and modification of other predisposing factors such as edema, obesity, eczema, and venous insufficiency can decrease the risk of recurrent cellulitis.

Bibliography

Stevens DL, Bisno AL, Chambers HF, Dellinger EP, et al. Practice guidelines for the diagnosis and management of skin and soft tissue infections: 2014 update by the Infectious Diseases Society of America. Clin Infect Dis. 2014 Jul 15;59(2):e10-52. [PMID: 24973422]

Item 21   Answer: B

Educational Objective: Manage recalcitrant actinic keratosis.

The most appropriate management for this lesion is biopsy. Actinic keratoses are red scaly papules and plaques that occur in sun-exposed areas, most often in those over age 50. They have a "gritty" texture, and early lesions are often easier to palpate than to see. Diagnosis is usually made clinically rather than with biopsy. Individual lesions are often treated with cryotherapy. In patients with a large number of actinic keratoses, areas with multiple lesions are best treated with topical preparations (such as 5-fluorouracil or imiquimod); photodynamic therapy may also be performed.

If traditional therapies do not eradicate the lesions, there is a possibility that the clinical diagnosis is incorrect. In this case, the lesion is now indurated, which is not compatible with the diagnosis of actinic keratosis. Possible alternative diagnoses include basal cell and squamous cell carcinomas. Histologic diagnosis would give definitive diagnosis and guide treatment options.

Repeated cryotherapy may treat the superficial portion of the lesion, while the deeper portion of the tumor may continue to grow. Cryosurgery can be used to treat basal cell carcinomas; however, the targeted depth and the temperature of the lesion need to be carefully monitored. However, a definitive diagnosis is required before this therapy can be considered.

Topical imiquimod is an interferon inducer, and it can treat actinic keratosis by producing an immunologic reaction against the lesion. It is also used to treat some basal cell carcinomas; it is an effective treatment and approved only for the superficial pathologic subtype of basal cell carcinoma. However, a biopsy of the lesion is the first step in the proper management of this patient.

Standard treatment for most basal cell carcinomas is wide local excision; however, some histologic types and body locations require more aggressive management. Biopsy prior to excision is important because the histopathologic diagnosis should be used to guide treatment.

KEY POINT

- Actinic keratoses that do not resolve with cryotherapy or other appropriate therapy will require a biopsy to rule out an invasive neoplasm.

Bibliography

Siegel JA, Korgavkar K, Weinstock MA. Current perspective on actinic keratosis: a review. Br J Dermatol. 2016. [PMID: 27500794] doi:10.1111/bjd.14852

Item 22   Answer: A

Educational Objective: Diagnose basal cell carcinoma.

The patient has a basal cell carcinoma, the most common type of skin cancer. The lesion demonstrates typical findings with a translucent (pearly) papule and arborizing telangiectasias. It typically appears on sun-exposed areas in fair-skinned persons with a history of extensive sun exposure. It is usually asymptomatic and enlarges slowly over time. Although it rarely metastasizes, basal cell carcinoma can cause significant local tissue destruction if not removed.

Melanocytic nevi, often referred to as "moles," are found in persons of all ages. They are benign collections of melanocytes and histologically consist of nests of melanocytes occurring at the dermal-epidermal junction and dermis. They occur most commonly in sun-exposed areas. Junctional nevi are flat and often dark brown in color. Compound nevi are raised (papules) and may be irregularly pigmented. Dermal nevi are soft and flesh-colored and may resemble skin tags. This patient's translucent papule with telangiectasias is not consistent with the findings of a dermal nevus.

Keratoacanthomas tend to be rapidly growing pink nodules with a crusted hyperkeratotic core or central crater of crust and scale ("volcaniform"). Keratoacanthomas usually stabilize after a period of rapid growth and then slowly involute, eventually resolving completely. Since some lesions fail to resolve completely and may persist, they are usually treated with surgical excision. A rapidly growing nodule with a hyperkeratotic core is not consistent with this patient's findings.

Melanoma is a neoplasm of the pigment-making cells, melanocytes. The clinical features that suggest melanoma are represented by the mnemonic "ABCDE," where "A" stands for Asymmetry, "B" for irregular Border, "C" for multiple Colors, "D" for Diameter greater than 6 mm, and "E" for Evolution, meaning increasing size. Melanoma may be further classified into several different subtypes. Nodular melanomas are the most aggressive subtype and have an invasive component from the beginning. A nodular melanoma appears as a darkly pigmented, pedunculated, or polypoid nodule. Amelanotic variants do occur but are rare. The patient's translucent nodule is not consistent with the typical findings of a nodular melanoma.

Squamous cell carcinoma is the second most common type of skin cancer and the most common skin cancer in persons who are immunocompromised following solid organ transplant. Squamous cell carcinoma appears as a pink hyperkeratotic papule or nodule. Compared with basal cell carcinoma, it usually has scale and does not have that translucent, pearly appearance.

Bibliography

Rubin AI, Chen EH, Ratner D. Basal-cell carcinoma. N Engl J Med. 2005;353:2262-9. [PMID: 16306523]

Item 23   Answer: B

Educational Objective: Diagnose lupus pernio.

This patient has lupus pernio, a variant of sarcoidosis that involves granulomatous inflammation of the skin around the nares. Histopathology of sarcoidosis shows granulomatous inflammation of the affected tissue with noncaseating granulomas and minimal lymphocytic infiltration.

The term "lupus pernio" is a source of potential confusion. "Lupus" generally refers to systemic lupus erythematosus; "pernio" generally refers to a condition of purple papules on the distal digits exacerbated by cold and moisture; and lupus vulgaris is a form of tuberculosis of the skin. Lupus pernio has little to do with these, however. The typical appearance of lupus pernio includes violaceous subcutaneous plaques or nodules of the central face, often with some overlying scaling, most commonly seen in black persons. Patients with lupus pernio tend to have a chronic, refractory course, and extracutaneous disease. A careful evaluation for the presence of extracutaneous disease is necessary in any patient with cutaneous sarcoid, and treatment depends on other organ involvement and the severity of the clinical disease.

Lepromatous leprosy may consist of erythematous macules, papules, and nodules or occasionally simply diffuse infiltration and palpable thickening of the skin. The condition is often generalized in distribution at diagnosis. There is frequent involvement of the nasal mucosa resulting in nasal stuffiness and eventually a saddle-nose deformity. The patient's localized skin findings are most consistent with lupus pernio.

The classic findings of lupus vulgaris, a chronic, progressive form of cutaneous tuberculosis, include multiple discrete, red-brown papules that subsequently coalesce to form a slowly growing asymptomatic plaque most typically found on the head and neck. Histopathology will show granulomas with a variable degree of central caseating necrosis; this finding is absent in this patient, making lupus vulgaris an unlikely diagnosis.

The most specific skin manifestations of systemic lupus erythematosus are variations on interface dermatitis, with pink-to-violet macules or plaques and varying scale or atrophy. One example is acute cutaneous lupus erythematosus (ACLE), also known as malar or butterfly rash. ACLE consists of erythema and edema over the cheeks and bridge of the nose and sometimes the forehead and chin. Granuloma formation is not a feature of lupus-specific skin disease.

KEY POINT

- Lupus pernio is sarcoidosis of the nose and central face, manifesting as violaceous subcutaneous plaques or nodules, often with some overlying scale.

Bibliography

Wanat KA, Rosenbach M. Cutaneous Sarcoidosis. Clin Chest Med. 2015;36:685-702. [PMID: 26593142] doi:10.1016/j.ccm.2015.08.010

Item 24   Answer: C

Educational Objective: Treat high-risk basal cell carcinoma.

The most appropriate treatment for this lesion is Mohs micrographic surgery. Mohs micrographic surgery is a specialized surgical procedure that provides margin control while sparing as much normal skin as possible. Indications for Mohs micrographic surgery include tumors with aggressive histologic subtypes (micronodular, morpheaform, infiltrative, perineural involvement), high-risk and cosmetically sensitive locations (face, genitals), large tumors or tumors arising in scar tissue, and in patients who are immunosuppressed. Because this patient has a high-risk tumor that is located in a cosmetically sensitive location, Mohs surgery is the most appropriate treatment.

Small noninfiltrating basal cell carcinomas can be treated with cryotherapy; however, other surgical methods are more commonly used. To treat basal cell carcinomas appropriately with cryotherapy, the target temperature is –50 °C using liquid nitrogen as the cryogen and this requires local anesthesia. Hypopigmentation is often seen after cryotherapy. The histologic subtype and location of the basal cell carcinoma make cryotherapy inappropriate for this patient.

Electrodesiccation and curettage is a widely used treatment for noninfiltrating basal cell carcinomas on low-risk anatomic sites (trunk and extremities). High-risk infiltrative and micronodular basal cell carcinomas are not appropriate for electrodesiccation and curettage. Additionally, because it may result in a cosmetically unappealing scar on the nose, it should not be used for this patient.

Topical therapies including 5-fluorouracil and imiquimod are most effective for superficial basal cell carcinomas. Superficial basal cell carcinomas are well-demarcated, irregularly bordered red patches; they tend to enlarge radially rather than invading into deeper structures. Topical therapies are not effective for more aggressive histologic subtypes of basal cell carcinomas.

Vismodegib is an oral medication that inhibits the hedgehog signaling pathway. It is reserved for locally advanced or metastatic basal cell carcinomas. There are significant side effects including dysgeusia, alopecia, and muscle cramps.

KEY POINT

- Mohs surgery, a form of margin-controlled surgery that minimizes loss of normal tissue, is particularly useful for basal cell tumors in areas such as the head and neck, for large or recurrent tumors, for histologically high-risk tumors, or when cosmetic outcome is crucial.

Bibliography

Connolly SM, Baker DR, Coldiron BM, Fazio MJ, Storrs PA, Vidimos AT, et al; American Academy of Dermatology. AAD/ACMS/ASDSA/ASMS 2012 appropriate use criteria for Mohs micrographic surgery: a report of the American Academy of Dermatology, American College of Mohs Surgery, American Society for Dermatologic Surgery Association, and the American Society for Mohs Surgery. Dermatol Surg. 2012;38:1582-603. [PMID: 22958088] doi:10.1111/j.1524-4725.2012.02574.x

Item 25   Answer: B

Educational Objective: Diagnose erythema multiforme major.

Erythema multiforme (EM) features the development of characteristic tricolored targetoid plaques, as this patient demonstrates on the extremities and face. In EM major, these targetoid plaques are accompanied by mucous membrane involvement. The most common cause of EM is infection, and herpes simplex virus 1 and 2 are the most commonly recognized, followed by *Mycoplasma pneumoniae*. The treatment of EM major is supportive, and most cases resolve in a week. Suppressive therapy may be necessary for patients who have relapses of EM with herpes outbreaks.

Patients with disseminated gonococcal infection and bacteremia present with vesiculopustular or hemorrhagic macular skin lesions, fever, chills, and polyarthralgia. Knees, elbows, and distal joints are typical sites of involvement. Tenosynovitis of the dorsa of the hands and/or feet is a characteristic feature. Gonococcemia does not cause targetoid plaques or mucositis.

Stevens-Johnson syndrome (SJS) and toxic epidermal necrolysis (TEN) are typically medication reactions. Mucous membrane involvement and targetoid lesions occur as well. Unlike EM, however, the targetoid lesions in SJS and TEN lack the true tricolor appearance and are thus labeled atypical targetoid plaques. Like EM, SJS can sometimes be triggered by infection, but unlike EM, SJS is characterized by necrosis and sloughing of the skin. SJS and TEN have systemic manifestations such as acute kidney injury and elevated liver chemistry tests, whereas EM does not.

KEY POINT

- Erythema multiforme major is recognized by targetoid lesions accompanied by mucous membrane involvement; a drug or infection (herpes simplex virus or *Mycoplasma pneumoniae*) can trigger erythema multiforme.

Bibliography

Stoopler ET, Houston AM, Chmieliauskaite M, Sollecito TP. Erythema Multiforme. J Emerg Med. 2015;49:e197-8. [PMID: 26281815] doi:10.1016/j.jemermed.2015.06.018

Item 26   Answer: E

Educational Objective: Diagnose actinic purpura.

Actinic purpura is a common incidental finding in elderly persons, and no intervention is needed at this time; however, reassurance should be provided to the patient and caregiver.

A myriad of changes occur in the skin over time; these can be due to chronologic aging alone or influenced by the cumulative effects of ultraviolet light exposure. Actinic purpura is caused by age-related capillary fragility and bleeding under atrophic skin. Minor trauma can cause impressive purpuric macules and patches, most commonly on the forearm. It is not a sign of vasculitis, a bleeding disorder, or nutritional deficiency, and it does not require additional evaluation with coagulation studies or therapy. Often associated with actinic purpura are stellate pseudoscars, jagged or linear atrophic scars that primarily occur on the forearms of patients with chronic actinic damage. Patients may or may not recall antecedent trauma. There is no treatment for actinic purpura. Good skin care measures such as emollient moisturizers can help reduce dryness and protect the skin from minor trauma such as scratching.

It is unnecessary to biopsy this lesion. There is no indication that it is a new growth or that this is an undiagnosed inflammatory skin condition or vasculitis.

Although it is good to be alert for abusive situations, in this case the findings are typical for actinic purpura.

Triamcinolone is a medium-potency glucocorticoid. Although initial application of the ointment will not harm the patient, chronic application of a medium-potency glucocorticoid on normal skin will result in thinning of the already thin skin, the development of striae and purpura, pigmentary changes, acneiform eruptions, and an increased risk for infection, resulting in more damage.

> **KEY POINT**
>
> - Actinic purpura is caused by age-related capillary fragility and bleeding under atrophic skin; minor trauma can cause impressive purpuric macules and patches, most commonly on the forearm.

Bibliography

Blume-Peytavi U, Kottner J, Sterry W, Hodin MW, Griffiths TW, Watson RE, et al. Age-associated skin conditions and diseases: current perspectives and future options. Gerontologist. 2016;56 Suppl 2:S230-42. [PMID: 26994263] doi:10.1093/geront/gnw003

Item 27   Answer: E
Educational Objective: Diagnose stasis dermatitis.

This patient has stasis dermatitis with the characteristic findings of bilateral edema, erythema, scaling, and pruritus of the bilateral lower legs. Crusting and erosions may also be seen. This is due to chronic venous insufficiency or other causes of chronic lower extremity edema. When secondary to chronic venous insufficiency, varicosities, telangiectasias, ulcers, and brown discoloration may also be noted. Symptomatic treatment with topical glucocorticoids and emollients should be used; however, the edema must be addressed with compression stockings and leg elevation for significant improvement to occur.

Allergic contact dermatitis is common in patients with stasis dermatitis. It commonly occurs due to the application of topical medications such as over-the-counter triple antibiotic ointment. This patient denies applying any topical medication or emollient to her legs, so her diagnosis would not be allergic contact dermatitis. In patients exposed to potential allergens, a clue to the diagnosis of contact dermatitis is the failure of the patient to respond to appropriate therapy for stasis dermatitis. In these patients, patch testing is often necessary to determine if a secondary allergic contact dermatitis is present.

Stasis dermatitis is often misdiagnosed as cellulitis. It would be unusual for cellulitis to present bilaterally. Unlike stasis dermatitis, cellulitis is typically tender and not pruritic. Cellulitis is usually hot to the touch and involves less scaling than stasis dermatitis.

Leukocytoclastic vasculitis is inflammation of the small vessels of the skin; it typically presents with nonblanching, violaceous papules (palpable purpura), and macules on the lower extremities. Leukocytoclastic vasculitis can be idiopathic, but it is usually associated with an infection or is often drug induced. Other causes of leukocytoclastic vasculitis include connective tissue disease, inflammatory bowel disease, and malignancies.

Psoriasis is characterized by well-demarcated, erythematous plaques with silvery scale. It commonly appears on the knees, elbows, and scalp. There can be associated nail changes (nail pits, onycholysis). This patient's clinical presentation is not consistent with psoriasis.

> **KEY POINT**
>
> - Stasis dermatitis is typically characterized by edema, erythema, scaling, and pruritus on the lower legs and occurs in patients with venous insufficiency or other causes of chronic lower extremity edema.

Bibliography

Eberhardt RT, Raffetto JD. Chronic venous insufficiency. Circulation. 2014 Jul 22;130(4):333-46. [PMID: 25047584]

Item 28   Answer: A
Educational Objective: Treat an epidermal inclusion cyst.

This patient has an epidermal inclusion cyst (sometimes called epidermoid cyst), and the most appropriate treatment is excision. The diagnosis of epidermal inclusion cysts is clinical. Epidermal inclusion cysts range from a few millimeters to several centimeters in size and are subepidermal, freely movable nodules with an epithelial lining and a core of accumulated keratin debris. They are most commonly found on the trunk. Epidermal inclusion cysts are often incorrectly referred to as "sebaceous cysts," a term that is erroneous because they possess keratin rather than sebum. Often they have a central punctum by which foul-smelling material can be expressed; the odor is derived from the presence of anaerobic bacteria. Epidermal inclusion cysts are benign but are frequently removed if they become bothersome to the patient. In this case, treatment is by excision with removal of the entire cyst wall.

When epidermal inclusion cysts rupture, they may become tender, inflamed, and occasionally infected. Ruptured cysts are often mistaken for furuncles or infectious abscesses. Ruptured cysts are treated with incision and drainage, and intralesional glucocorticoid injections may be used to reduce the inflammation.

Incision, as well as incision with drainage, can lead to temporary improvement of an inflamed epidermal cyst; however, recurrences are common as the epithelial lining must be removed for complete treatment. Therefore, these are not the preferred treatment.

Antibiotics are rarely required; they should only be used when there is concern for secondary infection.

KEY POINT

- Excision is the most appropriate treatment for bothersome epidermal inclusion cysts since the epithelial lining must be removed for complete treatment.

Bibliography
Higgins JC, Maher MH, Douglas MS. Diagnosing common benign skin tumors. Am Fam Physician. 2015;92:601-7. [PMID: 26447443]

Item 29   Answer: D

Educational Objective: Treat telogen effluvium.

This patient has telogen effluvium, and the most appropriate management is reassurance. Telogen effluvium is the most common cause of diffuse alopecia in adult women. Telogen effluvium is a generalized nonscarring alopecia that presents with excessive shedding of normal telogen club hairs. It is due to premature conversion of anagen hair follicles into the telogen, or final, phase of hair development after a physically or psychologically traumatic event such as surgery, parturition, or fever, commonly occurring 3 to 5 months after the event. It is particularly common after pregnancy. No specific therapy is required, and most cases will resolve spontaneously in about 6 to 12 months. Prognosis is especially good if the event causing the alopecia is identifiable.

Intralesional glucocorticoids are the treatment of choice for localized alopecia areata. This tends to present as rapid and complete loss of hair in well-demarcated round or oval patches. There may be some exclamation point hairs at the periphery.

In properly selected patients, finasteride is used to treat androgenic alopecia. Dihydrotestosterone (DHT) binds to androgen receptors in hair follicles, transforming terminal hair follicles to miniaturized hair follicles. Finasteride inhibits the conversion of testosterone to DHT and slows the process of androgenic alopecia. In androgenic alopecia the pattern of hair loss reflects the sensitivity of the hair follicle to DHT. Typically male-pattern hair loss starts with anterior hair line recession with eventual biparietal and vertex hair loss. In contrast, in women the top of the head is affected, and balding is not complete. A classic examination finding is a widening of the central part compared with the occipital part. Finasteride is contraindicated (FDA category X) in pregnant women

because it is known to cause birth defects in the male fetus. Women who are or may potentially be pregnant should not take finasteride and should avoid contact with crushed or broken tablets because it can be absorbed through the skin.

Topical minoxidil can be used for male or female patterned hair loss. Minoxidil prolongs the duration of anagen, shortens telogen, and enlarges miniaturized follicles. Like finasteride, minoxidil is ineffective (and unnecessary) in hair loss caused by telogen effluvium.

KEY POINT

- Telogen effluvium is a generalized nonscarring alopecia triggered by a physically traumatic event such as surgery, parturition, or fever; it usually spontaneously resolves in about 6 to 12 months if the trigger is removed or treated.

Bibliography
Mubki T, Rudnicka L, Olszewska M, Shapiro J. Evaluation and diagnosis of the hair loss patient: part II. Trichoscopic and laboratory evaluations. J Am Acad Dermatol. 2014;71:431.e1-431.e11. [PMID: 25128119] doi: 10.1016/j.jaad.2014.05.008

Item 30   Answer: B

Educational Objective: Diagnose melasma.

This patient has melasma, an acquired hypermelanotic condition most commonly affecting women of childbearing age. It presents as tan-brown reticulated patches in the centrofacial, malar, and mandible areas. Pigmentation can develop rapidly, often over weeks. Melasma is more apparent or more frequent in patients with darker skin and who live in sunny areas. The pathogenesis is unknown. Common causes are hormonal factors such as pregnancy and oral contraceptives, ultraviolet light, and genetic predisposition. While melasma has no medical significance, it can be very distressing to patients. Treatment is challenging and involves strict sun avoidance and topical depigmenting agents and chemical peels.

Irritant contact dermatitis is caused by a direct toxic effect on the epidermis from exposure to a chemical such as a cleaning agent, other caustic substances, or repeated wetting and drying. For example, excessive washing with harsh soap will often lead to dry irritated skin, which is not immune mediated. This patient's skin findings include primarily hyperpigmentation without evidence of dry irritated skin, making irritant contact dermatitis unlikely.

Morbilliform (meaning measles-like) drug eruption is characterized by a sudden generalized symmetrical appearance of bright red macules and papules most prominently on the trunk and extremities. Systemic symptoms include pruritus and sometimes low-grade fever. Eruptions typically start within 1 week of starting a new medication. This patient's brown pigmentation on her face without systemic symptoms is not compatible with a morbilliform drug reaction.

Postinflammatory hyperpigmentation is a darkening of the skin resulting from cutaneous inflammation. Common causes include acne vulgaris and eczematous dermatoses.

The duration of postinflammatory pigmentary changes varies, depending on the location and degree of inflammation. Hyperpigmentation on the lower legs can take several years to fade. Some postinflammatory pigment changes are permanent. Treatment of postinflammatory pigment changes includes treatment of any underlying skin inflammation, sun avoidance or sun protection, and consideration of a bleaching cream. The patient had no history of a previous inflammatory skin condition making postinflammatory hyperpigmentation an unlikely diagnosis.

KEY POINT

- Melasma is an acquired hypermelanotic condition most commonly affecting women of childbearing age; it is characterized by tan-brown reticulated patches in the centrofacial, malar, and mandible areas.

Bibliography

Sheth VM, Pandya AG. Melasma: a comprehensive update: part I. J Am Acad Dermatol. 2011;65:689-97; quiz 698. [PMID: 21920241] doi:10.1016/j.jaad.2010.12.046

Item 31   Answer: D

Educational Objective: Diagnose HIV-associated seborrheic dermatitis.

This patient has new-onset seborrheic dermatitis that is unresponsive to typical therapy, and he should be tested for HIV. Seborrheic dermatitis presents as erythematous patches with greasy scale on the scalp, nasolabial folds, and chest. This condition is extremely common in HIV patients, and most patients with AIDS have some evidence of seborrheic dermatitis. The incidence and severity of seborrheic dermatitis is also increased in patients with neurologic conditions, in particular Parkinson disease. Patients with new or explosive onset of seborrheic dermatitis, or seborrheic dermatitis that is severe or extensive, found in unusual locations, or is resistant to treatment, should be evaluated for HIV infection.

Patients with diabetes mellitus can develop a wide range of skin findings such as hyperpigmentation of acanthosis nigricans, which tends to present in the intertriginous areas, particularly in the axillae, in obese persons with diabetes. Patients with type 1 diabetes are at increased risk for development of vitiligo. Patients with diabetes may develop orange, atrophic plaques on their anterior shins (necrobiosis lipoidica). Other cutaneous findings associated with diabetes are bullous diabeticorum (large, asymptomatic, noninflammatory bullae on the lower extremities) and scleredema (an uncommon skin finding characterized by edematous induration of the upper back). Diabetic dermopathy (multiple hyperpigmented macules on the anterior shins) is one of the most common cutaneous findings. Seborrheic dermatitis is not associated with diabetes.

Hyperlipidemia may be associated with xanthomas. Xanthomas are localized lipid deposits in organs and their cutaneous manifestations include several subtypes, most commonly eruptive xanthomas, tuberous xanthomas, tendinous xanthomas, and plane xanthomas. The subtype of xanthoma can often predict the most likely associated underlying disorder. Seborrheic dermatitis is not associated with hyperlipidemia.

Chronic hepatitis C infection is associated with porphyria cutanea tarda and lichen planus. Porphyria cutanea tarda presents with small, transient, easily ruptured vesicles in sun-exposed areas, mainly on the hands. Hypertrichosis may be seen on the tops of the hands or cheeks. Lichen planus is an acute eruption of purple, pruritic, polygonal papules that most commonly develops on the flexural surfaces, especially the wrists and ankles. Lichen planus can also occur in the mucous membranes appearing as white plaques. Seborrheic dermatitis is not associated with hepatitis C infection.

KEY POINT

- Patients with new or explosive onset of seborrheic dermatitis, or seborrheic dermatitis that is severe or extensive, found in unusual locations, or is resistant to treatment, should be evaluated for HIV infection.

Bibliography

Tschachler E. The dermatologist and the HIV/AIDS pandemic. Clin Dermatol. 2014;32:286-9. [PMID: 24559565] doi:10.1016/j.clindermatol.2013.08.012

Item 32   Answer: D

Educational Objective: Diagnose transient acantholytic dermatosis.

Transient acantholytic dermatosis, also known as Grover disease, is a benign common eruption that is most often seen in middle-aged to elderly men. The eruption presents as small discrete papules, some of which may be scaly, and papulovesicles on the trunk. Symptomatically there are varying degrees of pruritus. Although the cause and pathogenesis are unknown, a very common association is xerosis. The eruption is frequently triggered by excessive sweating. Skin biopsy shows acantholytic dyskeratosis. Transient acantholytic dermatosis is typically self-limited, but therapy with topical glucocorticoids or moisturizers may be effective.

Allergic contact dermatitis is a pruritic eruption of patches and plaques with variable vesiculation. The eruption is found in areas of allergen exposure and typically worsens with subsequent exposures. In exuberant cases, the localized inflammation can lead to a secondary "id" reaction, a generalized acute cutaneous reaction in which pinpoint flesh-colored to red papules develop diffusely on the body. The absence of a known sensitizer and a pruritic rash that is worsened with heat and sweating is not consistent with allergic contact dermatitis. Histologic studies show spongiotic dermatitis with eosinophils.

Although atopic dermatitis is pruritic and associated with xerosis, it is clinically distinguished from transient acantholytic dermatosis by the presence of scaly eczematous patches with variable degrees of lichenification. Also, atopic dermatitis in adults appears in the flexures of the extremities rather than the torso. Finally, the prevalence of atopic dermatitis decreases with age, whereas transient acantholytic dermatosis is more common in middle-aged to elderly men. On skin biopsy, there are variable degrees of spongiosis.

Lichen planus (LP) is characterized by pruritic, purple, polygonal papules that may coalesce into plaques characteristically involving the ankles and flexor surfaces of the wrist. Fine white lines may be visible on the surface of the papules or plaques. LP can also occur in the mucous membranes (mouth, vaginal vault, and penis) with white plaques that, if uncontrolled, may ulcerate. The eruption can also develop in the nails, leading to thickening and distortion of the nail plate. LP is most commonly idiopathic but may be induced by medications or possibly infection. The purple polygonal papules and plaques of LP are not consistent with this patient's rash. A skin biopsy shows lichenoid dermatitis.

KEY POINT

- Transient acantholytic dermatosis is characterized by red pruritic papules on the chest, flanks, and back associated with dry skin, heat, and sweating.

Bibliography

Berger TG, Shive M, Harper GM. Pruritus in the older patient: a clinical review. JAMA. 2013;310:2443-50. [PMID: 24327039] doi:10.1001/jama. 2013.282023

Item 33   Answer: D

Educational Objective: Diagnose melanotic macule.

Melanotic macule or mucosal lentigo is a small, well-circumscribed, brown-to-black macule. The most common location is the lower mucosal lip, but they can occur on any mucosal surface. They are the mucosal counterpart of a lentigo on the skin. They are typically solitary, but multiple macules can occur. Numerous mucosal lentigines are associated with various syndromes such as Peutz-Jeghers and Laugier-Hunziker syndromes. Peutz-Jeghers syndrome is an autosomal dominant hamartomatous polyposis syndrome characterized by hamartomatous polyps in the gastrointestinal tract, mucocutaneous pigmentation, and an increased risk of cancer. Laugier-Hunziker syndrome is an acquired, benign disorder characterized by lentigines on the lips and buccal mucosa. It not associated with any systemic disorder.

Actinic cheilitis appears as chronic red-to-tan scaly patches with erosions and characteristically involves the lower lip. Actinic cheilitis is a premalignant condition and is considered the precursor to squamous cell carcinoma in situ. Treatment with topical chemotherapy agents (5-fluorouracil), imiquimod, laser therapy, photodynamic therapy, or cryotherapy is recommended. Actinic cheilitis differs from angular cheilitis, which is inflammation involving one or both corners of the mouth and often related to a bacterial or fungal infection.

Amalgam tattoos are the most common source of localized pigmentation on the buccal mucosa. Amalgam dental fillings contain metals that can become implanted into the adjacent mucosa at the time of application. They appear as blue-gray macules and do not change over time. The typical location for amalgam tattoos is the buccal mucosa, not the lip. Diagnosis can be made clinically, or confirmation can be made with biopsy and pathology. No treatment is necessary.

Although it can arise anywhere in the skin or mucous membranes, malignant melanoma most commonly occurs in sun-exposed areas. The back is the most common location in men, and the legs are the most common location in women. The clinical features that suggest melanoma are asymmetry, irregular border, multiple colors, diameter greater than 6 mm, and changing size. The more of these features a pigmented lesion possesses, the more worrisome it is for malignant melanoma or melanoma in-situ, and these entities must be excluded with an excisional biopsy. This patient's lesion is small, round, well-circumscribed and has no worrisome features of a melanoma.

KEY POINT

- Melanotic macules are well-circumscribed, brown-to-black macules that most commonly occur on the lower lip, although they may be seen on the gingiva, buccal mucosa, or tongue.

Bibliography

Müller S. Melanin-associated pigmented lesions of the oral mucosa: presentation, differential diagnosis, and treatment. Dermatol Ther. 2010;23:220-9. [PMID: 20597941] doi:10.1111/j.1529-8019.2010.01319.x

Item 34   Answer: C

Educational Objective: Diagnose localized scleroderma (morphea).

This patient has localized scleroderma, or morphea. Localized scleroderma is one of the scleroderma spectrum disorders, a group of diseases sharing the feature of skin hardening. The scleroderma spectrum disorders include systemic sclerosis (SSc), localized scleroderma, and scleroderma-like conditions. SSc is further characterized as two distinct subsets based on skin involvement: limited SSc and diffuse SSC. In limited SSc, scleroderma is restricted to the fingers and hands and, to a lesser extent, the face and neck. Scleroderma involving the fingers and hands, chest, abdomen, forearms, upper arms, and shoulders indicates diffuse SSc. Morphea is a localized form of scleroderma limited to one or more indurated plaques confined to the torso and proximal extremities. Although histologic findings of morphea are identical to those seen in patients with SSc, visceral manifestations and Raynaud phenomenon are absent. This patient has a generalized variant of morphea called pansclerotic morphea, which often appears in areas of friction and pressure, such as the waistband area or inframammary regions. Diffuse and limited SSc involve the fingers first, and sclerosis proceeds proximally, sometimes very rapidly.

Scleredema has a variable clinical presentation but is most easily recognizable as large, noninflammatory woody-indurated plaques over the shoulder girdle, neck, and upper extremities. In adults, scleredema occurs most commonly as a complication of diabetes mellitus but may be seen following a streptococcal infection in children or as a complication of monoclonal gammopathy.

Scleromyxedema is characterized by deposition of mucin with large numbers of stellate fibroblasts in the dermis, presenting as waxy yellow-red papules overlying thickened skin. It affects the face, upper torso, and upper extremities. The condition is rare but is most frequently associated with paraproteinemia and may therefore occur in the setting of multiple myeloma or AL amyloidosis. In a few patients, a mild inflammatory myopathy may accompany the disorder.

KEY POINT

- Localized scleroderma (morphea) is characterized as isolated sclerotic circumscribed plaques; it is not associated with Raynaud phenomenon or systemic disease and does not include sclerodactyly.

Bibliography
Sperber K, Ash J, Gutwein F, Wasserrman A, Rao V, Tratenberg M. Localized scleroderma: a clinical review. Curr Rheumatol Rev. 2016. [PMID: 27604889]

Item 35   Answer: B

Educational Objective: Diagnose lentigo maligna.

This patient has a melanoma in situ, lentigo maligna subtype. The clinical features that suggest melanoma are represented by the mnemonic "ABCDE," where "A" stands for Asymmetry, "B" for irregular Border, "C" for multiple Colors, "D" for Diameter greater than 6 mm, and "E" for Evolution, meaning increasing size. The more of these features a pigmented lesion possesses, the more worrisome it is for melanoma. Unfortunately, melanomas do not always adhere to these criteria; they may be red or flesh colored, smaller than 6 mm, perfectly symmetric, or homogeneously colored. Thus, a low threshold for biopsy should be present for any atypical-appearing skin lesion, changing or symptomatic nevus, or any mole that stands out from the background nevi pattern of the particular patient.

Melanoma may be further classified into several different subtypes. Lentigo maligna is a subtype of melanoma in situ that tends to arise on the head and neck region of elderly persons, especially those with a long history of sun damage. They are more indolent and slow growing. As the name would imply, it clinically often resembles a benign solar lentigo. A biopsy would provide the definitive diagnosis.

Melanocytic nevi are benign growths of melanocytes commonly referred to as "moles." The junctional component of the term indicates where the melanocytic nests are located. In junctional melanocytic nevi, the melanocytic nests are located in the dermal-epidermal junction. They clinically appear as brown-to-black uniform macules during early childhood and can increase in number through middle age. It is very rare for a new melanocytic nevus to appear at the age of 69.

Nodular melanoma is the most aggressive form of malignant melanoma. It is rapid growing and begins with an invasive vertical growth phase. It appears as blue-black, smooth, or eroded nodules, occurring anywhere on the body. Nodular melanomas are responsible for most deaths from melanoma.

Solar lentigines are brown, well-demarcated macules and patches that occur on the sun-exposed skin of older persons, particularly the face and dorsal hands. Previously, they were often referred to as "liver spots" because their color resembles that of the liver. Although benign, they are a marker for someone who has relatively fair skin and has received a significant amount of sun exposure over the years. They frequently occur near more worrisome lesions such as actinic keratoses or skin cancers. Lentigines with atypical features or broad, growing lentigines (particularly on the face of older, light-skinned persons) should be biopsied to rule out lentigo maligna. This patient has had extensive sun exposure and now has a growing lesion making lentigo maligna a more likely diagnosis. A biopsy is required to establish the correct diagnosis.

KEY POINT

- Melanoma in situ, lentigo maligna subtype is typically found on the head and neck region of older persons; it is associated with frequent chronic ultraviolet light exposure.

Bibliography
Longo C, Pellacani G. Melanomas. Dermatol Clin. 2016;34:411–419. [PMID: 27692447] doi:10.1016/j.det.2016.05.004

Item 36   Answer: D

Educational Objective: Treat mild inflammatory acne in pregnancy.

The patient has some mild inflammatory and comedonal acne that would be best treated with topical erythromycin. There are two main types of acne lesions: inflammatory and noninflammatory. The prototypical lesion of noninflammatory acne is the comedone, which results from follicular plugging by keratin. Comedones can be open ("blackheads") or closed ("whiteheads"). Acne typically starts with closed comedones that are visible as subtle small 1- to 2-mm flesh-colored papules. Inflammatory acne consists of erythematous pustules, nodules, or cysts (deeper and often painful) that occur later and are the result of inflammation in and around the hair follicle. Lesion morphology should guide treatment. It is also important to consider the safety of medications used for acne treatment during pregnancy. Topical erythromycin is pregnancy category B and can be used safely during pregnancy. To reduce the incidence of bacterial resistance, topical erythromycin can be combined with topical benzoyl peroxide, also safe in pregnancy.

Doxycycline is pregnancy category D and can cause dental staining and enamel hypoplasia when used in the second and third trimesters; it is not to be used during pregnancy.

Isotretinoin is a teratogen (pregnancy category X) and can cause fetal loss, especially when used in the first trimester. It can also cause severe head and cardiac defects. Oral isotretinoin is reserved for the treatment of severe nodulocystic acne and gram-negative folliculitis in nonpregnant patients. Patients must be monitored carefully once therapy with isotretinoin is initiated and participation in the risk prevention program iPLEDGE is mandated for all patients, providers, and dispensing pharmacies. Mandatory office visits are required every 30 days with regular monitoring for pregnancy and medication side effects.

Acne in women, particularly those whose acne flares around menses, may respond to spironolactone. Spironolactone is pregnancy category C, and in rat studies has caused delayed sexual maturation in female rats and feminization of male rat fetuses.

Topical retinoids are appropriate for comedonal and mild inflammatory acne. Tazarotene is a topical retinoid, but is rated pregnancy category X and should not be used in this patient.

KEY POINT

- Management of dermatologic conditions during pregnancy with topical agents should be considered before prescribing systemic medications because they are lower risk, with the exception of tazarotene (category X).

Bibliography

Murase JE, Heller MM, Butler DC. Safety of dermatologic medications in pregnancy and lactation: Part I. Pregnancy. J Am Acad Dermatol. 2014;70:401.e1-14; quiz 415. [PMID: 24528911] doi:10.1016/j.jaad. 2013.09.010

Item 37   Answer: B

Educational Objective: Diagnose morbilliform drug reaction.

This patient is experiencing a classical morbilliform, or exanthematous, drug eruption, which is the most common form of cutaneous adverse drug reaction. Morbilliform eruptions begin 4 to 14 days after the initiation of a new medication. Characteristic skin findings begin as coalescing fine monomorphic papules on the trunk and spread distally and symmetrically. Peripheral eosinophilia or leukocytosis may be seen, but other signs of systemic involvement are not present. The therapy is to stop the medication and treat symptomatically with antihistamines and medium-potency topical glucocorticoids for a brief time while the reaction resolves.

Drug reaction with eosinophilia and systemic symptoms (DRESS) is another severe cutaneous adverse reaction. Its onset is notably remote from initiation of the offending agent, often by as much as 2 to 6 weeks. While eosinophilia is a feature of DRESS syndrome, DRESS is associated with other signs of systemic involvement such as liver chemistry abnormalities. DRESS may manifest a morbilliform appearance, but typical features also include skin pain and pronounced facial edema that are absent in morbilliform drug eruption.

Stevens-Johnson syndrome results in necrosis and sloughing of the epidermis. Skin pain and involvement of mucous membranes is a key feature. Rare cases of Stevens-Johnson syndrome are precipitated by an infection, but this patient's skin findings are more consistent with morbilliform eruption.

Viral exanthem may appear identical in morphology to a morbilliform drug eruption. However, the appearance of this rash should be closer to the onset of symptoms of the infection, as opposed to 3 weeks later. In this case, a common cause of morbilliform reaction and development of rash within 4 days of starting the medication makes morbilliform reaction more likely.

KEY POINT

- Characteristic findings of morbilliform drug reaction include erythematous papules coalescing into plaques, often with some pruritus, and no accompanying systemic symptoms.

Bibliography

Ferner RE. Adverse drug reactions in dermatology. Clin Exp Dermatol. 2015;40:105-9; quiz 109-10. [PMID: 25622648] doi:10.1111/ced.12572

Item 38   Answer: D

Educational Objective: Diagnose vitiligo.

The patient has vitiligo, an autoimmune disease that causes the loss of melanocytes and subsequent depigmentation of the skin. It usually presents in childhood or young adulthood with a peak onset between 10 and 30 years. The most commonly affected areas involve the extensor surfaces such as the dorsal hands, elbows, and knees, and the periorificial areas such as around the mouth, eyes, rectum, and genitals, and it is often bilaterally symmetrical. It appears as completely white, well-demarcated regular macules or patches with no scale. Its onset is insidious and asymptomatic, starting as smaller macules and gradually enlarging. Treatment is challenging and typically starts with topical glucocorticoids or immunomodulators. Vitiligo can be associated with other autoimmune conditions such as diabetes mellitus, alopecia areata, or Hashimoto thyroiditis.

Pityriasis alba is characterized by hypopigmented patches and is most often seen on the face and upper arms of dark-pigmented children. Lesions typically manifest some border irregularity and are associated with a fine scale. The cause is unknown and considered a mild eczematous process. The irregular borders and scale of pityriasis alba are not consistent with vitiligo.

Tinea versicolor is a superficial fungal infection caused by *Malassezia furfur* and is most common in warm, humid environments. It presents as hypopigmented, hyperpigmented, or pink patches that are dry and slightly scaly. Although the patches can occur anywhere, the neck, upper back, and chest, with extension to the abdomen or extremities, are commonly affected. These areas often become more noticeable after exposure to the sun because the organism prevents the skin from tanning. Scaly patches are not consistent with vitiligo.

Tuberous sclerosis is an inherited disorder with the classic triad of angiofibromas, mental deficiency, and epilepsy. Other associated features include ash-leaf hypomelanotic macules, periungual fibromas, collagenomas, and café-au-lait macules. Hypomelanotic macules range in number and are found in about 85% of tuberous sclerosis cases. They are present at birth or develop during childhood. The appearance of this patient's depigmented lesions at age 20 and absence of epilepsy and mental deficiency makes tuberous sclerosis an unlikely diagnosis.

KEY POINT

- Vitiligo is an autoimmune disease that causes the loss of melanocytes and subsequent depigmentation of the skin appearing as completely white, regular, well-demarcated macules or patches with no scale.

Bibliography

Alikhan A, Felsten LM, Daly M, Petronic-Rosic V. Vitiligo: a comprehensive overview Part I. Introduction, epidemiology, quality of life, diagnosis, differential diagnosis, associations, histopathology, etiology, and work-up. J Am Acad Dermatol. 2011;65:473-91. [PMID: 21839315] doi:10.1016/j.jaad.2010.11.061

Item 39   Answer: D

Educational Objective: Diagnose hidradenitis suppurativa.

This patient has hidradenitis suppurativa, a chronic inflammatory disease that predominantly affects the apocrine-gland–bearing areas of the skin. The common sites are the axillae, breasts and inframammary creases, inguinal folds, and gluteal cleft. It is recognized by its characteristic inflammatory abscesses, sinus tracts (with foul-smelling drainage), and scarring in intertriginous areas. The pathogenesis of hidradenitis begins with follicular occlusion but not infection or inflammation of the apocrine glands. Following occlusion, secretions build up in the follicular duct and result in rupture and a subsequent inflammatory reaction that resembles a bacterial abscess. Following this, an acute inflammatory reaction is triggered in the surrounding tissue. The role of bacteria is controversial and is likely a secondary colonization since lesions are initially sterile, and antibiotics are not entirely effective in preventing new lesions. Hidradenitis is associated with smoking, obesity, and metabolic syndrome. The chronic and recurrent nature of hidradenitis helps distinguish it from other infectious causes. Treatment is difficult. Clindamycin-rifampin combination antibiotics, infliximab, and surgical excision have the greatest evidence of effectiveness. It is important to recognize hidradenitis suppurativa early in order to initiate management to reduce scarring and progression of the disease.

Carbuncles can present as tender nodules with purulent drainage; however, these typically respond well to antibiotics and are not chronic in nature. Recurrent carbuncles or abscesses should raise suspicion for possible hidradenitis. Sinus tracts are not typically involved with carbuncles.

Chancroid is a sexually transmitted disease caused by *Haemophilus ducreyi*. It presents with one or more painful ulcerations, typically on the penis or labia. Inguinal lymphadenopathy may be present, but sinus tracts and inflammatory abscesses are not seen.

Epidermal inclusion cysts are benign nodules with a central punctum and a chamber containing keratinaceous material. When punctured, they often eject a copious amount of foul-smelling keratinaceous material. The cyst wall may occasionally rupture, leading to the formation of a tender red swollen nodule that resembles a furuncle. Epidermal inclusion cysts are typically solitary lesions with no sinus tract involvement and minimal scarring.

KEY POINT

- Hidradenitis suppurativa is characterized by inflammatory abscesses, sinus tracts, and scarring in intertriginous areas; it is associated with smoking, obesity, and the metabolic syndrome.

Bibliography

Micheletti RG. An update on the diagnosis and treatment of hidradenitis suppurativa. Cutis. 2015 Dec;96(6 Suppl):7-12. [PMID: 27051885]

Item 40   Answer: C

Educational Objective: Diagnose pyoderma gangrenosum.

This patient has pyoderma gangrenosum (PG). PG is an autoimmune neutrophilic dermatosis in which neutrophils invade and fill the dermis, leading to marked tissue edema and possible ulceration. PG may also present with bullous lesions, pustulonodules, and vegetative plaques. The typical history is a small pustule or red nodule that may develop after trauma and rapidly expands causing an edematous, infiltrated, actively inflamed border and a painful, exudative wet ulcer. Classically the border is described as violaceous or "gun-metal gray" and, because of the nature of the inflammation, the epidermis often overlies the ulcer, with a "hanging border" or residual thin anastomosing strands of epidermis remaining over the expanding ulcer. These lesions also display pathergy, a worsening/expansion of a lesion after trauma. Because of this characteristic, debridement should be avoided in these lesions.

Although pyoderma gangrenosum can be idiopathic, it is most commonly associated with inflammatory bowel disease (Crohn disease and ulcerative colitis). It is also associated with several other conditions including leukemia, myeloma, hepatitis C, and systemic lupus erythematosus. Management starts with investigating and treating the underlying

CONT.

cause. Depending on the severity of disease, treatment also includes application of potent topical glucocorticoids, systemic glucocorticoids, and immunosuppressive agents such as azathioprine, cyclosporine, and infliximab.

Acrodermatitis enteropathica (AE) is an inherited or acquired metabolic disorder characterized by perioral and acral (in the extremities) erythematous and vesiculobullous dermatitis and alopecia related to zinc deficiency. AE has been associated with Crohn disease, but not ulcerative colitis. This patient's ulcer is not consistent with AE.

Clinically, lesions of calciphylaxis are exquisitely painful subcutaneous nodules or plaques with overlying red-brown discoloration and often superimposed angulated purpuric patches, often with central necrosis. Patients with advanced calciphylaxis may have ulceration or large, thick, black eschar formation. Given this patient's lack of kidney disease, her history of inflammatory bowel disease, and the description of the ulceration, pyoderma gangrenosum is the most likely diagnosis.

Venous stasis ulcers tend to be associated with chronic venous insufficiency and arise on the medial aspects of the lower legs. They are typically shallow and lack the characteristic undermined borders of PG. This patient also did not have the background venous stasis changes such as edema, varicosities, and pigmentary changes seen in venous stasis ulcerations.

> **KEY POINT**
>
> - Pyoderma gangrenosum presents as a painful, exudative ulcer with a purulent base and ragged, edematous, violaceous, "overhanging" border; it may be idiopathic but it can be associated with an underlying disease.

Bibliography
Pompeo MQ. Pyoderma gangrenosum: recognition and management. Wounds. 2016 Jan;28(1):7-13. [PMID: 26779805]

Item 41   Answer: A

Educational Objective: Treat psoriasis with narrow-band ultraviolet B (UVB) therapy.

Narrowband ultraviolet B (UVB) therapy has become the standard form of phototherapy used in the initial treatment of psoriasis. The light source emits a narrow band of UVB radiation, in this case 311 nm of ultraviolet light. This wavelength was chosen for its efficacy and the fact that this wavelength of light is not absorbed by DNA. The theory is that if the light is not absorbed by DNA, less skin damage will occur, and there will be far fewer skin cancers as a side effect of the therapy. Broadband UVB was the mainstay of therapy until the advent of narrowband UVB. Broadband is still used in some centers today. Broadband UVB emits light in the 280 to 320 nm range; 260 nm is the wavelength of light with the maximum absorption by DNA. DNA absorption of UVB drops off dramatically after 290 nm. Broadband UVB contains wavelengths of light capable of causing DNA damage, leading to ultraviolet skin damage and ultimately skin cancer.

Photodynamic therapy is not used for the treatment of psoriasis, but rather for the treatment of actinic keratoses. Aminolevulinic acid, a chemical precursor of the heme synthesis pathway, is applied to the skin before its exposure to visible blue light. Aminolevulinic acid is used as a photosensitizer and is absorbed by the actinically damaged skin cells; upon exposure to light it causes necrosis of the actinically damaged skin by producing reactive oxygen species. It can be extremely painful for patients to undergo photodynamic therapy.

Psoralen plus ultraviolet A (PUVA) therapy is now used almost exclusively for the treatment of cutaneous T-cell lymphoma. It is effective for treating psoriasis, but it has been shown to cause an increase in the risk of nonmelanoma and melanoma skin cancer. For these reasons, it is not used as first-line therapy for psoriasis.

Oral retinoid (acitretin) plus PUVA therapy, also called RePUVA, has been used in the past for treating psoriasis and cutaneous T-cell lymphoma. It is highly efficacious, but has the highest side effect profile of the various forms of phototherapy and is not used frequently today. Short-term complications of RePUVA include profound nausea in some and risk of treatment-related burns. Long-term complications include an 11-fold increase in cutaneous squamous cell carcinoma and slight increase in the risk for basal cell carcinoma, melanocytic atypia, and melanoma.

Ultraviolet A (UVA) alone is rarely used in the dermatology clinic. Morphea (localized scleroderma) has been shown to benefit from exposure to UVA phototherapy.

> **KEY POINT**
>
> - Narrowband ultraviolet B (UVB) is the standard form of phototherapy used in the treatment of extensive psoriasis.

Bibliography
Lim HW, Silpa-archa N, Amadi U, Menter A, Van Voorhees AS, Lebwohl M. Phototherapy in dermatology: A call for action [Editorial]. J Am Acad Dermatol. 2015;72:1078-80. [PMID: 25981004] doi:10.1016/j.jaad.2015. 03.017

Item 42   Answer: D

Educational Objective: Diagnose cutaneous-only polyarteritis nodosa.

This patient has the cutaneous-only variant of polyarteritis nodosa (PAN). PAN is a medium-vessel vasculitis not associated with the development of ANCAs. The skin may be the only organ involved (cutaneous-only PAN) or it may be involved as part of a systemic disease. Biopsy of an affected organ will show medium-vessel vasculitis.

Patients with cutaneous-only PAN experience tender subcutaneous nodules from vascular inflammation, stellate erosions, or ulcerations from ischemia in the watershed of the affected vessels, and they may develop livedo reticularis or livedoid purpura. Cutaneous-only disease treatment is guided by symptoms and may include systemic antihistamines, colchicine, dapsone, or immunosuppressants such

CONT.

as azathioprine. Symptoms of systemic PAN may include abdominal pain or gastrointestinal bleeding (if the mesenteric vessels are affected), hypertension (if the renal vessels are affected), neuropathy (typically mononeuritis multiplex), and constitutional symptoms. Biopsy of an affected organ will show a medium-vessel vasculitis. Although patients with systemic PAN are frequently found to have preceding chronic viral hepatitis, most patients with cutaneous-only PAN are not usually virally infected.

Granulomatosis with polyangiitis (GPA) and microscopic polyangiitis (MPA) are ANCA-associated small- and medium-vessel vasculitides. Skin findings can include palpable purpura; tender subcutaneous nodules; or necrosis of digits, nose, tongue, or genitals. Typical organ involvement includes the upper respiratory tract (including sinuses and ears), lungs, and kidney. GPA is associated with positive enzyme-linked immunosorbent assay (ELISA) for anti-proteinase 3 antibodies, and MPA is associated with anti-myeloperoxidase antibodies. Biopsy will usually show small-vessel involvement (not present in this case). Although a minority of patients with GPA and MPA may be ANCA-negative, the lack of any other characteristic systemic involvement in the ANCA-negative setting makes it extremely unlikely that this patient has an ANCA-associated vasculitis.

Leukocytoclastic vasculitis (LCV) is a finding, not a diagnosis. It manifests as palpable purpura (not present in this case) and is always secondary to another condition. Infections, autoimmune conditions such as systemic lupus erythematosus or rheumatoid arthritis, or medications may precipitate LCV. It lacks the tender nodules, stellate ulcerations, and livedoid skin changes of a medium-vessel vasculitis.

Takayasu arteritis is a large-vessel vasculitis that typically does not have skin findings; Takayasu arteritis should be suspected in patients under 40 years with unexplained systemic inflammation and/or signs and symptoms of large-vessel impairment.

KEY POINT

- Patients with cutaneous-only polyarteritis nodosa experience tender subcutaneous nodules from vascular inflammation, stellate erosions, or ulcerations from ischemia in the watershed of the affected vessels, and may develop livedo reticularis or livedoid purpura.

Bibliography

Alibaz-Oner F, Koster MJ, Crowson CS, Makol A, Ytterberg SR, Salvarani C, et al. The clinical spectrum of medium-sized vessel vasculitis. Arthritis Care Res (Hoboken). 2016. [PMID: 27564269] doi:10.1002/acr. 23007

Item 43   Answer: B

Educational Objective: Evaluate erythema nodosum with chest radiography.

This patient needs a chest radiograph to complete the evaluation of her erythema nodosum (EN). EN is the most common form of panniculitis, or inflammation of the fat, with most inflammation concentrated on the intralobular septae. Because the inflammation is deep under the skin, the clinical manifestation seen on the surface is often tender, ill-defined erythema with some substance on palpation, which may fade from an active inflammatory red-pink to dull brown. Most commonly, EN occurs bilaterally and symmetrically on the anterior shins; however, it may also appear in any fatty area. Although lesions will often come and go, most resolve over 4 to 6 weeks. EN is a nonspecific reaction pattern occurring in response to some systemic process. EN can be idiopathic, but the most common associations are streptococcal infection, hormones (including oral contraceptives, hormone replacement therapy, or pregnancy), inflammatory bowel disease, sarcoidosis, lymphoma, and medication reactions. The diagnosis of EN can be clinically based on the acute onset of tender nodules on the bilateral shins typically in a young woman. Biopsy is not necessary in typical lesions.

Most authorities recommend a chest radiograph in the evaluation of EN to assess for the presence of lymphoma, sarcoidosis, tuberculosis, and fungal infection such as coccidioidomycosis.

In the absence of gastrointestinal symptoms, a colonoscopy for inflammatory bowel disease is unlikely to reveal a causative diagnosis. Patients with disseminated gonococcal infection and bacteremia manifest vesiculopustular or hemorrhagic macular skin lesions, not tender subcutaneous nodules as seen in this patient.

Patients with disseminated gonococcal infection present with dusky pustules or purpura, fever, chills, and polyarthralgia. Knees, elbows, and distal joints are typical sites of involvement. Subcutaneous nodules are not features of this infection

KEY POINT

- A chest radiograph is recommended in the evaluation of erythema nodosum to assess for the presence of lymphoma, sarcoidosis, tuberculosis, and fungal infection such as coccidioidomycosis.

Bibliography

Chowaniec M, Starba A, Wiland P. Erythema nodosum - review of the literature. Reumatologia. 2016;54:79-82. [PMID: 27407284] doi:10.5114/reum.2016.60217

Item 44   Answer: D

Educational Objective: Diagnose pitted keratolysis.

Pitted keratolysis is a bacterial infection most commonly caused by *Kytococcus sedentarius*. The key features are waxy or scaly plaques, thickening of the plantar skin (keratoderma), small punctate erosions in the plaques that may coalesce to form broader erosions, and odor. Risk factors for infection include excess sweating (hyperhidrosis) and prolonged occlusion of the feet in footwear. Usually symptoms are minimal, with most complaints directed toward odor, but minor itching can occur. Treatment is best accomplished with topical antibiotics and keeping the feet dry, including the use of topical antiperspirants.

Aquagenic keratoderma presents with wrinkling, translucency, and scaling of the palmar hands and plantar feet shortly after exposure to water and is associated with carrier status of the cystic fibrosis gene. Aquagenic keratoderma does not feature pitting.

Erythrasma is also a bacterial infection that tends to involve intertriginous areas such as the axillae and the crural folds. Skin may develop a finely wrinkled, cigarette paper texture, but would not feature pitting. Erythrasma will fluoresce to a coral red color with a Wood lamp examination because of bacterial porphyrin production.

Keratoderma blenorrhagicum is a keratoderma of the palms or soles associated with reactive arthritis. With this rash, patients develop psoriasiform red plaques with lamellar scale. Patients may have other features of reactive arthritis such as asymmetric monoarthritis or oligoarthritis in the lower extremities, enthesopathy, dactylitis, and sacroiliitis.

Tinea pedis can cause scaling and itching of the feet. Patients typically develop pink or red scaly plaques with a serpiginous or arcuate discrete border. Scale is often emphasized at the edge of plaques. Pustules may be present at hair follicles, but pitting and strong odor are not typical. Potassium hydroxide preparation of skin scrapings should reveal fungal elements, except in partially treated cases.

KEY POINT

- Pitted keratolysis is a superficial bacterial infection characterized by small pits and punctate erosions primarily on the plantar aspects of the feet; risk factors include increased perspiration (hyperhidrosis) and prolonged occlusion of the feet.

Bibliography
Leung AK, Barankin B. Pitted Keratolysis. J Pediatr. 2015;167:1165. [PMID: 26316369] doi:10.1016/j.jpeds.2015.07.056

Item 45   Answer: A
Educational Objective: Treat venous stasis ulcers with compression therapy.

This patient has a venous stasis ulcer, and the most appropriate additional management is compression therapy. Venous stasis ulcers are the most common leg ulcers. Most patients have a history of stasis dermatitis and often have some level of scarring and dyspigmentation on the bilateral lower extremities. Venous stasis ulcers usually occur on the distal lower leg, particularly the medial aspect of the ankle, and may result from a minor trauma, a medical procedure, or an acute stasis dermatitis flare. The symptoms vary from negligible discomfort to significant pain. The ulcers tend to have an irregular border and surrounding hyperpigmentation, and the skin and subcutaneous tissues are thickened, resulting in lipodermatosclerosis (fibrosing panniculitis of the subcutaneous tissue). Patients often have varicose veins and peripheral edema. Treatment is directed toward three main areas: reducing the

peripheral edema, creating a wound environment that is conducive to healing, and treating any secondary infection that may be present. Reduction of peripheral edema is achieved by the use of compression stockings, pneumatic compression boots, and compression dressings (Unna boots). Compression is the key to venous ulcer healing.

Oral cephalexin is a treatment for cellulitis and other skin infections. Clues to suggest active infection are rapidly expanding ulcer size, worsening pain, heat, swelling and increased surrounding erythema, and copious exudate; these findings are absent and indicate that oral antibiotics should not be used. Furthermore, the inappropriate use of antibiotics can result in the emergence of resistant organisms.

Oral cilostazol is used to increase peripheral blood flow for the treatment of intermittent claudication. It is sometimes used in the treatment of arterial insufficiency ulcers, but evidence supporting its effectiveness is sparse. Because this patient has a venous stasis ulcer, oral cilostazol would not be used.

The use of topically applied antiseptics, such as hydrogen peroxide, povidone iodine, acetic acid, and sodium hypochlorite, is not supported by evidence. Some animal studies have demonstrated that the cellular toxicities of these agents exceed their bactericidal activities. Therefore, topical antiseptics should not be used in the management of venous ulcers.

KEY POINT

- The mainstay of venous ulcer treatment consists of compression therapy.

Bibliography
Kirsner RS, Vivas AC. Lower-extremity ulcers: diagnosis and management. Br J Dermatol. 2015 Aug;173(2):379-90. [PMID: 26257052]

Item 46   Answer: B
Educational Objective: Diagnose erythroderma following systemic glucocorticoid therapy.

Psoriasis vulgaris can flare to erythroderma following use of systemic glucocorticoids. The most common cause of erythroderma, or redness over 80% body surface area, is a preexisting condition. Peripheral edema, erosions from excoriations due to severe pruritus, and scaling are common findings. Owing to compromise of the skin barrier, affected patients are at risk for dehydration, electrolyte abnormalities, protein loss, heat loss, and infection, which can be fatal. Short courses of systemic glucocorticoids in a patient with psoriasis can result in a striking increase in skin disease upon abrupt cessation. The presence of lamellar scale that bleeds when peeled away (Auspitz sign) and nail pitting support the diagnosis of erythrodermic psoriasis.

Drug reaction with eosinophilia and systemic symptoms (DRESS) can also present with erythroderma. This represents a delayed response to a medication several weeks after initiation. Patients present with rash, striking facial edema, peripheral eosinophilia (or less common atypical

CONT.

lymphocytosis), lymphadenopathy, and evidence of organ involvement such as acute kidney injury or abnormal liver chemistry tests.

Sézary syndrome is an acute leukemic variant of cutaneous T-cell lymphoma. Patients often present with erythroderma, ectropion, and lymphadenopathy. The absence of a preceding history of cutaneous T-cell lymphoma makes this diagnosis unlikely.

Stevens-Johnson syndrome may cause erythroderma, but it manifests as epidermal necrosis with dusky plaques that slough rather than scale. Mucous membrane involvement is a keystone of diagnosis and is absent in this patient. Most cases of Stevens-Johnson syndrome are caused by a medication.

KEY POINT

- Psoriasis can flare to erythroderma following brief use of systemic glucocorticoids.

Bibliography
Mistry N, Gupta A, Alavi A, Sibbald RG. A review of the diagnosis and management of erythroderma (generalized red skin). Adv Skin Wound Care. 2015;28:228-36; quiz 237-8. [PMID: 25882661] doi:10.1097/01.ASW.0000463573.40637.73

Item 47   Answer: A

Educational Objective: Evaluate an annular, scaly patch with a potassium hydroxide examination.

The most appropriate diagnostic test to perform on this patient is the potassium hydroxide (KOH) examination. This patient's skin lesions are erythematous annular patches with noticeable surface scale. When confronted with an annular scaly patch, the most common diagnosis is tinea from a dermatophyte infection. Direct microscopic examination of KOH-prepared specimens is the simplest, cheapest method used for the diagnosis of dermatophyte infections of the skin. After scraping the leading edge of scale with a number 15 blade or the edge of the glass slide, apply 2 to 3 drops of KOH on the debris and then apply a coverslip. Evaluate the specimen initially with 10 power magnification. Tinea is confirmed by the presence of septated branching hyphae.

A scabies preparation is used when the patient has burrows. Burrows are pathognomonic for a scabies infection and are most frequently found along the wrists, fingers, and palms. To obtain the specimen, place a drop of mineral oil on the burrow and scrape the area with a number 15 blade. After placing the specimen on a glass slide, apply the coverslip, and examine with 10 power magnification to identify mites, eggs, and/or feces.

A Tzanck preparation should be performed on patients when the skin findings are concerning for a herpes virus infection. Grouped vesicles on an erythematous base or tender vesicles in a dermatomal distribution are both primary skin findings in which a Tzanck preparation can be performed. This is done by deroofing the blister and scraping the base of the blister. The scraping is smeared on a glass microscope slide and stained with an appropriate stain (Tzanck or Giemsa). The presence of multinucleated giant cells is diagnostic for herpes viral infections. This finding, however, cannot distinguish the responsible virus. Viral culture or direct immunofluorescence can be used to identify the specific virus, if needed.

A Wood lamp is an ultraviolet light source that can be used to evaluate hypo- and depigmentation lesions as seen in vitiligo. Vitiligo will appear bright white and sharply delineated when examined with a Wood light and is most helpful in fair-skinned persons where depigmentation may not otherwise be visible. A Wood lamp can also detect skin fluorescence associated with erythrasma and the urine fluorescence in patients with porphyria cutanea tarda.

KEY POINT

- Diagnosis of dermatophyte infection can be performed by examination of the scale with potassium hydroxide; the presence of branching hyphae is diagnostic.

Bibliography
Levitt JO, Levitt BH, Akhavan A, Yanofsky H. The sensitivity and specificity of potassium hydroxide smear and fungal culture relative to clinical assessment in the evaluation of tinea pedis: a pooled analysis. Dermatol Res Pract. 2010;2010:764843. [PMID: 20672004] doi:10.1155/2010/764843

Item 48   Answer: A

Educational Objective: Diagnose calciphylaxis.

This patient has calciphylaxis. Patients with calciphylaxis present with angulated, lacy, or netlike retiform purpuric patches with areas of central dusky or black necrotic tissue that may form bullae, ulcerate, and leave a hard eschar. For unknown reasons, calcium is deposited in the medial layer of small arteries, which leads to thrombus, infarction of the overlying skin, and significant pain. The thighs and lower abdomen have been reported as the most frequent areas of involvement. Calciphylaxis typically occurs in patients who have underlying end-stage kidney disease; however, only 1% to 2% of patients on dialysis will develop calciphylaxis. Persons with calciphylaxis will usually have a corrected calcium-phosphorus product greater than 60 to 70 mg^2/dL^2.

Therapy is difficult and multifactorial. It includes surgery to debride any areas of potential infection and parathyroidectomy in those patients with hyperparathyroidism. Medical therapies are dialysis, intravenous sodium thiosulfate, decreasing calcium intake, bisphosphonates, and meticulous wound care. Infection leading to sepsis is the leading cause of death. Prevention of infection is critically important.

Kyrle disease is most frequently seen in persons with diabetes and end-stage kidney disease. It can present with an individual papule or numerous widespread hyperpigmented papules. The papules have an umbilicated central core. Kyrle disease is caused by collagen extrusion from the dermis into and through the epidermis.

CONT.

Nephrogenic systemic fibrosis is characterized by yellowish, thickened papules and nodules with progressive skin tightening and sclerosis. If biopsied, the skin findings mimic those of scleromyxedema. This condition has been seen in patients undergoing dialysis for end-stage kidney disease who were exposed to gadolinium-containing contrast dyes.

Progressive systemic sclerosis presents similarly to nephrogenic systemic fibrosis. It is an autoimmune disease with cutaneous and systemic findings. The cutaneous findings are thickening of the skin, which results in lack of joint mobility, dilated periungual capillary loops, Raynaud phenomenon, digital ulcerations, and digital infarcts.

Ulcerations and eschar formation on the upper thighs do not occur in Kyrle disease, nephrogenic systemic sclerosis, or progressive systemic sclerosis.

KEY POINT

- Calciphylaxis lesions are intensely painful, angulated, retiform purpuric patches with areas of black necrotic tissue that may form bullae, ulcerate, and leave a hard, firm eschar in patients with end-stage kidney disease.

Bibliography

Nigwekar SU, Kroshinsky D, Nazarian RM, Goverman J, Malhotra R, Jackson VA, et al. Calciphylaxis: risk factors, diagnosis, and treatment. Am J Kidney Dis. 2015;66:133-46. [PMID: 25960299] doi:10.1053/j.ajkd.2015.01.034

Item 49   **Answer: B**

Educational Objective: Treat a cutaneous abscess.

This patient has an abscess with no systemic signs of infection, so the most appropriate treatment would be incision and drainage. Gram stain and culture of pus from carbuncles and abscesses are strongly recommended, but treatment without these studies is reasonable in typical cases. Treatment with antibiotics is not indicated unless there are systemic signs of infection including fever (38 °C [100.4 °F]), tachycardia (>90/min), tachypnea (>24/min), an abnormal leukocyte count (>12,000/µL or <400/µL), or immunocompromise. This patient does not present with any of these indications for antibiotic therapy. If antibiotic therapy is indicated, empiric treatment of purulent skin and soft tissue infection (furuncle, carbuncle, and abscess) should include an agent that is active against methicillin-resistant *Staphylococcus aureus* (MRSA), for example, trimethoprim-sulfamethoxazole or doxycycline.

Antibiotic therapy based on culture results is an inappropriate choice for this cutaneous abscess. Bacterial cultures should be obtained from the abscess, but treatment with incision and drainage should proceed before the culture results return. Antibiotics should be added to incision and drainage if there are systemic symptoms. If antibiotic therapy is indicated, it should be initiated empirically prior to obtaining culture results. The culture results can be used to modify the antibiotic selection if necessary.

Incision and drainage plus oral cephalexin should not be used for abscesses without systemic signs of infection. In addition, if antibiotic therapy were indicated, cephalexin lacks MRSA activity and would be an inappropriate antibiotic selection for an abscess.

Oral trimethoprim-sulfamethoxazole would be an appropriate choice for an abscess if antibiotic therapy were indicated. Because this patient's skin and soft tissue infection is categorized as mild (no systemic signs or symptoms), antibiotic therapy is not indicated.

KEY POINT

- Primary treatment for abscess with no systemic signs of infection is incision and drainage; antibiotics should be added only if systemic symptoms or signs are present.

Bibliography

Stevens DL, Bisno AL, Chambers HF, Dellinger EP, et al. Practice guidelines for the diagnosis and management of skin and soft tissue infections: 2014 update by the Infectious Diseases Society of America. Clin Infect Dis. 2014 Jul 15;59(2):e10-52. [PMID: 24973422]

Item 50   **Answer: C**

Educational Objective: Diagnose halo nevus.

This patient has a halo nevus. Halo nevi are benign melanocytic nevi that are in the process of being attacked and eliminated by the immune system. They are characterized by a pigmented macule or papule with a surrounding "halo" of hypopigmented or depigmented skin. The halo gradually enlarges, and the mole shrinks until all that is left is a depigmented area on the skin that resembles a small area of vitiligo. These lesions are particularly common on the back in children, teenagers, and young adults.

Melanocytic nevi are benign neoplasms comprising melanocytes, commonly referred to as "moles." They vary in clinical appearance depending on the location of melanocytes within the skin. Junctional nevi are flat and often dark brown in color. Compound nevi are raised (papules) and may be irregularly pigmented. Dermal nevi are soft and flesh-colored and may resemble skin tags. The terms "junctional," "compound," and "dermal" refer to the location of the melanocytic nests: junctional nevi have nests located at the dermal-epidermal junction, compound nevi have nests at the dermal-epidermal junction and in the dermis, and dermal nevi have nests in the dermis. Nevi undergo a benign maturation process from junctional to compound to dermal over a period of many years.

Dysplastic nevi can display one or more of the identifying characteristics of melanoma, making an accurate clinical diagnosis difficult; however, a biopsy of the lesion can typically exclude melanoma. They are often asymmetric, irregularly bordered, and more than one shade of brown, and they may be quite large in diameter. Many dysplastic nevi have a dark brown center and a surrounding ring of light brown, a pattern that is often referred to as a "fried egg" appearance. Patients with multiple dysplastic nevi are at risk for developing melanoma and should be monitored closely. Melanoma can arise within any melanocytic nevi including dysplastic nevi; therefore, biopsy should be limited to clinically worrisome or changing lesions.

Malignant melanoma presents as macules, papules, or plaques typically larger than 6 mm in diameter and shows asymmetry and irregular boarders, as well as color variation within the lesion. The surrounding skin can show erythema or hypopigmentation.

KEY POINT

- Halo nevi are benign pigmented macules or papules with a surrounding "halo" of hypopigmented or depigmented skin, most frequently presenting on the back of teenagers and young adults.

Bibliography

Weyant GW, Chung CG, Helm KF. Halo nevus: review of the literature and clinicopathologic findings [Letter]. Int J Dermatol. 2015;54:e433-5. [PMID: 26146814] doi:10.1111/ijd.12843

Item 51   Answer: C

Educational Objective: Diagnose inverse psoriasis.

Based on the finding of the well-demarcated, erythematous plaques in intertriginous areas, this patient has inverse psoriasis. Psoriasis is a chronic inflammatory dermatosis that manifests with scaling, variably pruritic plaques that may be recalcitrant to topical therapy. There are many different patterns of psoriasis including classic psoriasis vulgaris (erythematous patches with a thick, adherent scale), inverse psoriasis (red, thin plaques with variable amount of scale in the axillae, under the breasts or pannus, intergluteal cleft, and perineum), sebopsoriasis (red, thin plaques in the scalp, eyebrows, nasolabial folds, central chest, and pubic area), and guttate psoriasis (0.5- to 2-cm red plaques that erupt suddenly on the trunk often after a group A streptococcal infection). Psoriasis can also involve the nails presenting as pit-like indentations and "oil spots" often involving multiple nails. Inverse psoriasis can be difficult to diagnosis because it often lacks the classic silvery scale. It also resembles other common dermatologic conditions such as tinea, intertrigo, and allergic contact dermatitis.

Allergic contact dermatitis, while possible in these locations, would be less likely without history of exposure to an allergen. Allergic contact dermatitis does not explain the patient's erythematous plaques with scale on the scalp.

Candida is frequently found in the flexures of obese patients, but typically presents with a bright red plaque with satellite papules and pustules. *Candida* would also respond to topical antifungal treatment.

Seborrheic dermatitis can be found in the scalp, face, chest, and groin. It is more prevalent in those with HIV/AIDS or neurologic diseases such as Parkinson disease. This rash usually has a greasy, sometimes yellow scale and improves with antifungal medications.

Tinea cruris is also commonly found in the inguinal folds. It typically presents as an annular plaque with an active, scaly border. The lack of scale and lack of response to antifungal therapy makes tinea cruris an unlikely diagnosis.

KEY POINT

- Inverse psoriasis is characterized by red, thin plaques with variable amounts of scale in the axillae, intergluteal cleft, and perineum, and under the breasts and pannus.

Bibliography

Omland SH, Gniadecki R. Psoriasis inversa: A separate identity or a variant of psoriasis vulgaris? Clin Dermatol. 2015 Jul-Aug;33(4):456-61. [PMID: 26051061]

Item 52   Answer: B

Educational Objective: Treat dermatitis herpetiformis.

This patient has dermatitis herpetiformis (DH), and the most appropriate treatment is a gluten-free diet and dapsone. DH is a subepidermal autoimmune bullous disorder that is extremely pruritic. There are small tense vesicles and papules, which are rarely intact, so the usual presentation is excoriations on the elbows, knees, and buttocks. The diagnosis can be confirmed with skin biopsy for routine and direct immunofluorescence testing. Deposition of granular IgA in the dermal papillary tips is pathognomonic of dermatitis herpetiformis. While dapsone is effective in inducing a clinical remission of DH, a gluten-free diet is the preferred long-term therapy. DH has a strong association with celiac disease. Dapsone will successfully treat the skin symptoms of dermatitis herpetiformis, but does not treat the associated gastrointestinal disease. A gluten-free diet treats both the cause and the symptoms of both diseases. In patients with celiac disease, failure to maintain a gluten-free diet increases the risk for small bowel lymphoma. Prior to initiating therapy with dapsone, patients should be checked for glucose-6-phosphate dehydrogenase deficiency because these patients have a high risk of hemolysis on dapsone therapy.

Potent topical glucocorticoids, such as betamethasone valerate, may help alleviate pruritus associated with DH but are not adequate monotherapy and should always be used in combination with dapsone and a gluten-free diet. Long-term side effects of topical glucocorticoids include cutaneous atrophy, striae, and hypopigmentation.

Numerous oral antihistamines are available for the treatment of pruritus, and anecdotal experience suggests that the more sedating antihistamines such as diphenhydramine may have a better antipruritic effect than the less-sedating products. However, DH is not a histamine-mediated disease, and the use of antihistamines for this condition is not very effective and may result in intolerable sedation in some patients.

In addition to the significant complications associated with the long-term use of prednisone, it is not effective in inducing or maintaining clinical remission in patients with DH and should not be used.

For patients who cannot tolerate dapsone, other sulfon-amide drugs are a potential treatment option for DH. Case reports suggest that sulfasalazine is effective. While sulfa-salazine does not cause hemolysis, there is an increased risk for agranulocytosis and hypersensitivity reactions. As with dapsone, periodic laboratory monitoring for significant side effects is recommended.

KEY POINT

- Dapsone should be used in conjunction with a gluten-free diet as first-line treatment of dermatitis herpeti-formis.

Bibliography

Jakes AD, Bradley S, Donlevy L. Dermatitis herpetiformis. BMJ. 2014;348:g2557. [PMID: 24740905] doi:10.1136/bmj.g2557

Item 53 Answer: A

Educational Objective: Manage contact dermatitis in the setting of stasis dermatitis.

The most appropriate initial management is to discontinue application of the neomycin/polymyxin B/bacitracin oint-ment. This patient has contact dermatitis from the topical antibiotic in the setting of chronic stasis dermatitis with venous stasis ulcerations. Neomycin and bacitracin are usu-ally the causative agents. Topical antibiotics applied to venous stasis ulcers commonly lead to the development of aller-gic contact dermatitis. This often presents with worsening erythema and weeping of the lower extremities. It is often mistaken for cellulitis.

Intravenous vancomycin is an antibiotic used for the treatment of severe skin infections. It is often combined with surgical debridement to treat hospitalized patients with complicated skin and soft tissue infection defined as deeper soft tissue infections, surgical/traumatic wound infection, major abscesses, cellulitis, and infected ulcers and burns. This patient does not have a complicated skin infection, and intravenous vancomycin is not needed.

Mild cellulitis (no focus of purulence or systemic symp-toms) can be treated with oral clindamycin, penicillin, dicloxacillin, or a cephalosporin. In this patient, the cause of the worsening erythema is most likely contact derma-titis and not infection, and discontinuation of the topical antibiotic is the best management before initiation of any antimicrobial therapy.

Oral terbinafine is the treatment for fungal infections such as tinea capitis or onychomycosis. There is reason to suspect a fungal infection in this patient.

Topical triamcinolone ointment is a glucocorticoid preparation commonly used in the treatment of stasis der-matitis and for allergic contact dermatitis; however, the best initial management in allergic contact dermatitis is removal of the offending agent. Adding a topical glucocorticoid with-out stopping the contact allergen is unlikely to result in clinical improvement. A topical glucocorticoid is often used as an adjunctive therapy after stopping the topical antibiotic.

KEY POINT

- Neomycin and bacitracin can cause allergic contact dermatitis that mimics a wound infection; the most appropriate initial management is to discontinue its use.

Bibliography

Spring S1, Pratt M, Chaplin A. Contact dermatitis to topical medicaments: a retrospective chart review from the Ottawa Hospital Patch Test Clinic. Dermatitis. 2012 Sep-Oct;23(5):210-3. [PMID: 23010827]

Item 54 Answer: D

Educational Objective: Treat hand dermatitis.

This patient has hand dermatitis likely caused by an irritant contact dermatitis from frequent water exposure, and the most appropriate management would be to minimize hand washing and to apply thick emollients such as petrolatum to repair the skin barrier. Hand dermatitis is character-ized by inflamed, scaling, and sometimes fissured skin on the palmar or dorsal hand. The most common causes are over-washing, allergic or irritant contact dermatitis, atopic dermatitis, dyshidrotic eczema (pompholyx), and tinea. Repeated or extended washing with soap causes hand der-matitis by friction, removal of the protective skin barrier, and irritation from the surfactant properties of the soap. People who are required to repeatedly wash their hands (such as medical professionals) or those who wash repeat-edly because of obsessive-compulsive or autism spectrum disorders often have extremely pronounced hand dermatitis. This type of irritant dermatitis will be especially marked on the dorsal hands where the stratum corneum is thinner than that of the palms. For irritant hand dermatitis due to over-washing, avoiding the irritant by washing less and moisturizing more can prevent development of a rash. Top-ical petrolatum jelly is an inexpensive and effective way of repairing the damaged skin barrier. A topical glucocorticoid may be necessary for a short period while the triggers are identified or if the skin is very inflamed.

Epicutaneous patch testing can be used to help deter-mine causes of hand dermatitis due to allergic contact der-matitis. In this patient, the most likely cause is hand derma-titis from frequent hand washing, so patch testing would not be the most appropriate management. It could be considered if there was no improvement after minimizing hand wash-ing and the application of emollients.

Oral fluconazole is a treatment for fungal infec-tions such as candidiasis. It can be effective in cases of tinea manuum. "Two feet, one hand" tinea is a common presentation of concomitant tinea pedis and tinea manuum. In this patient, the potassium hydroxide was negative and her feet were clear, so treatment with antifungal therapy would be inappropriate.

Oral prednisone can improve acute flares of hand der-matitis but often results in relapses of chronic hand derma-titis. Because there are also significant side effects of oral prednisone, it would not be the most appropriate initial treatment for this patient.

> **KEY POINT**
> - Treatment of hand dermatitis includes topical emollients such as petrolatum to repair the skin barrier; hand washing should be minimized.

Bibliography

Perry AD, Trafeli JP. Hand Dermatitis: A review of etiology, diagnosis, and treatment. J Am Board Fem Med. 2009 May-Jun;22(3): 325-30. [PMID: 19429739]

Item 55 Answer: D

Educational Objective: Treat comedonal acne.

This patient has comedonal acne and should be treated with a topical retinoid. Treatment begins by considering the types and distribution of lesions, as well as the pregnancy status of the female patient. Interventions are selected with the goal of modifying the main causal factors, such as follicular occlusion, sebum production, *Propionibacterium acnes* proliferation, and inflammation. Comedonal acne consists of open and closed comedones (blackheads and whiteheads, respectively) with no inflammatory papules or pustules. First-line treatment for most patients with comedonal acne is topical retinoid. Topical retinoids are the only choice that is comedolytic and normalizes keratinization of the hair follicle. Topical retinoids are also effective in treating inflammatory acne. Because retinoids are preventive, they need to be applied to the entire acne-prone area and not used as a spot treatment. The most common adverse effects are dryness and irritation.

Isotretinoin is an oral retinoid used to treat severe nodulocystic acne with scarring or when other traditional therapies have failed. This patient does not have evidence of scarring or cystic lesions and has not previously failed any other prescription therapies. Isotretinoin is teratogenic, and use requires that providers, patients, and pharmacies must be registered in the iPLEDGE program, an FDA-approved regulatory program to prevent birth defects, and complete monthly reports. Patients must use two forms of birth control in order to be eligible for isotretinoin therapy.

Oral contraceptive pills are more effective in inflammatory and adult acne, which is characterized by inflammatory papules and cystic lesions along the jawline. Oral contraceptive pills have been shown to reduce comedones, but are not as effective as topical retinoids for comedonal acne.

Topical antibiotics are important in inflammatory acne when pustules and inflammatory papules are present. They work to inhibit *P. acnes* and decrease inflammation. They are not comedolytic and would not be effective in treating comedonal acne. Owing to the increased incidence of antibiotic resistance, topical antibiotics should not be used as monotherapy. Benzoyl peroxide is available over the counter and is an excellent complement to treatment with an oral or topical antibiotic, as it reduces the development of bacterial resistance.

> **KEY POINT**
> - Topical retinoids are first-line treatment for comedonal acne because they are comedolytic and normalize keratinization of the hair follicle.

Bibliography

Zaenglein AL, Pathy AL, Schlosser BJ, et al. Guidelines of care for the management of acne vulgaris. J Am Acad Dermatol. 2016 May;74(5):945-973. e33. [PMID: 26897386]

Item 56 Answer: A

Educational Objective: Treat postscabetic pruritus.

This patient has postscabetic pruritus, which follows an infestation caused by the ectoparasite *Sarcoptes scabiei* resulting in intense pruritus. Treatment of the patient and close contacts is required to eliminate the original infestation. Topical application of permethrin 5% cream is a first-line therapy. The cream is applied overnight to the entire body surface from neck to toes, including genitals and under fingernails. The lotion is removed by showering or bathing 8 to 14 hours following application. Repeat treatment in 7 to 10 days is usually recommended. Clothing, linens, and anything that has had contact with skin within the preceding 1 to 2 weeks must be thoroughly washed. Itching can persist for several weeks following treatment, and this alone does not constitute a treatment failure; however, treatment failure or reinfestation should be considered if new lesions continue to develop. The persistence of pruritus in the absence of reinfection or treatment failure, termed "postscabetic pruritus" can be treated with antihistamines, topical glucocorticoids, and, if severe, oral glucocorticoids can be used.

Two doses of oral ivermectin separated by 7 to 10 days appears to be as effective as permethrin but is contraindicated in pregnant and breastfeeding women. Safety in children has not been established. Ivermectin is often reserved for patients that are intolerant of other therapies, for treatment failures, and when topical application of permethrin is impractical such as outbreaks in nursing homes. Crusted scabies, a complication usually seen in patients with HIV or other immunodeficiencies, should be treated with both 5% permethrin and oral ivermectin.

Lindane 1% lotion has been associated with neurotoxicity and is typically reserved as third-line therapy in patients who cannot intolerant of other therapies or for treatment failures.

> **KEY POINT**
> - Itching can persist for several weeks following treatment of scabies and does not constitute a treatment failure; persistent itching can be treated with antihistamines, topical glucocorticoids, and, if severe, oral glucocorticoids.

Answers and Critiques

Bibliography

Rosamilia LL. Scabies. Semin Cutan Med Surg. 2014;33:106-9. [PMID: 25577847]

Item 57   Answer: C

Educational Objective: Diagnose ocular rosacea.

The most likely diagnosis is ocular rosacea. This patient presents with the facial erythema, telangiectasias, and papulopustules that are characteristic of rosacea. Rosacea is a common chronic condition of the facial skin characterized by pink papules, pustules, erythema, and telangiectasias. It is typically found in a bilaterally symmetric distribution on the convexities of the face, namely the forehead, cheeks, nose, and chin. Both acne and rosacea have inflammatory papules and pustules, but comedones are not seen in rosacea. Ocular rosacea is seen in more than 50% of patients with cutaneous rosacea. Symptoms are burning or a foreign body sensation in the eye. Blepharitis, chalazia, and chronic eye infections can develop. This patient has anterior blepharitis, which is characterized by anterior lid margin edema and hyperemia and accumulated squamous debris around the lash bases. Eyelid thickening and loss of eyelashes can be seen in chronic cases. An ophthalmology consultation is recommended, and treatments include topical ophthalmic cyclosporine, topical erythromycin, or systemic tetracyclines.

Anterior scleritis is inflammation of the superficial sclera and deep vessels of the episclera. It is often associated with systemic inflammatory disorders. Patients may present with severe ocular pain, photophobia, tearing, and vision changes. On examination, the sclera may have a blue or violet coloration and be tender to palpation.

Episcleritis is an abrupt localized inflammation of the superficial vessels of the episclera. The cause is often unclear, but occasional association with rheumatic diseases is noted. Patients with episcleritis frequently present without pain or decreased visual acuity. On examination, the inflammation appears more localized than with conjunctivitis, which is typically diffuse.

Viral conjunctivitis, typically caused by an adenovirus, is often acute, unilateral, and associated with antecedent upper respiratory tract infection and exposure to infected persons. Symptoms are itching, foreign body sensation, and crusting of the eyelids following sleep. Viral conjunctivitis typically resolves in 3 to 7 days. Viral conjunctivitis does not typically cause blepharitis.

Anterior episcleritis, scleritis, or viral conjunctivitis is not associated with rosacea.

KEY POINT

- Ocular rosacea is characterized by burning, itching, dryness, or a foreign body sensation; blepharitis, chalazia, and chronic eye infections can develop.

Bibliography

Webster G, Schaller M. Ocular rosacea: a dermatologic perspective. J Am Acad Dermatol. 2013 Dec;69(6 Suppl 1):S42-3. [PMID: 24229636]

Item 58   Answer: A

Educational Objective: Diagnose erythema nodosum.

This patient has erythema nodosum, a form of panniculitis that affects women more frequently than men. Patients present with tender pink-to-red nodules on their lower extremities, most frequently the anterior lower legs. Erythema nodosum has been associated with many different medical conditions, medications, and hormones, including pregnancy, oral contraceptive pills, and hormone replacement therapy. All women of childbearing age who present with erythema nodosum should be evaluated for pregnancy. Those taking oral contraceptive pills should discontinue use.

Other associations have been reported in persons with erythema nodosum, including tubercular, streptococcal, HIV, fungal infections (coccidioidomycosis), sarcoidosis, and inflammatory bowel disease. A thorough history, physical examination, and targeted testing should be done.

Most cases of erythema nodosum are self-limited and will resolve within 6 to 9 months. Patients benefit from compression stockings, NSAIDs, rest, and elevation. A saturated solution of potassium iodide has been used successfully, as has prednisone, dapsone, and colchicine.

Granuloma annulare is a chronic dermatosis of unknown cause consisting of erythematous annular non-scaling plaques usually on the dorsal hands, feet, elbows, and knees. Generalized granuloma annulare is associated with diabetes mellitus. Usually asymptomatic, this dermatosis will resolve spontaneously after several months to years.

Lipodermatosclerosis is a fibrosing panniculitis of the subcutaneous tissue associated with chronic venous insufficiency. Characteristic findings include a woody induration of the subcutaneous tissues in association with findings of chronic venous stasis including varicosities, edema, ulcerations, and brown discoloration of the skin.

Necrobiosis lipoidica presents as atrophic, orange-colored patches often associated with visible vasculature from skin thinning; the lesions may ulcerate. Necrobiosis lipoidica may develop in patients with diabetes mellitus, and when present may be a sign of end-organ damage, as such patients are more likely to have retinopathy or nephropathy.

Pyoderma gangrenosum is an uncommon inflammatory process that typically occurs on the pretibial aspects of the lower legs and is often associated with an underlying systemic disease, such as inflammatory bowel disease. The ulcers are very deep and painful, with a dusky or violet-colored undermined border.

KEY POINT

- Erythema nodosum, a form of panniculitis, is often triggered by hormones, including oral contraceptives, hormone replacement therapy, and pregnancy, as well as certain infections and other inflammatory diseases.

Bibliography

Acosta KA, Haver MC, Kelly B. Etiology and therapeutic management of erythema nodosum during pregnancy: an update. Am J Clin Dermatol. 2013;14:215–22. [PMID: 23625180] doi:10.1007/s40257-013-0024-x

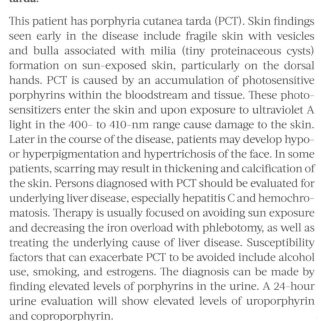

Item 59   Answer: D

Educational Objective: Treat arterial insufficiency ulcers.

This patient has an arterial insufficiency ulcer characterized by a well-demarcated painful ulcer with a dry wound bed; surgical revascularization will improve lower extremity circulation and facilitate wound healing. Arterial ulcers are most commonly found on the tips of and between the digits, but they can also form at sites of increased pressure, such as the lateral malleolus and metatarsal heads, or at sites of previous trauma. Arterial ulcers tend to be painful; discomfort may increase with elevation of the legs, compression, or any other maneuver that further limits circulation. Unlike venous stasis ulcers, which often have somewhat irregular borders and a significant amount of surrounding post-inflammatory hyperpigmentation, arterial insufficiency ulcers have a "punched out" appearance with surrounding erythema. The extremities as a whole often appear pale, and the skin is thin, taut, and shiny, and lacks hair. Pedal pulses are often difficult to appreciate; the toes are cold, and capillary refill is poor. If arterial insufficiency is suspected, diagnosis can be confirmed by measuring the ankle-brachial index (ABI). An ABI less than 0.9 is indicative of peripheral artery disease. Basic care of arterial ulcers includes debridement of necrotic tissue and proper dressings, but the most beneficial treatment is restoration of adequate circulation to the extremity. Surgical revascularization, percutaneous angioplasty, or stent placement are all options to restore blood flow to the affected area.

Compression stockings are a preferred treatment for venous stasis ulcerations. They should not be applied to a patient with arterial insufficiency ulcerations because of the risk of further ischemia.

Oral cilostazol is a phosphodiesterase inhibitor with antiplatelet activity and vasodilatory properties. When combined with a structured exercise program, cilostazol can improve maximum and pain-free treadmill-walking distance and quality-of-life measures in patients with peripheral artery disease. There is limited evidence of its benefit in arterial insufficiency ulcers.

Skin grafting is a procedure often used for the treatment of recalcitrant venous ulcers that fail to respond to compression and usual wound care. Revascularization, not skin grafting, is the primary treatment of arterial ulcers.

KEY POINT

- In patients with arterial insufficiency ulcers, surgical revascularization to improve the lower extremity circulation is often necessary to facilitate wound healing.

Bibliography

Kirsner RS, Vivas AC. Lower-extremity ulcers: diagnosis and management. Br J Dermatol. 2015 Aug;173(2):379–90. [PMID: 26257052]

Item 60   Answer: E

Educational Objective: Diagnose porphyria cutanea tarda.

This patient has porphyria cutanea tarda (PCT). Skin findings seen early in the disease include fragile skin with vesicles and bulla associated with milia (tiny proteinaceous cysts) formation on sun-exposed skin, particularly on the dorsal hands. PCT is caused by an accumulation of photosensitive porphyrins within the bloodstream and tissue. These photosensitizers enter the skin and upon exposure to ultraviolet A light in the 400- to 410-nm range cause damage to the skin. Later in the course of the disease, patients may develop hypo- or hyperpigmentation and hypertrichosis of the face. In some patients, scarring may result in thickening and calcification of the skin. Persons diagnosed with PCT should be evaluated for underlying liver disease, especially hepatitis C and hemochromatosis. Therapy is usually focused on avoiding sun exposure and decreasing the iron overload with phlebotomy, as well as treating the underlying cause of liver disease. Susceptibility factors that can exacerbate PCT to be avoided include alcohol use, smoking, and estrogens. The diagnosis can be made by finding elevated levels of porphyrins in the urine. A 24-hour urine evaluation will show elevated levels of uroporphyrin and coproporphyrin.

Bullous pemphigoid is the most frequent cause of autoimmune blistering disease. Patients will have pruritic urticarial red plaques that eventually develop large bullae. These blisters are subepidermal in nature, and milia may occasionally be seen. The blisters occur most frequently on the trunk and can be quite large and tense.

Bullous tinea is typically unilateral and associated with an annular scaly patch or patches. A potassium hydroxide examination will reveal fungal hyphae. The blisters are intraepidermal in nature, and milia will not be seen.

Dermatitis herpetiformis presents with tiny fragile vesicles or small erosions on the elbows, knees, or scalp. Itching is pronounced, and the condition is worsened by consumption of food containing gluten. Involvement of the dorsal hands would be an unusual clinical finding.

Persons with pemphigus vulgaris develop fragile vesicles and bulla without milia formation. The oral mucosa is frequently involved and is often the site of first involvement.

Patients with bullous pemphigoid, pemphigus vulgaris, and dermatitis herpetiformis do not develop hypertrichosis.

KEY POINT

- Porphyria cutanea tarda presents with skin fragility and small, transient, easily ruptured vesicles in sun-exposed areas, mainly on the hands; these eventually rupture, forming erosions, dyspigmentation, and scarring.

Answers and Critiques

Bibliography
Balwani M, Desnick RJ. The porphyrias: advances in diagnosis and treatment. Blood. 2012;120:4496-504. [PMID: 22791288] doi:10.1182/blood-2012-05-423186

Item 61   Answer: A
Educational Objective: Diagnose melanoma during pregnancy.

The patient has a changing mole that is very suspicious for melanoma on her left leg. It needs to be biopsied promptly as not to delay the diagnosis of melanoma. The skin biopsy is an important part of the diagnostic work-up for melanoma. Ideally, an atypical pigmented lesion should be removed using an excisional biopsy, in which the entire lesion is removed. Since this is not always practical or possible, additional options are sometimes used. These include punch biopsy, in which a sample of the lesion is removed using a cylindrical blade and sent for analysis. Although this type of biopsy generally provides a sample of adequate depth, there is concern about sampling error given that the area removed may not necessarily be representative of the remainder of the lesion. Similarly, although shave biopsies are often readily available and easy to perform, this technique carries the risk of transecting the melanoma if a deep enough sample is not taken. This would result in an underestimate of the true depth of the lesion, which could have implications regarding further work-up and management.

There is no reason to delay the biopsy in a suspicious melanocytic lesion during pregnancy. Lidocaine is classified by the FDA as pregnancy category B and can be safely used as local anesthesia during pregnancy. It is controversial to use epinephrine as it is FDA classified as category C. Although no adverse events have been documented in humans, in vitro studies of human uterine arteries have shown that in high doses, epinephrine can cause spasms and reduce flow through the uterine artery. Obtaining a biopsy from a changing mole in a pregnant woman should be done promptly as not to delay the diagnosis of melanoma.

It is not appropriate to treat a highly suspicious lesion with cryotherapy. The depth of invasion (Breslow depth) of a melanoma is the most important prognostic feature and correlates most strongly with the risk of recurrence and metastasis. Destruction of a pigmented lesion removes the possibility of making a proper diagnosis and prognosis for a potential melanoma.

Providing reassurance and thereby delaying diagnosis of melanoma could result in poor prognosis for the mother and child. Malignant melanoma is the most common malignancy during pregnancy. Studies show that changes in size in nevi during pregnancy occur on the front of the body owing to the stretching of the skin as the pregnancy progresses. Nevi on other locations, such as the leg, typically do not change during pregnancy, and this development is a red flag for possible melanoma.

Bibliography
Bieber AK, Martires KJ, Driscoll MS. Grant-Kels JM, Pomeranz MK, Stein JA. Nevi and pregnancy. J Am Acad Dermatol. 2016;75:661-6. [PMID: 27646736] doi:10.1016/j.jaad.2016.01.060

Item 62   Answer: C

Educational Objective: Treat pyoderma gangrenosum.

This patient has pyoderma gangrenosum, and a glucocorticoid, such as prednisone, is the preferred initial treatment. Typically required in doses of 1 mg/kg, prednisone is often effective in controlling pyoderma. To protect from long-term side effects of prolonged glucocorticoid use, steroid-sparing agents, immunosuppressants, intralesional glucocorticoids, or high-potency topical glucocorticoids are frequently used. Pyoderma gangrenosum is commonly associated with inflammatory bowel disease, hematologic abnormalities, and malignancies. The disease predominately affects the lower legs, but can be seen at any location. The beginning sign is often a tender pustule or red papule or nodule. This will quickly erode into an ulcer. Classic cases will have a rolled purplish border and undermined edges. As the ulcer resolves, it tends to heal with atrophic scarring in a cross-like or cribriform pattern. The ulcer is extremely painful. The diagnosis is one of exclusion, and other causes of ulceration need to be ruled out. Skin biopsies are not diagnostic. Surface cultures will grow myriad bacteria, which are most likely colonizing the ulcer and not causative.

Compression can be used in patients with extensive edema, but it is not a mainstay of therapy. Compression is often not tolerated because of pain. Good wound care with nonadherent dressings is important. Avoiding tape on the skin is necessary to prevent pathergy, the occurrence of lesions at sites of trauma, from the skin tape.

Dapsone has been used with some success, likely because of its anti-neutrophil effects, but it is not used as first-line treatment of pyoderma.

Pyoderma gangrenosum often occurs in the site of trauma (pathergy). For this reason, surgical debridement should be avoided unless a life-threatening infection is suspected. One exception is peristomal pyoderma gangrenosum. Surgical reanastomosis and closure of the ostomy site often results in healing of peristomal pyoderma. Relocating the stoma to another skin site will often result in resolution of the original peristomal ulcer; however, pyoderma will likely develop at the new ostomy site.

Potent topical glucocorticoids have been used for small lesions, but topical hydrocortisone is of no benefit as it is a low-potency glucocorticoid. Patients with underlying disease (inflammatory bowel disease, hematologic malignancy,

CONT.

rheumatoid disease) often improve with therapy that is directed at the underlying disease. Active pyoderma in persons with underlying disease often means that the underlying disease is not adequately controlled.

KEY POINT

- Prednisone is the preferred initial treatment for pyoderma gangrenosum.

Bibliography

Herberger K, Dissemond J, Hohaus K, Schaller J, Anastasiadou Z, Augustin M. Treatment of pyoderma gangrenosum: retrospective multicentre analysis of 121 patients [Letter]. Br J Dermatol. 2016;175:1070-1072. [PMID: 27060666] doi:10.1111/bjd.14619

Item 63   Answer: D

Educational Objective: Treat severe allergic contact dermatitis.

This patient has severe contact dermatitis from poison ivy (*Toxicodendron* genus), and the most appropriate treatment is a 21-day taper of oral prednisone. There are two types of contact dermatitis: allergic and irritant. Allergic contact dermatitis is a type IV delayed hypersensitivity reaction. With repeated exposure, a pruritic eczematous dermatitis develops on the exposed area. In exuberant cases, the localized inflammation can lead to a secondary "id" reaction, a generalized acute cutaneous reaction in which pinpoint flesh-colored to red papules develop diffusely on the body. Irritant contact dermatitis is caused by a direct toxic effect on the epidermis from exposure to a chemical such as a cleaning agent, other caustic substances, or repeated wetting and drying, and it is not mediated by the immune system. Urushiol is an allergen in the *Toxicodendron* genus of plants. Examples of these plants include poison ivy, poison oak, and poison sumac. Typically this rash presents with geometric lines or splatters of red papules and vesicles, with surrounding erythema, especially on exposed areas. In severe cases involving multiple body areas or the face, systemic glucocorticoids are the best treatment. Two- to 3-week courses of glucocorticoids are preferred over shorter courses in order to decrease the risk of rebound dermatitis.

A 7-day course of oral acyclovir is the treatment for herpes zoster. Herpes zoster typically presents with painful clusters of vesicles in a dermatomal distribution. The widespread clinical presentation of a pruritic vesicular rash is not consistent with herpes zoster.

Oral doxycycline is an antibiotic often combined with incision and drainage for the empiric treatment of moderate purulent skin infections such as furuncles, carbuncles, and abscesses. Although allergic contact dermatitis can become secondarily infected with *Staphylococcus aureus* or streptococcus, there is no evidence of infection in this patient (for example, extensive and spreading erythema, warmth, drainage, and increasing pain).

A 6-day taper of methylprednisolone would increase the risk of rebound dermatitis after completion of the short

taper. A longer 14- to 21-day taper of systemic glucocorticoids is preferred.

Hydrocortisone 1% is a low-potency topical glucocorticoid and would be ineffective for treating this severe case of contact dermatitis. High-potency glucocorticoids such as clobetasol propionate 0.05% or betamethasone dipropionate 0.05% can be helpful in early and localized disease.

KEY POINT

- Severe allergic contact eruptions such as those from poison ivy may necessitate a 2- to 3-week taper of systemic glucocorticoids; because of the risk of rebound dermatitis, shorter courses are not recommended.

Bibliography

Usatine RP1, Riojas M. Diagnosis and management of contact dermatitis. Am Fam Physician. 2010 Aug 1;82(3):249-55. [PMID: 20672788]

Item 64   Answer: A

Educational Objective: Treat tinea pedis.

Dermatophytosis or tinea of non–hair-bearing skin with limited involvement can be treated with imidazole cream applied once to twice daily for 2 to 4 weeks. Application should extend a few centimeters beyond the advancing border. For tinea pedis, the web spaces between the toes should be treated. Other topical agents including miconazole, clotrimazole, ketoconazole, ciclopirox, or terbinafine can also be used. Over-the-counter preparations are cost-effective options with good efficacy. Most infections will resolve but may recur and require retreatment. In immunosuppressed patients, recognition and treatment of superficial skin fungal infections is essential, as fungal infections can lead to epidermal breakdown and create a portal of entry for invasive pathogens. Tinea pedis is also a potential cause of recurrent bacterial cellulitis.

Dermatophytes do not respond to topical nystatin, which is used to treat infections caused by *Candida* species.

Oral antifungal therapy with terbinafine or an azole antifungal agent such as itraconazole or fluconazole may be necessary for treating tinea capitis, onychomycosis, Majocchi granuloma (a granulomatous response to dermatophyte infection in the dermis and hair follicles), or extensive infection. Oral ketoconazole no longer has an indication for superficial fungal infection because of severe and sometimes fatal idiosyncratic liver toxicity. In addition, ketoconazole is a potent inhibitor of CYP3A4 resulting in significant drug interactions. Prolonged use of ketoconazole also may result in adrenal gland suppression.

Combination therapy with potent topical glucocorticoids, such as betamethasone, and antifungal creams, such as clotrimazole, should be avoided because of an increased risk of treatment failures, development of skin atrophy with prolonged use, and increased cost without increased efficacy.

Bibliography

Darlenski R, Kazandjieva J, Tsankov N. Systemic drug reactions with skin involvement: Stevens-Johnson syndrome, toxic epidermal necrolysis, and DRESS. Clin Dermatol. 2015;33:538-41. [PMID: 26321400] doi:10.1016/j.clindermatol.2015.05.005

KEY POINT

- Treatment of tinea of non–hair-bearing skin includes topical antifungal agents such as imidazole, miconazole, clotrimazole, ketoconazole, ciclopirox, or terbinafine; topical nystatin is not effective, and oral ketoconazole should be avoided.

Bibliography

Jewell JR, Myers SA. Topical Therapy Primer for Nondermatologists. Med Clin North Am. 2015;99:1167-82. [PMID: 26476246] doi:10.1016/j.mcna.2015.06.001

Item 65   Answer: A

Educational Objective: Diagnose drug reaction with eosinophilia and systemic symptoms (DRESS).

This patient's symptoms are characteristic of drug reaction with eosinophilia and systemic symptoms (DRESS) or drug hypersensitivity syndrome. DRESS is a severe, life-threatening, idiosyncratic medication reaction. The most common culprit medications include sulfonamide antibiotics, allopurinol, and anticonvulsants, but many more have been implicated. DRESS is unique in that the onset is usually 2 to 6 weeks after exposure to a causative medication. Because of this delayed onset, DRESS is often underrecognized or misdiagnosed. The eruption is usually an exuberant morbilliform eruption with prominent facial edema, lymphadenopathy, fever, and, in severe cases, hypotension. Typical laboratory findings include leukocytosis with eosinophilia and increased serum alanine aminotransferase levels. Cessation of the causative agent and systemic glucocorticoids with a long taper are the best treatment. DRESS reactions with carbamazepine may cross-react with phenytoin and phenobarbital, but not levetiracetam or valproic acid.

The term *retiform purpura* describes the angulated or netlike configuration that reflects the underlying vascular structure in the skin. Various conditions can cause retiform purpura, many of which disrupt arterial blood flow such as thrombosis and embolization.

Stevens-Johnson syndrome (SJS) and toxic epidermal necrolysis (TEN) are both severe drug reactions, but these reactions happen closer to the start date of the offending agent than DRESS syndrome. SJS/TEN lack the facial edema of DRESS syndrome, and DRESS syndrome lacks the epidermal necrosis of SJS/TEN. DRESS can cause mucositis in the minority of cases. Both SJS/TEN and DRESS can result in liver or kidney function abnormalities, but eosinophilia is strongly indicative of DRESS.

KEY POINT

- Drug reaction with eosinophilia and systemic symptoms (DRESS) is a systemic drug hypersensitivity reaction that presents with rash, prominent facial edema, lymphadenopathy, and fever 2 to 6 weeks after the initiation of the causative drug.

Item 66   Answer: B

Educational Objective: Evaluate the cause of pruritus in the absence of skin findings.

The most appropriate initial management for this patient is to discontinue hydrochlorothiazide. Pruritus in the absence of skin findings should be evaluated for underlying systemic causes. These include kidney disease, hyperthyroidism, hepatobiliary diseases, HIV infection, lymphoproliferative disorders (lymphoma), and myeloproliferative disorders (polycythemia vera). Drug-induced pruritus should also be considered. This patient has a normal complete blood count, liver chemistry tests, thyroid-stimulating hormone levels, serum creatinine, and sedimentation rate, making many of the systemic diseases unlikely. However, this patient is taking hydrochlorothiazide for hypertension. Hydrochlorothiazide, calcium channel blockers, opiates, and NSAIDs are all medications that can cause generalized pruritus without skin findings. In patients taking multiple medications, it can be challenging to determine which drug(s) may be contributing to pruritus, as patients may develop medication-induced itch even after months or years on a drug. The most appropriate management in this patient would be to discontinue hydrochlorothiazide and monitor for 2 to 4 weeks to detect improvement of his pruritus.

Hodgkin lymphoma is the malignant disease most strongly associated with pruritus. CT of the chest and abdomen could be ordered to evaluate for Hodgkin disease, but he has no other symptoms to suggest lymphoma, such as fever or weight loss, and no lymphadenopathy on physical examination. The high cost of CT imaging and radiation exposure would make this an inappropriate initial management option for this patient. A plain chest radiograph would be a better initial imaging test if Hodgkin lymphoma were suspected.

Topical permethrin is prescribed for the treatment of scabies. Although scabies should be considered in any patient with pruritus, there are no skin findings to suggest scabies in this patient, such as erythematous papulonodules and scaling patches, especially in web spaces, wrists, axillae, nipples, waistline, and genitals.

Topical triamcinolone can be used for pruritus associated with inflammatory skin conditions, such as atopic dermatitis or psoriasis. This patient has no evidence of atopic dermatitis or psoriasis, such as inflamed, dry, red, itchy skin, or thick silvery scale on erythematous patches.

KEY POINT

- Pruritus in the absence of skin findings should be evaluated for underlying systemic causes; many medications such as hydrochlorothiazide, calcium channel blockers, opiates, or NSAIDs can also cause generalized pruritus without skin findings.

Bibliography

Silverberg JI. Practice gaps in pruritus. Dermatol Clin. 2016 Jul;34(3):257-601. [PMID: 27363881]

 Item 67 **Answer:** **A**

Educational Objective: Treat low-risk basal cell carcinoma.

Electrodesiccation and curettage (ED&C) is a widely used treatment for noninfiltrating basal cell carcinomas on low-risk anatomic sites (trunk and extremities). Treatment of basal cell carcinomas depends on many factors, including the histologic subtype, location, size, cosmetic considerations, and patient's age and comorbidities. Nodular and superficial basal cell carcinomas on the trunk and extremities are often treated with ED&C. Infiltrative and micronodular basal cell carcinomas, especially on the face, are not appropriate for ED&C. For this patient, his lesion is a small, histologically low-risk subtype of basal cell carcinoma on the back that can be treated with ED&C.

Mohs micrographic surgery is a specialized surgical procedure that provides margin control while sparing as much normal skin as possible. Indications for Mohs micrographic surgery include tumors with aggressive histologic subtypes (micronodular, morpheaform, infiltrative, perineural involvement); high-risk and cosmetically sensitive locations (face, genitals); large tumors or tumors arising in scar tissue; and tumors in patients who are immunosuppressed. This patient's lesion would not be an appropriate use of Mohs surgery.

Radiation therapy for skin cancers is appropriate for patients who refuse surgery or are not optimal surgical candidates. The patient will be able to tolerate an ED&C without any difficulty.

Vismodegib is an oral medication that inhibits the hedgehog signaling pathway; this signaling pathway is aberrant in most basal cell carcinomas. It is reserved for locally advanced or metastatic basal cell carcinomas.

KEY POINT

- Noninfiltrating basal cell carcinomas on low-risk areas such as the trunk and extremities are best treated with electrodesiccation and curettage.

Bibliography

Connolly SM, Baker DR, Coldiron BM, Fazio MJ, Storrs PA, Vidimos AT, et al; American Academy of Dermatology. AAD/ACMS/ASDSA/ASMS 2012 appropriate use criteria for Mohs micrographic surgery: a report of the American Academy of Dermatology, American College of Mohs Surgery, American Society for Dermatologic Surgery Association, and the American Society for Mohs Surgery. Dermatol Surg. 2012;38:1582-603. [PMID: 22958088] doi:10.1111/j.1524-4725.2012.02574.x

Item 68 **Answer:** **A**

Educational Objective: Diagnose alopecia areata.

This patient has alopecia areata, a patchy, nonscarring alopecia. It most often occurs in early adulthood and is associated with autoimmune disorders such as type 1 diabetes mellitus, thyroid disease, and vitiligo. Alopecia areata tends to have an acute onset. It appears as round or oval patches of hair loss with the periphery studded with exclamation point hairs. These are hair shafts that narrow as they approach the skin surface. The scalp is most often affected with severe 2- to 3-cm patches of hair loss. The clinical course of alopecia areata is variable and unpredictable with spontaneous recovery for most patients with localized disease. Treatment is dependent on the area involved. In localized disease, high-potency topical glucocorticoids are first-line treatment.

Discoid lupus erythematosus is a form of patchy scarring alopecia. It is characterized by oval plaques that may have a pink, active rim with a white atrophic center. A biopsy of the scalp would confirm the diagnosis. Local treatment involves high-potency topical or intralesional glucocorticoids.

Secondary syphilis can cause patchy nonscarring alopecia ("moth eaten"). Alopecia is seen in approximately 7% of patients with secondary syphilis. There are other syphilids in secondary syphilis such as copper-colored macules and papules on the trunk and extremities, including palms and soles. Serology would aid in diagnosis. Treatment involves intramuscular benzathine penicillin.

Tinea capitis is a superficial infection of the scalp, seen mostly in school-aged children. It can appear as a patchy, nonscarring alopecia with broken hair shafts. Occipital lymph nodes can often be palpated. As there is often scale, it can look like seborrheic dermatitis. A potassium hydroxide microscopic examination and culture of broken hairs can confirm the diagnosis. Treatment involves systemic antifungal agents.

Trichotillomania, alopecia from compulsive twisting and pulling, is in the differential diagnosis for patchy nonscarring alopecia; however, on physical examination, the patches are often more irregular and ill-marginated with broken hairs. Patients with trichotillomania often have a history of psychiatric conditions and anxiety.

KEY POINT

- Alopecia areata is a chronic autoimmune disease that results in smooth, hairless patches of skin, most commonly appearing on the scalp.

Bibliography

Mubki T, Rudnicka L, Olszewska M, Shapiro J. Evaluation and diagnosis of the hair loss patient: part I. History and clinical examination. J Am Acad Dermatol. 2014;71:415.e1-415.e15. [PMID: 25128118] doi:10.1016/j.jaad.2014.04.070

Item 69 **Answer:** **A**

Educational Objective: Diagnose amyloidosis.

This patient likely has amyloidosis. Amyloid light chain amyloidosis is the most common type of amyloidosis; it is a plasma cell dyscrasia-related disease characterized by end-organ damage secondary to tissue deposition of monoclonal free λ or κ light-chain fibrils. Clinical symptoms and manifestations vary and are dictated by the tissue tropism of the amyloidogenic light chain. If amyloid deposits are identified on tissue biopsy, other types of amyloidosis should be excluded by typing, which can be done by κ/λ light-chain immunohistochemistry. Major clinical manifestations include proteinuria with worsening kidney function, restrictive cardiomyopathy, and hepatomegaly. Neurologic findings include a symmetric, distal sensorimotor neuropathy, carpal tunnel syndrome, and autonomic neuropathy with orthostatic hypotension. Skin manifestations are present in 30% to 40% of patients and include generalized waxy appearance, ecchymoses with minor pressure ("pinch purpura"), ecchymoses around the eyes ("raccoon eyes"), yellow waxy papules and plaques especially in a periorbital location, dystrophic nails, and macroglossia. Bleeding caused by acquired factor X deficiency may also occur.

A pathognomonic cutaneous feature of dermatomyositis is a heliotrope rash, a distinctive purple or lilac erythema of the eyelids that may be accompanied by edema. It is not yellow or papular as seen in this patient.

Xanthelasma is a type of plane xanthoma localized to the periorbital area, most commonly on the upper medial eyelid, and it is characterized by soft, nontender, nonpruritic plaques. Xanthelasma can occur without hyperlipidemia, particularly in older persons, but it is often associated with familial dyslipidemias when seen in a younger person. This patient's periorbital lesions are not consistent with xanthelasma.

Classic cutaneous sarcoidosis appears as violaceous papules around the nose including the ala, or periorbitally and around the oropharynx and nasal openings. This patient's yellow periorbital papules are not consistent with sarcoidosis.

The combination of the patient's periorbital skin findings, easy bruising and bleeding, hepatomegaly, and proteinuria cannot be explained by dermatomyositis, hyperlipidemia, or sarcoidosis.

KEY POINT

- Skin manifestations of amyloid light chain amyloidosis are present in 30% to 40% of patients and include generalized waxy appearance, ecchymoses with minor pressure ("pinch purpura"), ecchymoses around the eyes ("raccoon eyes"), yellow waxy papules and plaques especially in a periorbital location, dystrophic nails, and macroglossia.

Bibliography

Wechalekar AD, Gillmore JD, Hawkins PN. Systemic amyloidosis. Lancet. 2016;387:2641-54. [PMID: 26719234] doi:10.1016/S0140-6736(15)01274-X

Item 70   Answer: C

Educational Objective: Diagnose eruptive xanthoma-associated hypertriglyceridemia.

This patient has eruptive xanthomas, which are characterized by a rapid onset of numerous yellow papules with surrounding erythema found primarily on the extensor surfaces of the extremities and buttocks. Xanthomas are localized lipid deposits whose presence is suggested by characteristic cutaneous papules, plaques, or nodules.

Cutaneous xanthomas can be idiopathic and not associated with an underlying disorder or an indication of a primary

dyslipidemia, hyperlipidemia secondary to another disorder, medication effect (estrogens, prednisone, protease inhibitors), or hematologic disease. The ability to diagnose the xanthoma subtype will direct the proper testing and treatment. When necessary, diagnosis can be confirmed with a skin biopsy that shows lipid-laden macrophages in the dermis. Eruptive xanthomas are pathognomonic of hypertriglyceridemia, and a vast number of these patients also have a diagnosis of diabetes mellitus. Eruptive xanthomas have also been reported as a complication of hypertriglyceridemia-induced pancreatitis.

Tuberous xanthomas are associated with markedly elevated low-density lipoprotein levels (familial hypercholesterolemia) and elevated intermediate-density lipoprotein and triglyceride levels (familial dysbetalipoproteinemia). Tuberous xanthomas present as yellow to red papules or nodules up to 3 cm in size located over joints and extensor surfaces of the elbows and knees. The location and size of tuberous xanthomas distinguish them from eruptive xanthomas.

Tendinous xanthomas are skin-colored nodules most commonly located over the Achilles tendon. They are smooth, firm, and mobile and are attached to and move with the tendon. Tendon xanthomas are typically associated with familial hypercholesterolemia and familial defective apo B-100. The location, size, and color of these tumors distinguish them from eruptive xanthomas.

Plane xanthomas may occur in the absence of lipid disorders in approximately 50% of adults or can be associated with familial dysbetalipoproteinemia, homozygous familial hypercholesterolemia, and hypercholesteremia associated with primary biliary cirrhosis. Plane xanthomas are recognized as yellow thin plaques most commonly found around the eyelids (xanthelasma), neck, trunk, shoulders, axillae, and in some cases, palms. The flat plaque-like appearance and location of plane xanthomas distinguishes them from eruptive xanthomas.

KEY POINT

- Eruptive xanthomas, characterized by yellow papules with surrounding erythema, are pathognomonic of hypertriglyceridemia, with a number of these patients also having a diagnosis of diabetes mellitus.

Bibliography

Roga G, Jithendriya M. Eruptive xanthoma: Warning sign of systemic disease. Cleve Clin J Med. 2016;83:715-716. [PMID: 27726830] doi:10.3949/ccjm.83a.15126

Item 71   Answer: B

Educational Objective: Diagnose dermatofibroma.

Dermatofibromas are benign, fibrohistiocytic lesions common on the extremities of young adults, in particular women, but they also occur on the trunk in both men and women. Diagnosed clinically, dermatofibromas are tan-to-brown or reddish discrete papules about the size of a pencil eraser. They "dimple" when lateral pressure is applied to the lesion with the thumb and first finger as shown (see top of next page).

Multiple lesions may be present in some persons. They are thought to arise from minor injury, including insect

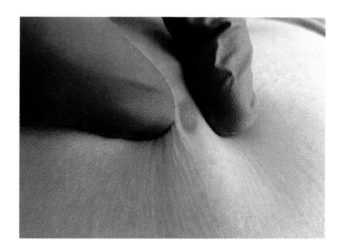

bites, shaving injuries, or folliculitis. Dermatofibromas are benign and do not require treatment.

Acrochordons or "skin tags" are skin-colored, pedunculated papules. They are most commonly seen on the neck and skin folds in older adults. They are harmless but often bothersome from a cosmetic standpoint. They may also occasionally become tender when traumatized. The presence of numerous lesions, particularly in the setting of obesity and acanthosis nigricans, is associated with insulin resistance.

Neurofibromas are asymptomatic, benign nerve sheath tumors that present as soft skin-colored papules, which show invagination of the papule with lateral pressure ("buttonhole" sign). Isolated lesions are common in the general population and are not associated with any underlying disease. The presence of numerous neurofibromas suggests a diagnosis of neurofibromatosis type 1. Additional findings that suggest this diagnosis include multiple café-au-lait macules, Lisch nodules (raised, pigmented hamartomas of the iris), and axillary freckling. Neurofibromas are benign and do not require treatment.

Pyogenic granulomas are bright red vascular lesions that arise suddenly and grow rapidly; they often appear during pregnancy or in the setting of certain medications (such as antiretroviral therapy). The name is misleading, as they are neither pyogenic nor granulomatous. They resemble cherry hemangiomas, but are often more friable and tend to bleed more easily. They are benign lesions that do not have any systemic disease associations; they are treated with biopsy or electrocautery.

KEY POINT

- Dermatofibromas are benign firm brown or reddish papules about the size of a pencil eraser that most commonly occur on the lower extremities; they "dimple" when lateral pressure is applied to the lesion with the thumb and first finger.

Bibliography
Higgins JC, Maher MH, Douglas MS. Diagnosing Common Benign Skin Tumors. Am Fam Physician. 2015;92:601-7. [PMID: 26447443]

Item 72   Answer: A

Educational Objective: Evaluate the cause of acanthosis nigricans.

This patient has acanthosis nigricans (AN), and he should be screened for insulin resistance with a fasting blood glucose measurement. AN presents as velvety-to-verrucous, gray-to-brown thickening with accentuation of skin marking seen in the intertriginous folds and neck. AN is more common in persons of color. It can be benign and associated with diabetes or present as a paraneoplastic syndrome. Benign AN is characteristically seen in patients with type 2 diabetes mellitus and obesity; however, it can be seen in patients with other endocrine abnormalities that involve insulin resistance. Therefore, a diagnosis of AN should prompt screening for diabetes. If symptoms are extensive and of acute onset, in particular involving the palms and tongue, a screening for malignancy is indicated with a thorough review of systems and a complete physical examination.

Acanthosis nigricans is associated with endocrinopathies other than diabetes that can cause insulin resistance, including Cushing syndrome. This patient has some elements of Cushing syndrome including obesity and truncal acne, but the absence of hypertension and striae make this diagnosis less likely, and a 24-hour urine cortisol measurement is therefore not the next diagnostic test.

A thyroid-stimulating hormone and serum thyroxine measurement should be performed in patients with pretibial myxedema. Pretibial myxedema presents with firm nodules and plaques with a "'peau d'orange" appearance on the pretibial area. Pretibial myxedema is almost always associated with the signs and symptoms of hyperthyroidism. Extrathyroidal manifestations of Graves disease include Graves orbitopathy, pretibial myxedema (thyroid dermopathy), and acropachy. Acropachy is swelling of the soft tissues on the hands and feet with digital clubbing. This patient has no findings consistent with pretibial myxedema.

Erythrasma is a superficial infection with *Corynebacterium minutissimum*. Its growth is encouraged by a warm, moist environment, such as intertriginous areas. Erythrasma causes well-defined, pink-to-brown patches with fine scale, located in the axillae, groin, or inframammary regions. A unique feature of this infection is that it fluoresces a bright coral-red color when illuminated with a Wood lamp. The location, morphology, and color of this patient's skin findings are not consistent with erythrasma.

KEY POINT

- Acanthosis nigricans presents as skin thickening and darkening of the intertriginous areas, particularly the axillae and neck; it can be associated with insulin resistance or present as a paraneoplastic syndrome.

Bibliography
Murphy-Chutorian B, Han G, Cohen SR. Dermatologic manifestations of diabetes mellitus: a review. Endocrinol Metab Clin North Am. 2013;42:869-98. [PMID: 24286954] doi:10.1016/j.ecl.2013.07.004

Answers and Critiques

Index

Note: Page numbers followed by f and t indicates figure and table respectively. Test questions are indicated by Q.

A

ABCDEs, of melanoma, 42
ABDs. *See* Autoimmune bullous diseases (ABDs)
Abscesses, bacterial, 22–23, 22f
Acantholytic dermatosis, transient, 11–12, 11f
Acanthosis nigricans (AN), 60t, 62–63, 62f, Q72
Acitretin
    in pregnancy, 83t
    for psoriasis, 9
Acne, 17–19
    adult, 19
    clinical features of, 17, 17f, 18f
    differential diagnosis of, 18t
    grading system, 18–19
    nodulocystic/recalcitrant, 19, Q12
    pathogenesis of, 18
    treatment of, 18–19, 18f
Acneiform eruptions
    acne, 17–19, 17f, 18f
    hidradenitis suppurativa, 21, 21f, 21t
    rosacea, 19–21, 19f, 20f, 20t
    types of, 18t
Acne keloidalis nuchae, 72, 73f
Acquired hypertrichosis lanuginosa, 69t
Acral lentiginous melanoma, 43, 43f. *See also* Melanoma
Acrochordons, 37, 37f
Acroosteolysis, 54
Actinic cheilitis, 78
Actinic keratosis, 41, 41f, Q21
Actinic purpura, 84, 84f, Q26
Acute febrile neutrophilic dermatosis. *See* Sweet syndrome
Acute generalized exanthematous pustulosis (AGEP),
        68, 68f
Acute seroconversion syndrome, 63
Acyclovir
    for herpes zoster, 30
    for HSV infection, 29
Adalimumab, Q19
    for hidradenitis suppurativa, 21
Adapalene, for acne, 19
AGEP. *See* Acute generalized exanthematous pustulosis (AGEP)
Aging, skin conditions during, 81, 83–84
    actinic purpura, 84, 84f
    changes due to aging, 84t
    chronic wounds, 84
    dryness, 83–84, 84f
    infection, 84
Albendazole, for cutaneous larva migrans, 34
Allergic contact dermatitis, 5, Q63
    causes of, 5–6, 6f
    patch testing for, 5, 5f
Alopecia, 70–73. *See also specific type*
    localized/generalized, 70
    management of, 71t
    nonscarring, 70, 71t, 72f
    scarring, 70
Alopecia areata, 70, 71t, 72f, Q68
Aluminum hydroxide, for pitted keratolysis, 25
Amalgam tattoo, 76
Ammonium lactate, for acanthosis nigricans, 63
Ampicillin, for folliculitis, 22
Amyloidosis, 60t, 61–62, 62f, Q69
    macroglossia in, 62f
    periorbital purpura in, 62f
    pinch purpura in, 61, 62f
Amyopathic dermatomyositis, 53, Q13. *See also* Dermatomyositis
Anaphylaxis, 16
Androgenetic alopecia, 70, 71t, 72f

Angioedema, 46
    mast cell-associated, 46
Angiolipomas, 39
Anthropophilic dermatophytes, 26. *See also* Tinea
Antibiotics
    oral
        for acne, 19
        for cellulitis in immunocompetent patients, 25
        for erythrasma, 25, 26f
        for hidradenitis suppurativa, 21
        for impetigo, 24
        for rosacea, 20
    topical, 3t, 4
        for acne, 19
        for impetigo, 24
        side effects, 4
        for wounds, 34
Antifungal agents
    for paronychia, 73
    topical, 3t, 4
Antifungal powder, for intertrigo, 7
Antihistamines
    for postscabetic pruritus, Q56
    for pruritus, 45
Anti-Jo1, 53
Antimalarial agents
    for cutaneous lupus, 52, 52t
    for dermatomyositis, 53
Antiparasitic medications, 3t
Antiperspirants, for pitted keratolysis, 25
Antisynthetase syndrome, 53, 54f
Antiviral therapy
    for erythema multiforme, 65
    for HSV infection, 29
Aphthous ulcers, 77, 77f
Apoptotic epidermolysis syndrome, 50
Apremilast, for psoriasis, 9
Arterial insufficiency ulcers, 79–80, 80f, Q59
Asteatotic eczema. *See* Xerotic eczema
Atopic dermatitis, 4–5, 5f, Q3
    in HIV/AIDS, 63
Atopic triad, 4
Atrophy, 1t
Autoimmune bullous diseases (ABDs), 46–50, Q1
    characteristics of, 47t–48t
    diagnosis of, 48
    drug-induced, 49t
    intraepidermal, 46
    management of, 50
    subepidermal, 48
Azathioprine, for dermatomyositis, 53
Azelaic acid, for rosacea, 20

B

Bacitracin, 34
    and allergic dermatitis, 6
Bacterial skin infections, 21–25
    abscesses/furuncles/carbuncles, 22–23, 22f
    cellulitis/erysipelas, 24–25, 24f, 24t
    erythrasma, 25, 26f
    folliculitis, 21–22, 22f
    impetigo, 23–24, 23f, 24f
    MRSA infections, 23
    pitted keratolysis, 25, 25f
Balsam of Peru, 6t
Basal cell carcinoma (BCC), 39–41, 40f, Q22, Q67
    diagnosis of, 40
    follow-up skin examination, 40
    nodular, 40
    pigmented, 40
    sclerotic, 40

Basal cell carcinoma (BCC) (*Continued*)
    superficial, 40
    treatment of, 40, Q24
    UV light exposure and, 39
Bazex syndrome, 60t
BCC. *See* Basal cell carcinoma (BCC)
Beau lines, 74t
Bed bugs, 32
    bites, 32, 33f
    treatment of, 32t
Benzophenones, 6t
Benzoyl peroxide
    for acne, 18f, 19
    for pitted keratolysis, 25
Biologic agents, for psoriasis, 9
Biopsy. *See also* Skin biopsy
    for actinic keratoses, 41, Q21
    for basal cell carcinoma, 40
Birt-Hogg-Dube syndrome, 61t
Bisphosphonates, in calciphylaxis, 57
Bites and stings
    fleas, 34, 34f
    hymenoptera, 33
    spiders, 33, 33f
    worms, 34, 34f
Black hairy tongue, 78, 78f
Blue nails, 74t
Body lice, 32, 32t
Bowen disease (squamous cell carcinoma in situ), 41, 42f
Breast, Paget disease of, 60t
Brimonidine, for rosacea, 20
Brown recluse spider (*Loxosceles reclusa*), 33, 33f
Bulla, 1t
Bullous lupus, 50
Bullous pemphigoid, 47t, 48, 49f, Q16. *See also* Autoimmune bullous
        diseases (ABDs)
Burns, 34–35
    first-degree burn, 34f
    grading of, 35t
    rule of 9s, 34
    thermal, 34
Burrow, 1t

C
Calcineurin inhibitors, for atopic dermatitis, 5
Calciphylaxis, 57, 57f, 65t, 81t, Q48
Callus, 36
Candidiasis, 28, 28f
Canker sores. *See* Aphthous ulcers
Carbuncles, 22–23, 22f
Carcinoid syndrome, 60t
Cat flea (*Ctenocephalides felis*), 34
Celiac disease, 58, 59
Cellulitis, 8, 24–25
    causes of, 25
    clinical presentation of, 24, 24f
    differential diagnosis of, 24t
    in immunocompetent patients, 25
    recurrent, Q20
    treatment of, 25
Central centrifugal cicatricial alopecia, 71t
Cephalexin, for impetigo, 24
Charcot foot, 80
Chemical peels, for melasma, 14
Chemotherapy
    for actinic keratoses, 41
    for basal cell carcinoma, 40
    for squamous cell carcinoma, 42
    for stage IV melanoma, 44
    topical, 3t
Cherry angiomas, 37, 37f
Chest radiography, for erythema nodosum, Q43
Chickenpox, 29, 29f
Chilblains/pernio, 51, 52f
Chloasma. *See* Melasma
Chlorhexidine
    for folliculitis, 22
    for hidradenitis suppurativa, 21
    for MRSA infection, 23
Cicatricial pemphigoid, 47t, 49t. *See also* Autoimmune bullous diseases (ABDs)
Ciprofloxacin, for folliculitis, 22
Cirrhosis, 58

CLE. *See* Cutaneous lupus erythematosus (CLE)
Clindamycin, for pitted keratolysis, 25
Cocamidopropyl betaine, 6t
Colchicine, for pyoderma gangrenosum, 59
Comedo, 1t
Comedonal acne, topical retinoids for, Q55
Compound melanocytic nevus, 35f, 35t
Compression therapy, for venous stasis ulcers, 79, Q45
Condyloma acuminata (genital warts), 30, 31f. *See also* Warts
Contact allergens, 6t
Contact dermatitis, 5–6, 5f, 6f, 6t, 8, 24t, Q63
    allergic, 5
    causes of, 5–6, 6f
    epicutaneous patch testing for, 5, 5f
    irritant, 5
    in setting of stasis dermatitis, Q53
    treatment of, 6
Corns, 36
Corynebacterium minutissimum, 25
Cowden syndrome, 61t
Crust, 1t
Cryoglobulinemia, 56
Cryoglobulinemic vasculitis, 56
Cryotherapy
    for acrochordon, 36
    for actinic cheilitis, 78
    for actinic keratoses, 41
    for basal cell carcinoma, 40
    for cutaneous larva migrans, 34
    for seborrheic keratosis, 35
    for warts, 31
Cutaneous larva migrans, 34, 34f
Cutaneous lupus erythematosus (CLE), 50. *See also* Lupus erythematosus (LE)
    acute CLE (ACLE), 50–51, 50f, 51f
        maculopapular variant, 50
        malar butterfly rash, 50, 51f
    chronic CLE (CCLE), 50, 50f, 51, 51f, 52
        discoid lupus, 51, 51f, 52f
    subacute CLE (SCLE), 50, 50f, 51, 51f, 51t
        annual and polycyclic macules and plaques, 51, 51f
        drug induced, 51t
        psoriasiform scaly plaques, 51
Cuts and scrapes, 34
Cyclosporine
    for cutaneous lupus, 52, 52t
    for dermatomyositis, 53
    for psoriasis, 9
    for pyoderma gangrenosum, 59
Cyst, 1t

D
Dapsone
    for cutaneous lupus, 52, 52t
    for dermatitis herpetiformis, 50, 59, Q52
    for pyoderma gangrenosum, 59
Daptomycin, for abscesses/furuncles/carbuncles, 22
Deep venous thrombosis, 24t
Demodex folliculitis, 22
Depigmentation therapy, 13
Dermatitis
    atopic, 4–5, 5f
    contact, 5–6, 5f, 6f, 6t
    hand, 7, 7f
    intertrigo, 6–7, 7f
    seborrheic, 10–11, 10f
    stasis, 8, 8f
Dermatitis herpetiformis, 48, 48t, 50, 50f, 58, 59, Q52. *See also*
        Autoimmune bullous diseases (ABDs)
    and gluten-sensitive enteropathy, 59
    sites of involvement, 59
Dermatofibromas, 37, Q71
    dimple sign, 37, 37f
Dermatologic conditions. *See also specific condition*
    differential diagnosis of, 1
    growths, 1
    rashes, 1
Dermatology
    approach to patient in, 1–2
    diagnostic tests, 2
    emergencies in, 2, 2t
    physical examination, 2
    skin lesions, types of, 1, 1t

skin, structure of, 1, 1f
therapeutic principles in, 3–4
general considerations, 3, 3t
phototherapy, 4
topical antibiotics, 4
topical antifungal agents, 4
topical glucocorticoids, 3, 4t
topical immunomodulators, 4
topical retinoids, 4
vehicles for topical medications, 3t
Dermatomyositis, 53–54, 60t
amyopathic, 53, Q13
and cutaneous lupus erythematosus, 53
Gottron papules, 53, 53f
heliotrope rash, 53
nailfold capillary beds in, 53
shawl sign, 53, 53f
treatment of, 53
V-sign, 53
Dermatophytosis. *See* Tinea
Dermatoscope, 2
DHS. *See* Drug hypersensitivity syndrome (DHS)
Diabetes
and acanthosis nigricans, 62–63, Q72
and necrobiosis lipoidica, 63
Dicloxacillin, for impetigo, 24
Digital myxoid cysts, 39
Direct immunofluorescence (DIF), 48
Discoid eczema. *See* Nummular eczema
Discoid lupus erythematosus, 51, 51f, 52f
on scalp, 71t, 72, 72f
Distal subungual onychomycosis, 73
Dorsal pterygium, 9
Doxycycline
for abscesses/furuncles/carbuncles, 22
for rosacea, 20
DRESS. *See* Drug reaction with eosinophilia and systemic symptoms (DRESS)
Drug hypersensitivity syndrome (DHS), 67–68
Drug reactions, 14–17
fixed, 15t, 16, 16f
hypersensitivity vasculitis, 15t, 17
morbilliform/exanthematous, 14, 15t, 16f
photosensitivity disorders, 15t, 16–17, 17f
treatment, 17
types of, 14, 15t
urticarial reactions, 14, 15t, 16, 16f
Drug reaction with eosinophilia and systemic symptoms (DRESS), 67–68, 67t, 68f, Q65
Dry river bed sign, eosinophilic fasciitis, 55
Dry skin, 63. *See also* Xerosis
and pruritus, 44, 45
xerotic dermatitis and, 7, 7f
Dyshidrotic eczema, 7
Dysplastic nevi, 35–36, 36f
excision of, 36
fried egg appearance, 35
and melanoma risk, 36, 36f
Dysplastic nevus syndrome, 36

E
Ecthyma, 23, 24f
Ectopic ACTH syndrome, 60t
Eczema. *See also* Eczematous dermatoses
dyshidrotic, 7
nummular, 8, 8f
xerotic, 7–8, 7f
Eczema craquelé. *See* Xerotic eczema
Eczematous dermatoses, 4
atopic dermatitis, 4–5, 5f
contact dermatitis, 5–6, 5f, 6f, 6t
hand dermatitis, 7, 7f
intertrigo, 6–7, 7f
lichen simplex chronicus, 6, 6f
nummular eczema, 8, 8f
stasis dermatitis, 8, 8f, Q27
xerotic eczema, 7–8, 7f
Eflornithine cream, 70
Electrodesiccation and curettage (ED&C), for basal cell carcinoma, 40, Q67
EM. *See* Erythema multiforme (EM)
Emergencies, dermatologic, 2, 2t

acute generalized exanthematous pustulosis, 68
drug hypersensitivity syndrome/DRESS syndrome, 67–68
erythema multiforme, 65–66
erythroderma, 68–69
retiform purpura, 64–65
Stevens-Johnson syndrome and toxic epidermal necrolysis, 66–67
Emollients
for hand dermatitis, 7, Q54
for pruritus, 45
End-stage kidney disease, skin disease with, 57
calciphylaxis, 57, 57f
Kyrle disease, 57–58, 58f
nephrogenic systemic fibrosis, 58
Eosinophilic fasciitis, 55
Eosinophilic folliculitis, 63
Ephelides, 37
Epidermal inclusion cysts, 38–39, 38f, Q28
Epidermolysis bullosa acquisita, 47t, 48. *See also* Autoimmune bullous diseases (ABDs)
Eruptive xanthoma-associated hypertriglyceridemia, Q70
Eruptive xanthomas, 62, Q70
Erysipelas, 24–25
Erythema multiforme (EM), 65–66, 67t
EM major, 65, Q25
EM minor, 65
targetoid lesions of, 65, 65f
Erythema nodosum, 64, 64f, Q58
chest radiography for, Q43
Erythrasma, 25, 26f
Erythroderma, 68–69
causes of, 68t
management of, 69
prednisone and, Q46
with redness and scaling, 68f
Erythrodermic psoriasis, Q46
Erythromycin
for acne in pregnancy, Q36
for pitted keratolysis, 25
Erythroplakia, 76
Exclamation point hairs, 70, 72f
Excoriation, 1t
Extramammary Paget disease, 60t

F
Famciclovir
for herpes zoster, 30
for HSV infection, 29
Finasteride, for hirsutism, 70
Fire ants (*Solenopsis invicta*), 33
Fissure, 1t
Fixed drug reactions, 15t, 16, 16f
Fleas, 34, 34f
Fluconazole
for folliculitis, 22
for oropharyngeal candidiasis, 77
5-fluorouracil, for actinic cheilitis, 78
Folliculitis, 21–22, 22f
diagnosis of, 22
hot tub, 21, 22f
infectious, 21–22
noninfectious, 21
treatment for, 22
Foot and lower leg ulcers, 79
arterial insufficiency ulcers, 79–80, 80f, Q59
neuropathic ulcers, 80, 80f
rarer causes of, 80, 81t
venous stasis ulcers, 79, 79f, Q45
Fragrances, and allergic dermatitis, 6
Freckles, 37
Frontal fibrosing alopecia, 71t
Fungal infections, 25–28
candidiasis, 28, 28f
pityriasis versicolor, 27–28, 28f
tinea, 25–27, 26f, 27f
Furuncles, 22–23, 22f

G
Gabapentin, for pruritus, 45
Generalized pustular psoriasis of pregnancy, 82t
Geographic tongue, 78, 79f
Geophilic dermatophytes, 27. *See also* Tinea

Glucocorticoids, 3, 3t, 4t
    for acute generalized exanthematous pustulosis, 68
    for atopic dermatitis, 5, Q3
    for autoimmune bullous diseases, 50
    for contact dermatitis, 6
    for cutaneous sarcoidosis, 64
    for dermatomyositis, 53
    for eosinophilic fasciitis, 55
    for erythema multiforme, 66
    for lichen planus, 78
    for paronychia, 73
    for postscabetic pruritus, Q56
    potency and examples of, 4t
    in pregnancy, 83t
    for pruritus, 45
    for psoriasis, 9
    in PUPPP, 81, Q10
    for pyoderma gangrenosum, 58, Q62
    side effects, 3
    for SJS/TEN, 66
    and topical antifungal agents, 4
    for vitiligo, 13
Gluten-free diet, in dermatitis herpetiformis, 50, 59
Gram-negative folliculitis, 22
Graves disease, and pretibial myxedema, 63
Green nail syndrome, 74t
Grover disease. *See* Transient acantholytic dermatosis
Guttate hypomelanosis, 12–13, 13f
Guttate psoriasis, 9

H
Hair disorders
    alopecia, 70–73
    hypertrichosis/hirsutism, 69–70, 69t, 70f
Half and half (Lindsey) nails, 74t
Halo nevi, 36, 36f, Q50
Hand dermatitis, 7, 7f, Q54
    differential diagnosis of, 7
    treatment of, 7
Head lice, 32, 32t, 33f
Heat rash. *See* Miliaria
Hepatic uroporphyrinogen decarboxylase (UPDC), 59
Herald patch, 10
Hereditary angioedema, 46
Herpes gestationis. *See* Pemphigoid gestationis
Herpes simplex virus, 28–29, 29f
    classic presentation of, 28–29, 29f
    diagnosis of, 29, 29t
    site of infection, 28
    treatment of, 29
    types 1 (HSV1) and 2 (HSV2), 28
Herpes zoster, 24t, 29–30, 30f, Q6
    ophthalmicus, 30
Herpetic folliculitis, 22
Hidradenitis suppurativa, 21, 21f, Q39
    nodules in, 21f
    risk factors, 21f
    treatment for, 21, 21t
Hirsutism, 69–70, 69t, 70f
HIV-associated eosinophilic folliculitis, 21
HIV-associated primary dermatologic disorders, 63
HIV-associated seborrheic dermatitis, 10, Q31
Hives. *See* Urticaria
Hookworm, 34. *See also* Cutaneous larva migrans
Household cleansers, and allergic dermatitis, 6
Human papillomavirus (HPV), 30. *See also* Warts
    subtypes, 30t
    vaccination, 31
Hydrochlorothiazide, Q66
Hydroquinone, for melasma, 13–14
Hydroxychloroquine
    for cutaneous lupus, 52, 52t
    for porphyria cutanea tarda, 60
Hymenoptera stings, 33
Hypersensitivity vasculitis, 14, 17
Hypertrichosis, 69–70, 69t
Hypertrophic scars, 37, 38f

I
Idiopathic guttate hypomelanosis, 12–13, 13f
Id reaction, 5

IgA pemphigus, 47t. *See also* Autoimmune bullous diseases (ABDs)
Imidazole creams
    for dermatophytosis, 27
    for tinea pedis, Q64
Imiquimod, for actinic cheilitis, 78
Immunomodulators, topical, 4
Immunotherapy, for stage IV melanoma, 44
Impetigo, 23–24
    bullous, 23, 23f
    ecthyma, 23, 24f
    nonbullous, 23, 23f
    topical mupirocin for, 24, Q17
    treatment, 24
Impetigo herpetiformis, 82t
Incisional biopsy, for melanoma, 43
Incision and drainage, for abscesses/furuncles/carbuncles, 22, Q49
Infection
    in elderly, 84
    nail, 73
Infestations
    bed bugs, 32, 33f
    lice, 31–32, 33f
    scabies, 31, 32f, 32t
Inflammatory bowel disease, 58
Inflammatory dermatosis, 73, 75, 75f
Infliximab, for pyoderma gangrenosum, 59
Ingrown toenail, 75, 75f
Injectable epinephrine pen, 33
Interdigital intertrigo, Q20
Interleukin-17 inhibitors, for psoriasis, 9
Interleukin-12/interleukin-23 inhibitors, for psoriasis, 9
Intertrigo, 6–7, 7f, 28, Q20
    and *Candida* infection, 7, 28
    predisposing conditions, 6–7
    treatment of, 7
Intradermal melanocytic nevus, 35t
Intrahepatic cholestasis of pregnancy, 82t
Intravenous immunoglobulin
    in dermatomyositis, 53
    for pyoderma gangrenosum, 59
    for SJS/TEN, 66
Inverse psoriasis, 9, Q51
Ipilimumab, for stage IV melanoma, 44
IPLEDGE program, 19
Isotretinoin
    for acne, 19, Q12
    for folliculitis, 22
    in pregnancy, 83t
    for transient acantholytic dermatosis, 12
Itching. *See* Pruritus
Itraconazole
    for dermatophytosis, 27
    for onychomycosis, 73
    for pityriasis versicolor, 28
Ivermectin
    for cutaneous larva migrans, 34
    for *Demodex* folliculitis, 22
    for rosacea, 20

J
JAK/STAT inhibitors, for dermatomyositis, 53
Junctional melanocytic nevus, 35t

K
Keloids, 37–38
Keratoacanthoma, 42
    volcaniform appearance, 42, 42f
Ketoconazole
    for pityriasis versicolor, 28
    for seborrheic dermatitis, 11
Koilonychia (spoon nails), 74t
Kyrle disease, 57–58, 58f

L
Lactation, skin conditions during, 81, 82t
Laser therapy
    for actinic cheilitis, 78
    for rosacea, 20
LE. *See* Lupus erythematosus (LE)
Leg ulcers. *See* Foot and lower leg ulcers
Lentigo maligna, 43, 43f, Q35. *See also* Melanoma

Leprosy, 12
Leser-Trélat sign, 60t
Lesions, skin, 1, 1t
Leukoderma, 13
Leukoplakia, 76, 77f
Lice, 31–32, 33f
    body, 32
    head, 32, 33f
    pubic, 32
    treatment of, 32t
    types of, 31–32
Lichenification, 1t
Lichen planopilaris, 71t, 72, 73f
Lichen planus, 9–10, 10f, 77–78, 77f
    and nail plate dystrophy, 75, 75f
Lichen sclerosus, 78, 78f
Lichen simplex chronicus, 6, 6f
Linear IgA bullous dermatosis, 48t, 49t. *See also* Autoimmune bullous
    diseases (ABDs)
Linezolid, for abscesses/furuncles/carbuncles, 22
Lipomas, 39
Livedo reticularis, 56, 56f
Liver spots. *See* Solar lentigines
Lobular capillary hemangiomas. *See* Pyogenic granulomas
Löfgren syndrome, 64
Lupus erythematosus (LE), 50–53
    cutaneous, 50
    lupus-nonspecific skin disease, 50
    lupus-specific skin disease, 50
        acute cutaneous lupus erythematosus (ACLE), 50–51, 50f, 51f
        chronic cutaneous lupus erythematosus (CCLE), 50, 50f, 51, 51f, 52
        division of, 50, 50f
        subacute cutaneous lupus erythematosus (SCLE), 50, 50f, 51, 51f,
            51t, Q19
    systemic, 50
    therapy for, 52, 52t
Lupus hair, 52
Lupus panniculitis, 51
Lupus pernio, 64, Q23

M

Maculae ceruleae, 32
Macule, 1t
Malar butterfly rash, 50, 51f
Malassezia folliculitis, 22
Malignancy, cutaneous manifestations of, 60–61, 60t, 61t. *See also specific*
    syndrome
Malignant melanoma. *See* Melanoma
Malignant ulcer, 81t
Mask of pregnancy. *See* Melasma
Melanocytic nevi, 35, 35f
    clinical appearance, 35, 35f
    types of, 35t
Melanoma, 42–44, 43f
    ABCDEs of, 42
    acral lentiginous, 43, 43f
    biopsy of, 43, Q61
    clinical subtypes, 42
    lentigo maligna, 43, 43f, Q35
    nodular, 43, 43f
    staging of, 44
    superficial spreading, 42, 43f
    treatment of, 44
Melanonychia, 75–76, 76f, Q7
Melanotic macule, 76, 76f, Q33
Melasma, 13–14, 14f, Q30
    differential diagnosis, 13
    treatment, 13–14
Methacrylate, 6t
Methicillin-resistant *Staphylococcus aureus* (MRSA), 22
    in hospitalized patients, 23
Methotrexate
    for cutaneous lupus, 52, 52t
    for dermatomyositis, 53
    for eosinophilic fasciitis, 55
    in pregnancy, 83t
    for psoriasis, 9, Q9
    for pyoderma gangrenosum, 59
Methylisothiazolinone, 6t
Metronidazole, for rosacea, 20
Milia, 59

Miliaria, 11, Q11
    crystallina, 11, 11f
    pustulosa, 11, 11f
    rubra, 11
Mineral oil, 2
Mohs micrographic surgery
    for basal cell carcinoma, 40, Q24
    for squamous cell carcinoma, 42
Moles. *See* Melanocytic nevi
Molluscum contagiosum, 31, 31f, Q15
Monobenzyl ether of hydroquinone, 13
Morbilliform drug eruption, 14, 15t, 16f, Q37
Morphea, 54, 55, 55f, Q34
MRSA. *See* Methicillin-resistant *Staphylococcal aureus* (MRSA)
Mucous membranes, disorders of
    actinic cheilitis and squamous cell carcinoma, 78
    amalgam tattoo, 76
    aphthous ulcers, 77, 77f
    black hairy tongue, 78, 78f
    geographic tongue, 78, 79f
    leukoplakia and erythroplakia, 76, 77f
    lichen planus, 77–78, 77f
    lichen sclerosus, 78, 78f
    melanotic macule, 76, 76f, Q33
    oral candidiasis, 77, 77f
Muir-Torre syndrome, 61t
Mupirocin, 23, 34
    for impetigo, 24, Q17
Mycophenolate mofetil
    for cutaneous lupus, 52, 52t
    for dermatomyositis, 53
    in pregnancy, 83t
    for pyoderma gangrenosum, 59

N

Nail complex, 73. *See also* Nail disorders
Nail disorders, 73, 74t
    inflammatory dermatosis, 73, 75, 75f
    ingrown toenail, 75, 75f
    melanonychia, 75–76, 76f
    onychomycosis, 73, 74f
    paronychia, 73, 74f
    squamous cell carcinoma of nails, 76, 76f
Nail psoriasis, 9, 9f, 75, 75f
Narrowband ultraviolet B (UVB) phototherapy, for
    psoriasis, Q41
Nasal ulcerations, 52
Necrobiosis lipoidica, 63
Necrobiosis lipoidica diabeticorum, 81t
Necrobiotic xanthogranuloma, 60t
Necrolytic migratory erythema, 60t
Neomycin, 34
    and allergic dermatitis, 6
Neoplasms, benign
    acrochordons (skin tags), 37, 37f
    callus/corns, 36
    cherry angiomas, 37, 37f
    dermatofibromas, 37, 37f
    digital myxoid cysts, 39
    dysplastic nevi, 35–36, 36f
    epidermal inclusion cysts, 38–39, 38f, Q28
    halo nevi, 36, 36f
    hypertrophic scars and keloids, 37–38, 38f
    lipomas, 39
    melanocytic nevi, 35, 35f, 35t
    neurofibromas, 39, 39f
    pyogenic granulomas, 38, 38f
    sebaceous hyperplasia, 36, 36f
    seborrheic keratosis, 35, 35f
    solar lentigines and ephelides, 37, 38f
    xanthomas, 39, 39f
Nephrogenic systemic fibrosis, 58, 58f
Neurofibromas, 39
    buttonhole sign, 39
    in neurofibromatosis type 1, 39, 39f
Neuropathic ulcers, 80, 80f
Neutrophilic dermatoses, 60t
Nickel allergy, 5–6
Nivolumab, for stage IV melanoma, 44
Nodular melanoma, 43, 43f. *See also* Melanoma
Nodule, 1t

Nodulocystic acne, isotretinoin for, Q12
Nodulosis, accelerated, 55
Nummular eczema, 8, 8f

O

Oatmeal baths, 57
Ochronosis, drug-induced, 14
Ocular rosacea, Q57
Oil spots, 9, 9f
Onychogryphosis, 74t
Onychomadesis, 74t
Onychomycosis, 73, 74f
    in elderly, 84
Oral contraceptives, for acne, 19
Oral hairy leukoplakia, 76
Oral ulcerations, 52
Oropharyngeal candidiasis, 77, 77f
Oxymetazoline, for rosacea, 20

P

Paget disease of breast, 60t
Palmoplantar psoriasis, 9
Panniculitis, 24t
Papule, 1t
Papulosquamous dermatoses, 8
    lichen planus, 9–10, 10f
    pityriasis rosea, 10, 10f
    psoriasis, 8–9, 9f
    seborrheic dermatitis, 10–11, 10f
Paraneoplastic pemphigus, 47t, 60t. See also Autoimmune bullous diseases
    (ABDs)
Paraphenylenediamine, 6t
Paronychia, 73, 74f
    acute, 73
    chronic, 73, Q8
Patch, 1t
Patch testing, for contact dermatitis, 5, 5f
Peau d' orange appearance, pretibial myxedema, 63, 63f
Pembrolizumab, for stage IV melanoma, 44
Pemphigoid gestationis, 81, 82t, 83f
Pemphigus foliaceus, 47t, 48, 49f. See also Autoimmune bullous diseases
    (ABDs)
Pemphigus vulgaris, 47t, 48, 49f. See also Autoimmune bullous diseases (ABDs)
Perianal skin tags, 37
Periungual erythema, 74t
Petrolatum, for hand dermatitis, 7
Phlebotomy, in porphyria cutanea tarda, 60
Phosphodiesterase-4 inhibitor, for psoriasis, 9
Photoallergy, 17, 17f
Photodynamic therapy, for actinic cheilitis, 78
Photographs, 2
Photoprotection
    in dermatomyositis, 53
    in lupus erythematosus, 52
Photosensitivity disorders, 15t, 16–17, 17f
Phototherapy, 4
    for psoriasis, 9, Q41
    for uremic pruritus, 45
    for vitiligo, 13
Phototoxicity, 17
Physical examination, 2
Pigmentation, disorders of
    melasma, 13–14, 14f
    vitiligo, 12–13, 12f, 13f
Pimecrolimus
    for atopic dermatitis, 5
    for vitiligo, 13
Pitted keratolysis, 25, 25f, Q44
Pitted nails, 74t
Pityriasis alba, 12
Pityriasis rosea, 10, 10f
    herald patch, 10
    and secondary syphilis, 10
Pityriasis versicolor, 27–28, 28f, Q2
Plaque, 1t
Polyarteritis nodosa, 56, Q42
Polymorphous light eruption, 16–17
Porphyria cutanea tarda, 48t, 58, 59–60, Q60. See also Autoimmune bullous
    diseases (ABDs)
    cause of, 59–60
    diagnosis of, 60

epidermal erosions on sun-exposed skin, 59, 59f
    treatment of, 60
Postherpetic neuralgia, 30
Postinflammatory hyperpigmentation, 12, 14
Postscabetic pruritus, Q56
Potassium hydroxide (KOH), 2, Q47
Prednisone
    for autoimmune bullous diseases, 50
    for pyoderma gangrenosum, Q62
    for severe contact dermatitis, Q63
Pregnancy
    acne in, Q36
    dermatologic conditions during, 81
        treatment of, 81, 83t, Q36
    melanoma during, diagnosis of, Q61
    pemphigoid gestationis in, 81, 83f
    physiologic changes associated with, 82t
    PUPPP in, 81, 83f, Q10
Pretibial myxedema, 63, 63f
Prickly heat. See Miliaria
Primary biliary cirrhosis, 39
Primary skin lesions, 1, 1t
Propionibacterium acnes, 18, 19
Proximal subungual onychomycosis, 73
Prurigo of pregnancy, 82t
Pruritic urticarial papules and plaques of pregnancy (PUPPP), 81, 82t, 83f,
    Q10
Pruritus, 44–45
    in absence of skin findings, Q66
    cholestatic liver disease and, 44, 44f
    diagnosis of, 44–45
    end-stage kidney disease and, 57
    generalized, 44
    in HIV/AIDS, 63
    medications causing, 45, 45t
    neuropathic, 44, 45f
    and patient education, 45
    postscabetic, Q56
    psychogenic itch, 44, 45f
    in PUPPP, 81
    skin diseases and, 44
    systemic diseases with, 44
    treatment for, 45
Pseudofolliculitis barbae, 72
Pseudomonas folliculitis, 22
Pseudoporphyria, 48t, 49t
Psoralen with ultraviolet A (PUVA), 4
    for transient acantholytic dermatosis, 12
Psoriasis, 8–9, 9f
    and cardiovascular disease, 9
    clinical presentations, 8–9, 9f
    inverse, Q51
    nail pitting in, 75f
    smoking and, 9
    treatment of, 9, Q9, Q41
Psoriatic arthritis, 9
Pubic lice, 32, 32t
Punch biopsy, for basal cell carcinoma, 40
PUPPP. See Pruritic urticarial papules and plaques of pregnancy (PUPPP)
Pustule, 1t
Pyoderma gangrenosum, 58–59, 81t, Q40, Q62
    characteristics of, 58, 59f
    diagnosis of, 58
    management of, 58–59
    sites of involvement, 58
Pyogenic granulomas, 38, 38f

Q

Quaternium-15, 6t

R

Radiation therapy
    for basal cell carcinoma, 40
    for squamous cell carcinoma, 42
    for stage IV melanoma, 44
Ragged cuticles (Samitz sign), 74t
Ramsay Hunt syndrome, 30
Rashes, 1
    eczematous dermatoses, 4–8
    miliaria, 11
    papulosquamous dermatoses, 8–11

in persons with skin of color, 2
transient acantholytic dermatosis, 11–12
Raynaud phenomenon, 54, 54f
Recombinant zoster vaccine, 30
Red lunulae, 74t
Reed syndrome, 61t
Retapamulin, for impetigo, 24
Retiform purpura, 64–65
differential diagnosis for, 65t
on lower legs due to vasculitis, 64f
thrombotic and embolic causes, 64
ulceration and necrosis, 65f
Retinoids, 3t, 4
for acanthosis nigricans, 63
for acne, 19
for comedonal acne, Q55
for transient acantholytic dermatosis, 12
Rheumatoid arthritis, 55–56
rheumatoid nodules in, 55, 55f
rheumatoid vasculitis in, 56, Q18
Rhinophyma, 20, 20f
Rituximab, in pemphigus vulgaris, 50
Rodent ulcer, 40
Rosacea, 19–21
clinical presentations of, 19
erythema of, 20
erythrotelangiectatic, 19–20, 20f
gritty sensation in, 20
ocular, 20
papulopustular, 19, 19f
phymatous, 20
and rhinophyma, 20, 20f
treatment for, 20, 20t
Rubber accelerators, 6t

S

Salicylic acid, for acanthosis nigricans, 63
Sarcoidosis, 64
Satellite pustules, 7
Scabies, 31, 32f, 32t
characteristics of, 31, 32f
diagnosis of, 31, 32f
pruritus after, 31
treatment of, 32t
Scale, 1t
SCLE. *See* Subacute cutaneous lupus erythematosus (SCLE)
Sclerodactyly, 54, 54f
Scleromyxedema, 60t
Sclerosing disorders, 54–55
advanced diffuse systemic sclerosis, 54
cutaneous features of, 54, 54f
early diffuse systemic sclerosis, 54
eosinophilic fasciitis, 55
localized scleroderma, 54, 55f, Q34
Raynaud phenomenon in, 54, 54f
rhagades, lip atrophy and telangiectases in, 54, 55f
sclerodactyly, 54, 54f
Scoop biopsy, 43
SCORTEN scale, 66, 67t
Sebaceous cysts. *See* Epidermal inclusion cysts
Sebaceous hyperplasia, 36, 36f
Seborrheic dermatitis, 10–11, 10f
areas of involvement, 10
HIV-associated, Q31
in immunocompromised patients, 10–11
treatment of, 11
Seborrheic keratosis, 35, 35f
Secondary skin lesions, 1, 1t
Selenium sulfide
for pityriasis versicolor, 28
for seborrheic dermatitis, 11
Shave biopsy, for basal cell carcinoma, 40
Shingles. *See* Herpes zoster
Sickle cell disease, and ulcers, 81t
Skin
examination, 2
lesions, 1, 1t
structure of, 1, 1f
Skin biopsy
for amyloidosis, 62
for autoimmune bullous diseases, 48, Q1

for dermatitis herpetiformis, 59
for eosinophilic folliculitis, 63
for eruptive xanthomas, 62
for erythema multiforme, 65
for folliculitis, 22
for molluscum contagiosum, 31
for pemphigoid gestationis, 81
for pretibial myxedema, 63
for retiform purpura, 64
for seborrheic keratosis, 35
for small-vessel vasculitis, 56
for squamous cell carcinoma, 41
for transient acantholytic dermatosis, 12
for urticarial vasculitis, 46, Q4
Skin cancer, 39
actinic keratosis, 41, 41f
basal cell carcinoma, 39–41, 40f
keratoacanthoma, 42, 42f
malignant melanoma, 42–44, 43f
squamous cell carcinoma, 41–42, 41f, 42f
Skin infections. *See also specific type*
bacterial, 21–25
fungal, 25–28
viral, 28–31
Skin lesions
characteristics of, 1, 1t
morphology of, 1
primary, 1, 1t
secondary, 1, 1t
Skin tags. *See* Acrochordons
Sodium thiosulfate, in calciphylaxis, 57
Solar lentigines, 37, 38f
Sonidegib, for basal cell carcinoma, 40
Spider bites, 33, 33f
Spironolactone
for acne, 19
for hirsutism, 70
in pregnancy, 83t
Squamous cell carcinoma, 41–42, 41f, 42f
of lip, 78
of nails, 76, 76f
pink hyperkeratotic nodule, 41, 41f
poorly differentiated subtype, 41
risk factors for, 41
SCC in situ (Bowen disease), 41, 42f
Staphylococcus aureus, 5
Staphylococcus epidermis, 11
Stasis dermatitis, 8, 8f, 24t, Q27
Stevens-Johnson syndrome (SJS) and toxic epidermal necrolysis (TEN), 66–67, Q14
erythema multiforme and, 67t
medications leading to, 66t
SCORTEN scale, 66, 67t
systemic manifestations in, 66
treatment of, 66–67
Subacute cutaneous lupus erythematosus (SCLE), 50, 50f, 51, 51f, 51t, Q19
Sun exposure
basal cell carcinoma and, 40
lupus erythematosus and, 52
porphyria cutanea tarda and, 59
squamous cell carcinoma and, 41
Superficial spreading melanoma, 42, 43f. *See also* Melanoma
Surgical excision
for epidermal inclusion cyst, Q28
for melanoma, 44
for squamous cell carcinoma, 42
Surgical revascularization, arterial insufficiency ulcers and, Q59
Sweet syndrome, 61
associations with, 61, 61t
skin lesions in, 61, 61f
Systemic antibiotics, for folliculitis, 22
Systemic retinoids, for hidradenitis suppurativa, 21

T

Tacrolimus
for atopic dermatitis, 5
for vitiligo, 13
Tazarotene
for acne, 19
in pregnancy, 83t
Telangiectasia, 1t

Telogen effluvium, 70, 71t, Q29
Tendon xanthomas, 39
Terbinafine
    for dermatophytosis, 27
    for onychomycosis, 73
Terbinafine 1% and ciclopiroxolamine 0.77%, 27
Terry nails, 58, 74t
Tetracyclines
    for acne, 19
    for hidradenitis suppurativa, 21
    in pregnancy, 83t
Thalidomide
    for cutaneous lupus, 52
    for pyoderma gangrenosum, 59
Thyroid dermopathy, 63, 63f
Tinea, 25–27
    capitis, 26, 26f, 71t
    clinical presentation of, 27
    corporis, 8, 26, 27f
    cruris, 26, 26f
    diagnosis of, 27
    faciei, 26
    incognito, 27
    manuum, 25–26
    moccasin or glove distribution, 27, 27f
    pedis, 25, 26f, Q64
    treatment of, 27
Tinea versicolor, 12. See Pityriasis versicolor
Topical medications, 3. See also specific type
    effectiveness of, 3
    frequently used, 3t
    vehicles for, 3t
Toxic epidermal necrolysis (TEN), 66–67
    prognosis in, Q14
Trachyonychia, 74t
Transient acantholytic dermatosis, 11–12, 11f, Q32
Transverse indentations, 74t
Traumatic alopecia, 70, 71t
Tretinoin, for acne, 19
Triamcinolone cream, Q5
Trimethoprim-sulfamethoxazole
    for abscesses/furuncles/carbuncles, 22
    in pregnancy, 83t
Tripe palms, 60t
Tuberous sclerosis complex, 61t
Tumid lupus, 52, 52f
Tumor necrosis factor α inhibitors, for psoriasis, 9
Two feet–one hand syndrome, 7
Tzanck preparations, 2

U
Ulcers, 1t, 79
    arterial insufficiency, 79–80, Q59
    neuropathic, 80, 80f
    rarer causes of, 80, 81t
    venous stasis, 79, 79f
Ursodeoxycholic acid, for cholestatic pruritus, 45
Urticaria, 45–46
    and angioedema, 46
    causes of, 46
    diagnosis of, 46
    lesions of, 45–46, 46f
    physical, 46
Urticarial reactions, 14, 15t, 16, 16f
Urticarial vasculitis, 46, Q4
Urushiol, and allergic dermatitis, 5, 6f
U.S. Preventive Services Task Force (USPSTF), 2

V
Valacyclovir
    for herpes zoster, 30
    for HSV infection, 29

Vancomycin, for abscesses/furuncles/carbuncles, 22
Varicella. See Chickenpox
Varicella-zoster virus, 29–30, 30f
    chickenpox, 29, 29f
    herpes zoster/shingles, 29–30, 30f
    treatment, 30
Vasculitis, 56–57, 81t
    large-vessel, 56
    medium-vessel, 56, 56f
    rheumatoid, 56, Q18
    small-vessel, 56, 56f
Venous stasis ulcers, 79, 79f, Q45
Verruca plana (flat warts), 30, 30f. See also Warts
Verruca plantaris/palmaris, 30. See also Warts
Verruca vulgaris (common warts), 30. See also Warts
Vesicle, 1t
Viral skin infections, 28–31
    herpes simplex virus, 28–29, 29f
    molluscum contagiosum, 31, 31f
    varicella-zoster virus, 29–30, 30f
    warts, 30–31, 30f
Vismodegib, for basal cell carcinoma, 40
Vitamin D analogues, 3t
    for psoriasis, 9
Vitiligo, 12–13, Q38
    autoimmune conditions associated with, 12
    causes of depigmentation, 12–13
    clinical presentation, 12, 12f
    differential diagnosis
        leprosy, 12
        pityriasis alba, 12
        postinflammatory hyperpigmentation, 12
        tinea versicolor, 12
    history and physical examination, 13
    treatment for, 13
    Wood lamp examination, 13

W
Warts, 30–31, 30f
    common, 30
    flat, 30, 30f
    genital, 30, 31f
    HPV subtypes and, 30, 30t
    in immunocompromised persons, 31
    plantar/palmar, 30
    treatment of, 31
Wet mounting, 2
Wet ulcer, 58. See also Pyoderma gangrenosum
Wheal/Hive, 1t
Wickham striae, 77
Wide local excision, for stage IV melanoma, 44
Wood lamp, 2
Worms, 34

X
Xanthelasma, 39, 39f
Xanthomas, 39, 39f, Q70
    eruptive, 39
    plane, 39
    tendon, 39
Xerosis
    in aging population, 83–84, 84f
    end-stage kidney disease and, 57
    in HIV/AIDS, 63
Xerotic eczema, 7–8, 7f, 83–84, 84f

Y
Yellow nail syndrome, 74t

Z
Zinc gluconate, for hidradenitis suppurativa, 21
Zoophilic dermatophytes, 26–27. See also Tinea

A NAME AND ADDRESS (Please complete.)

Last Name _____ First Name _____ Middle Initial _____

Address _____

Address cont. _____

City _____ State _____ ZIP Code _____

Country _____

Email address _____

ACP ®
American College of Physicians
Leading Internal Medicine, Improving Lives

Medical Knowledge Self-Assessment Program® 18

TO EARN *CME Credits and/or MOC Points* YOU MUST:

1. Answer all questions.
2. Score a minimum of 50% correct.

===

TO EARN *FREE* INSTANTANEOUS *CME Credits and/or MOC Points* ONLINE:

1. Answer all of your questions.
2. Go to **mksap.acponline.org** and enter your ACP Online username and password to access an online answer sheet.
3. Enter your answers.
4. You can also enter your answers directly at **mksap.acponline.org** without first using this answer sheet.

To Submit Your Answer Sheet by Mail or FAX for a $20 Administrative Fee per Answer Sheet:

1. Answer all of your questions and calculate your score.
2. Complete boxes A–H.
3. Complete payment information.
4. Send the answer sheet and payment information to ACP, using the FAX number/address listed below.

B Order Number

(Use the 10-digit Order Number on your MKSAP materials packing slip.)

C ACP ID Number

(Refer to packing slip in your MKSAP materials for your 8-digit ACP ID Number.)

D Required Submission Information if Applying for MOC

Birth Month and Day
M M   D D

ABIM Candidate Number

COMPLETE FORM BELOW ONLY IF YOU SUBMIT BY MAIL OR FAX

Last Name _____ First Name _____ MI

Payment Information. Must remit in US funds, drawn on a US bank.
The processing fee for each paper answer sheet is $20.

☐ Check, made payable to ACP, enclosed

Charge to ☐ **VISA** ☐ **MasterCard** ☐ **AMERICAN EXPRESS** ☐ **DISCOVER**

Card Number _____

Expiration Date _____ / _____
MM   YY

Security code (3 or 4 digit #s) _____

Signature _____

Fax to: 215-351-2799

Mail to:
Member and Customer Service
American College of Physicians
190 N. Independence Mall West
Philadelphia, PA 19106–1572